Wheater's Functional Histology

DEDICATION

Paul Richard Wheater
1951–1989

Front cover photomicrograph
Elastic cartilage and overlying supporting tissue of external ear
(Elastic van Gieson × 120)

Back cover photomicrograph
Centrosome and microtubules
(EM × 30 000)

Wheater's Functional Histology
A TEXT AND COLOUR ATLAS

FIRST EDITION OF FUNCTIONAL HISTOLOGY BY

Paul R. Wheater

H. George Burkitt

Victor G. Daniels

THIRD EDITION BY

H. George Burkitt
BDSc Hons (Queensland), FRACDS, M Med Sci (Nottingham), MB BChir (Cambridge)
Family medical practitioner and medical author Sydney, New South Wales, Australia

Barbara Young
BSc Med Sci Hons (St. Andrews), PhD (Cambridge), MB BChir (Cambridge), MRCP (UK), FRCPA
Senior Lecturer in Pathology, The University of Newcastle, New South Wales, Australia

John W. Heath
BSc Hons (Melbourne), PhD (Melbourne)
Associate Professor of Anatomy, The University of Newcastle, New South Wales, Australia

Drawings by
Philip J. Deakin
BSc Hons (Sheffield), MB ChB (Sheffield)
General medical practitioner, Sheffield, UK

CHURCHILL
LIVINGSTONE

EDINBURGH LONDON NEW YORK PHILADELPHIA SYDNEY TORONTO 1993

CHURCHILL LIVINGSTONE
An imprint of Harcourt Brace and Company Limited

© Harcourt Brace and Company Limited 1999

⫸ is a registered trademark of Harcourt Brace and
Company Limited

First edition 1979
Second edition 1987
Third edition 1993
    Reprinted 1993
    Reprinted 1994
    Reprinted 1995
    Reprinted 1996
    Reprinted 1997
    Reprinted 1999

ISBN 0-443-04691-3

British Library Cataloguing in Publication Data
A catalogue record for this book is available from the British Library.

Library of Congress Cataloging in Publication Data
A catalogue record for this book is available from the Library of Congress.

For Churchill Livingstone:
Publisher
Timothy Horne

Project Editor
Jim Killgore

Production
Nancy Henry

Designer
Design Resources Unit

Sales Promotion Executive
Duncan Jones

The
publisher's
policy is to use
**paper manufactured
from sustainable forests**

Printed in Hong Kong
SWT/08

Preface to the Third Edition

The response from both students and teachers to the first and second editions of this book has been most gratifying. A new edition is now required to keep the subject matter up to date and further improve the quality of illustrations. Many of the major shortcomings of the first edition were addressed in the second edition, in which the contents were expanded by about 25 per cent including coverage of the vestibulo-auditory apparatus and major regional variations of the central nervous system. The subject matter was also rearranged and subdivided into three basic sections, namely 'The Cell', 'Basic Tissue Types' and 'Organ Systems', which correlate readily with the way in which the subject is learned.

The death of Paul Wheater cast a deep shadow over the preparation of this new edition, the book having become synonymous with his name, which is thus now incorporated in the title. His trailblazing photomicroscopic skills have led to the book becoming a widely used reference atlas of histology, with seven different language editions now in print. The role of the book as an atlas has been further developed with the involvement of Barbara Young and John Heath in the authorship team, each making particular contributions in their specialities of light and electron microscopy, respectively. One hundred and fourteen new colour micrographs and eighty new electron micrographs replace inferior pictures or expand the illustrative material. A comprehensive new section on the placenta has been added. In all, the book now contains seven hundred and ninety two illustrations, an expansion by a further 16 percent on the second edition.

The emphasis remains on human tissues, with animal tissues being used only where suitably fixed specimens of normal human tissue were not available. For light microscopy, we have continued the use of paraffin-embedded specimens in the majority of cases, as these will be comparable to the material in student histology and histopathology teaching collections. We would welcome the opinion of readers about the value of changing to acrylic-embedded sections for future editions. Many of the original electron micrographs have been replaced as befits the great improvement in electron microscope technology since the original edition was prepared over 15 years ago.

Although we recognise that the book is widely used as an altas and laboratory study guide, we have continued to see the captions as representing a comprehensive text pitched at the needs of medical and other undergraduate students for whom histology represents but a small part of their biological studies. The emphasis remains on important principles rather than esoteric details. In many respects the format reflects the approach used by teachers in the classroom situation where discussion is based around illustrations, with important principles being developed and reinforced with a variety of techniques; at the same time, more detail is constantly being added to the framework and correlated with tissue and organ function.

The text has been thoroughly revised and terminology updated. In this context, we have carefully considered the functional implications of the term 'connective tissue' and substituted the term 'supporting tissue' usually with some added description, e.g. 'loose collagenous supporting tissue', which we believe provides for much improved understanding. This follows the lead of Alan Stevens and James Lowe, our coauthors in *Basic Histopathology*, who have adopted this convention in their new book *Histology* (Gower, 1992). We have in the meantime applied to the International Anatomical Nomenclature Committee for formal recognition of this terminological change.

Newcastle, Australia, 1993

H.G. Burkitt
B. Young
J.W. Heath

Preface to the First Edition

Histology has bored generations of students. This is almost certainly because it has been regarded as the study of structure in isolation from function; yet few would dispute that structure and function are intimately related. Thus, the aim of this book is to present histology in relation to the principles of physiology, biochemistry and molecular biology.

Within the limits imposed by any book format, we have attempted to create the environment of the lecture room and microscope laboratory by basing the discussion of histology upon appropriate micrographs and diagrams. Consequently, colour photography has been used since it reproduces the actual images seen in light microscopy and allows a variety of common staining methods to be employed in highlighting different aspects of tissue structure. In addition, some less common techniques such as immunohistochemistry have been introduced where such methods best illustrate a particular point.

Since electron microscopy is a relatively new technique, a myth has arisen amongst many students that light and electron microscopy are poles apart. We have tried to show that electron microscopy is merely an extension of light microscopy. In order to demonstrate this continuity, we have included resin-embedded thin sections photographed around the limit of resolution of the light microscope; this technique is being applied increasingly in routine histological and histopathological practice. Where such less conventional techniques have been adopted, their rationale has been outlined at the appropriate place rather than in a formal chapter devoted to techniques.

The content and pictorial design of the book have been chosen to make it easy to use both as a textbook and as a laboratory guide. Wherever possible, the subject matter has been condensed into units of illustration plus relevant text; each unit is designed to have a degree of autonomy whilst at the same time remaining integrated into the subject as a whole. Short sections of non-illustrated text have been used by way of introduction, to outline general principles and to consider the subject matter in broader perspective.

Human tissues were mainly selected in order to maintain consistency, but when suitable human specimens were not available, primate tissues were generally substituted. Since this book stresses the understanding of principles rather than extensive detail, some tissues have been omitted deliberately, for example the regional variations of the central nervous system and the vestibulo-auditory apparatus.

This book should adequately encompass the requirements of undergraduate courses in medicine, dentistry, veterinary science, pharmacy, mammalian biology and allied fields. Further, it offers a pictorial reference for use in histology and histopathology laboratories. Finally, we envisage that the book will also find application as a teaching manual in schools and colleges of further education.

Nottingham, 1979

Paul R. Wheater
H. George Burkitt
Victor G. Daniels

Acknowledgements

We are indebted to many individuals who have made invaluable contributions in their specialised fields.

Most of the tissue preparation and photomicrography for the original edition was performed in the Departments of Pathology and Human Morphology of Queen's Medical Centre, University of Nottingham, and the authors are extremely grateful for the cooperation of Professors I.M.P. Dawson and R.E. Coupland who then headed those departments. Special thanks are due to Janet Palmer of the Department of Pathology who gave tireless assistance in the preparation of many of the tissues for light microscopy which were used in the first two editions. Similarly, thanks to Paul Beck of the Department of Human Morphology for producing a large number of valuable specimens. Many of the original electron micrographs were prepared by his colleagues John Kugler and Annette Tomlinson, to whom we are deeply indebted. From the Department of Biology, University of York, Peter Crosby provided most of the scanning electron micrographs, Brian Norman provided several light microscopic sections and Dr Robert Lang produced the freeze-etched preparation used in Figure 1.6(c). The otolith specimen used in Figure 21.27(c) was lent by Mr Roger Gray FRCS, Addenbrooke's Hospital, Cambridge and Professor N. Dilly, St. George's Hospital, Tooting. Donald Canwell of the Physiological Laboratory, University of Cambridge, contributed many sections from his personal collection, several of which enhanced the second edition. Dr Graham Robinson and Stan Terras of the Department of Pathology, University of Nottingham, each provided several electron micrographs, and with their colleague Linda Burns provided the thin resin sections used for light microscopy. Dr Terry Bennett of the Department of Physiology, University of Nottingham contributed Figure 7.11. Dr Pat Cooke of the Department of Genetics, City Hospital, Nottingham lent the chromosome preparation used in Figure 2.2. Pathologists Dr David Ansell of City Hospital, Nottingham, Drs Hugh Rice and Peter James of Nottingham General Hospital and Dr Pauline Cooper of Addenbrooke's Hospital, Cambridge, made available various tissue specimens and slides. Peter Squires and Hugh Pulsford of Huntingdon Research Centre, Cambridgeshire, were a great help in providing the primate tissues used when suitable human tissues were unavailable. To all of these kind and cooperative people we express our sincere thanks. Bill Brackenbury of the Department of Pathology, University of Nottingham, performed much of the macrophotography, and Leonard Beard of the Department of Medical Illustration, Hinchingbrooke Hospital, Huntingdon, photographed the two thin sections in black and white. The remaining colour photomicrographs in the first two editions were the work of the late Paul Wheater.

The new light micrographs in this edition were photographed on a Nikon Optiphot-2 photomicroscope supplied by FSE Australia. We gratefully acknowledge the help of the medical and scientific staff of the Division of Anatomical Pathology, Hunter Area Pathology Service, Newcastle, Australia, in particular Nancy Wilson and David Price. Special thanks to Debbie Pepperall for her work in tissue preparation and staining for light microscopy. Thanks also to Steven Medcalf of FSE, and Stephen McInally and colleagues of the Medical Communications Unit, Faculty of Medicine, University of Newcastle, for their technical assistance. A JEOL 100CX electron microscope was used for all of the new electron micrographs; we are most grateful to Gary Weber for his careful maintenance of this instrument. Special thanks also to Dr Grahame Kidd who photographed five of the new electron micrographs.

Typing the manuscript and pasting up were carried out with skill and great patience by Louise Morgan and Amanda Beisty who knew not what they were letting themselves in for; we cannot thank them enough. Finally, we thank our families for their forbearance and support throughout this challenging project which consumed much time which would otherwise have been spent with them.

Contents

The cell

1. Cell structure and function

Introduction

The cell is the functional unit of all living tissues, each cell having the capacity to perform all the essential life functions. Within the different tissues and organs of the body, the constituent cells exhibit a wide range of functional specialisations which are, nevertheless, merely amplifications of one or more of the fundamental cellular functions. Despite this extraordinary range of morphological forms, all cells conform to a basic structural model which is the subject of this chapter. The process by which cells assume specialised structure and function is known as *differentiation*.

Even with primitive light microscopy, it was evident that cells are divided into at least two components, the *nucleus* and the *cytoplasm*, and as microscopical techniques advanced it became increasingly obvious that both the cytoplasm and nucleus contain a number of subcellular elements called *organelles*.

The resolving power of the light microscope is limited to about 0.2 μm (200 nm) and the study of the ultrastructure of the cell had to await the advent of electron microscopy (EM). The capacity of electron microscopes in current use permits the resolution of structures as small as 1.0 nm (10 ångström units); this however, falls far short of many cellular processes which occur at the molecular level and which require biochemical methods of study. Nevertheless in recent years, light and electron microscopy have been successfully combined with biochemical and immunological techniques to define the location of many biological processes; these techniques are known as *histochemistry* and *immunohistochemistry* respectively.

Fig. 1.1 The cell *(illustration opposite; EM × 15 000)*

The basic structural features common to all cells are illustrated in this electron micrograph of a hormone-secreting cell from the pituitary gland. All cells are bounded by an external limiting membrane called the *plasma membrane* or *plasmalemma* **PM** which serves as a dynamic interface between the internal environment of the cell and its various external environments. In this particular example, the cell interacts with two types of external environment, adjacent cells **C** and intercellular spaces **IS**. Such interactions depend on the specialised function of the cell and include transfer of nutrients and metabolites, attachment of the cell to adjacent cells and other structures and intercellular communications.

The nucleus **N** is the largest organelle and its substance, often referred to as the *nucleoplasm*, is bounded by a membrane system called the *nuclear envelope* **NE**. The cytoplasm contains a variety of organelles most of which are also bounded by membranes. An extensive system of membrane-bound tubules, saccules and flattened cisterns, collectively known as the *endoplasmic reticulum* **ER**, is widely distributed throughout the cytoplasm. A more distended system of membrane-bound saccules, the *Golgi apparatus* **G**, is typically located close to the nucleus. Scattered free in the cytoplasm are a number of relatively large, elongated organelles called *mitochondria* **M** which have a smooth outer membrane and a convoluted inner membrane system. In addition to these major organelles, the cell contains a variety of other membrane-bound structures, an example of which are the numerous, electron-dense *secretory vacuoles* **V** (in this case containing hormone) seen in this micrograph.

Thus the cell is divided into a number of membrane-bound compartments each of which has its own particular biochemical environment. Membranes therefore serve to isolate incompatible processes. In addition, membranes incorporate enzyme systems as well as providing the site of many specific biochemical reactions.

The cytoplasmic organelles are suspended in a fluid medium called the *cytosol* in which much of the intermediary metabolism of the cell takes place. Within the cytosol, there is a network of minute tubules and filaments collectively known as the *cytoskeleton* which provides structural support for the cell and its organelles as well as providing a mechanism for cellular and intracellular movement; elements of the cytoskeleton are only visible with very high magnification.

The study of electron micrographs

To understand an electron micrograph, the first step is to identify individual cells (or parts thereof). The nucleus (if included in the plane of section) provides a good starting point and is a useful reference with respect to the size of other organelles. The plasma membrane is then identified and traced out, thus defining the limits of the cell. At times the membrane may appear to fade out; this is usually the product of an oblique plane of section which renders the membrane less easy to see. Other organelles such as mitochondria are then identified before more detailed examination is made of other organelles. From the relative proportions of organelles, much can then be deduced about the function of cells and thus the identity of the tissue.

(a)

(b)

POLAR

Nitrogenous compound

Phosphate bridge

Glycerol

NON-POLAR

Saturated fatty acid

Unsaturated fatty acid

(c)

Outer surface

Carbohydrate groups

Inner surface

Phospholipid bilayer

Extrinsic protein

Intrinsic protein

Transmembrane protein with pore

Cytoskeletal elements

Fig. 1.2 **Membrane structure** *(illustrations opposite)*

(a) EM × 210 000 (b) Phospholipid structure (c) Fluid mosaic model of membrane structure

Despite intensive investigation, the structure of cell membranes is still not known with certainty; however, a theoretical model has been progressively developed which satisfactorily incorporates much of the currently available biochemical and histological evidence.

Towards the end of the last century, it was observed that lipids rapidly gain entry into cells, and it was postulated that the 'cell boundary' was composed of lipid. In the 1920s, it was found that by measuring the minimum area that could be occupied by a monolayer of lipids extracted from a defined number of red blood cells, there was enough lipid present in the monolayer to cover each cell twice. From this it was concluded that cells were bounded by a double layer of lipid.

Later, it was proposed that cell membranes are symmetrical structures consisting of a bilayer of phospholipid molecules sandwiched between two layers of protein. This model, however, failed to explain the selective permeability of most cell membranes to molecules which are not lipid-soluble such as glucose, sodium ions and potassium ions. These theoretical difficulties were overcome by postulating the existence of 'pores' composed of protein through which hydrophilic molecules could be transported by passive or active mechanisms.

Electron microscopic studies in the 1950s revealed that all membranes have a three-layer (trilaminate) structure and this led to the concept of the *unit membrane* in which it was proposed that all cell membranes have a similar structure.

Fluid mosaic model of membrane structure

The current concepts of membrane structure derive from the work of Singer and Nicholson in the early 1970s. In this model, cell membranes consist basically of phospholipid molecules arranged as a bilayer.

Phospholipid molecules are *amphipathic*, i.e. they consist of a polar, hydrophilic (water-loving) head and a non-polar, hydrophobic (water-hating) tail. The polar heads are mainly derived from glycerol conjugated to a nitrogenous compound such as choline, ethanolamine or serine via a phosphate bridge as shown in diagram (b). The phosphate group is negatively charged whereas the nitrogenous group is positively charged. The non-polar tail of the phospholipid molecule consists of two long-chain fatty acids each covalently linked to the glycerol component of the polar head. In most mammalian cell membranes, one of the fatty acids is a straight-chain saturated fatty acid whilst the other is an unsaturated fatty acid which is 'kinked' at the position of the unsaturated bond. Because of their amphipathic nature, phospholipids in aqueous solution will spontaneously form a bilayer with the hydrophilic (polar) heads directed outwards and the hydrophobic tails forced together inwards. The weak intermolecular forces which hold the bilayer together allow individual phospholipid molecules to move relatively freely within each layer and sometimes to 'flip' between layers.

The fluidity and flexibility of the membrane is increased by the presence of unsaturated fatty acids which prevent close packing of the hydrophobic tails. Cholesterol molecules are also present in the bilayer in an almost one-to-one ratio with phospholipids. Cholesterol molecules themselves are amphipathic and have a kinked conformation, thus preventing too close packing of the phospholipid fatty acid tails whilst at the same time filling the gaps between the 'kinks' of the unsaturated fatty acid tails. Cholesterol molecules thus regulate the fluidity and stabilise the phospholipid bilayer.

Associated with the bilayer are a variety of protein molecules which make up almost half of the total mass of the membrane. Some proteins are incorporated within the membrane (*intrinsic* or *integral proteins*) whereas others are held to the inner or outer surface by weaker electrostatic forces (*extrinsic* or *peripheral proteins*). Some intrinsic proteins span the entire thickness of the membrane (*transmembrane proteins*) to be exposed to each surface, some functioning as 'pores' through which hydrophilic molecules are actively or passively transported across the membrane. Many proteins are not fixed but rather 'float' within the membrane such that they are freely mobile within the plane of the phospholipid bilayer. This has led to the use of the term *fluid mosaic model* of membrane structure. Whilst the lipid component of the membrane principally determines its mechanical properties, the dynamic functions of the membrane as an interface between biological compartments is a function of the membrane proteins. Other integral proteins may be fixed by attachment to elements of the cytoskeleton.

On the external surface of the plasma membranes of animal cells, many of the membrane proteins and some of the membrane lipids are conjugated with short chains of polysaccharide; these glycoproteins and glycolipids respectively project from the surface of the bilayer forming an outer coating which may be analogous to the cell walls of plants, bacteria and fungi. This polysaccharide layer has been termed the *glycocalyx* and appears to vary in thickness in different cell types; a similar layer is often also present on membrane surfaces within the cell which are not exposed to the cytosol (e.g. luminal aspects of membrane systems). The glycocalyx appears to be involved in cell recognition phenomena, in the formation of intercellular adhesions and in the adsorption of molecules to the cell surface; in some situations the glycocalyx also provides mechanical and chemical protection for the plasma membrane.

The electron micrograph in (a) provides a high magnification view of a plasma membrane **PM**, in this case of minute surface projections (microvilli) **MV** of a lining cell from the small intestine. The characteristic trilaminate appearance comprises two electron-dense layers separated by an electron-lucent layer. The outer dense layers are thought to correspond to the hydrophilic 'heads' of phospholipid molecules whilst the electron-lucent layer is thought to represent the intermediate hydrophobic layer mainly consisting of fatty acids and cholesterol. On the external surface of the plasma membrane is a fibrillar coat, called the '*fuzzy coat*', representing the glycocalyx **G**. This is an unusually prominent feature of small intestinal lining cells where it incorporates a variety of digestive enzymes.

Transport across plasma membranes

Plasma membranes mediate the exchange of molecules between the internal and external environments of the cell in four principal ways enabling the cell to control the quality of its internal environment with a high degree of specificity.

- **Passive diffusion.** This type of transport is entirely dependent on the presence of a concentration gradient across the plasma membrane. Lipids and lipid-soluble metabolites such as ethanol pass freely through plasma membranes which also offer little barrier to the diffusion of gases such as oxygen and carbon dioxide. The plasma membrane is, in general, impermeable to hydrophilic molecules. Nevertheless some small molecules including water and urea, and inorganic ions such as bicarbonate, are able to pass down osmotic and electrochemical gradients through the membrane via hydrophilic regions, the nature of which remains obscure.

- **Facilitated diffusion.** This type of transport is also concentration-dependent and involves the transport of larger hydrophilic metabolites such as glucose and amino acids. This process is strictly passive but requires the presence of so-called 'carriers' to which the metabolites bind specifically, but reversibly, in a manner analogous to the binding of substrate with enzyme.

- **Active transport.** This mode of transport is not only independent of concentration gradients but also often operates against extreme concentration gradients. The classic example of this form of transport is the continuous transport of sodium out of the cell by the 'sodium pump'; this process requires the expenditure of energy provided in the form of ATP. Active transport is mediated by 'dynamic pores' consisting of transmembrane protein systems. Both active and passive transport processes are enhanced if the area of the plasma membrane is increased by folds or projections of the cell surface as exemplified by the absorptive cells lining the small intestine (see Fig. 1.2).

- **Bulk transport.** This involves large molecules or small particles being engulfed by the plasma membrane, thus forming membrane-bound *vacuoles (vesicles)* within the cytoplasm. When the process involves the creation of small vacuoles it is known as *pinocytosis*, and when large vacuoles are formed it is called *phagocytosis*. The term *endocytosis*, encompassing both processes, is probably a more appropriate term for inwardly directed bulk transport. Endocytotic vesicles either discharge their contents directly into the cytoplasm or fuse with membrane-bound organelles called *lysosomes* which contain a variety of enzymes which are capable of degrading carbohydrates, lipids, proteins, nucleic acids and other organic molecules. Lysosomal enzymes digest engulfed material which is then made available for metabolic processes. In many secretory processes, bulk transport occurs in the opposite direction when it is termed *exocytosis*. In some tissues where cells form a barrier between two extracellular environments, bulk transport involving pinocytotic vesicles is used to transport large molecules from one side of the cell to the other without the involvement of lysosomes; this is described as *transcytosis*.

Histologically, the passive and active processes of transport can only be observed indirectly; for example, cells suspended in hypotonic solutions swell due to passive uptake of water whereas cells placed in hypertonic solutions tend to shrink due to outflow of water. Radio-isotope labelling techniques can be used to follow active transport processes. Bulk transport, however, is readily observable by microscopy (see Fig. 1.3).

(a) *(b)*

Fig. 1.3 Endocytosis *(a) Schematic diagram (b) EM × 11 750*

The diagram summarises the main steps in endocytosis of particulate matter.

The first stage of phagocytosis involves recognition of the matter to be ingested. This then becomes enveloped by plasma membrane which may involve the formation of cytoplasmic extensions called *pseudopodia*. When the particle is completely surrounded, the encompassing plasma membranes fuse and the membrane surrounding the engulfed particle forms a vesicle, known as a *phagosome* or *endocytotic vesicle*, which detaches from the plasma membrane to float freely within the cytoplasm. The phagosome is then in some way recognised by one or more lysosomes (*primary lysosomes*) which fuse with the phagosome to form a *secondary lysosome*. This exposes the engulfed material to a battery of lysosomal enzymes. When digestion is complete, the lysosomal membrane may rupture, discharging its contents into the cytoplasm.

Undigested material may remain within membrane-bound vesicles called *residual bodies*, the contents of which may be later discharged at the cell surface by exocytosis; alternatively residual bodies may accumulate in the cytoplasm. Membrane-bound organelles containing multiple small vesicles called *multivesicular bodies*, are also found in some cells and are thought to represent a form of secondary lysosome or residual body containing multiple pinocytotic vesicles or their remnants (see Fig. 1.4(a)).

Micrograph (b) illustrates a highly phagocytic white blood cell, a neutrophil, in the process of engulfing and destroying bacteria **B**. Note the manner in which pseudopodia **Pp**

embrace the bacteria before engulfment. Note also phagosomes **Ps** containing bacteria in various stages of degradation. Several primary lysosomes **L** are also visible.

Receptor-mediated endocytosis

Whilst some bulk transport may be relatively non-selective and driven by concentration gradients, much endocytosis is highly selective and mediated by specific receptors incorporated in the plasma membrane. The term *ligand* (ligare = to bind) is used to describe molecules taken up by such *receptor-mediated endocytosis*. The receptors are either located in small invaginations of the membrane called *coated pits* or drift laterally within the membrane to become localised within pits. Coated pits are so named for a coating on the inner (cytoplasmic) aspect of the membrane by a protein called *clathrin*; this mediates the engulfment process by formation of a curved lattice structure which governs the shape of the developing membranous vesicle. The *coated vesicles* so formed then lose this clathrin coating which is returned to the inner aspect of the surface membrane and reused in the formation of more coated pits.

Lysosomes are also involved in the degradation of cellular organelles, many of which have only a finite lifespan and are therefore replaced continuously; this lysosomal function is termed *autophagy*. Most autophagocytic degradation products accumulate and become indistinguishable from the residual bodies of endocytosis. With advancing age, residual bodies accumulate in the cells of some tissues and appear as brown *lipofuscin granules* (see Fig. 1.28).

(a)

(b)

(c)

Fig. 1.4 Lysosomes

(a) EM × 27 000 (b) EM × 60 000
(c) Histochemical method for acid phosphatase: EM × 50 000

These micrographs show the typical features of lysosomes and residual bodies. Micrograph (a) shows part of the cytoplasm of a liver cell. Primary lysosomes **Ly₁** vary greatly in size and appearance but they are recognised as membrane-bound organelles containing an amorphous granular material. Secondary lysosomes **Ly₂** are even more variable in appearance but are recognisable by their diverse particulate content some of which is extremely electron-dense. The distinction between residual bodies and secondary lysosomes is often difficult but one distinctive type of residual body, the multivesicular body **MB**, is seen in this micrograph. Note the size of lysosomes relative to mitochondria **M**.

Micrograph (b) shows two secondary lysosomes or residual bodies at higher magnification, allowing the limiting membrane to be visualised. Both contain electron dense particulate material and amorphous granular material.

The lysosomal enzymes comprise more than 40 different acid hydrolases which are optimally active at a pH of about 5.0. This may be a protective mechanism for the cell should lysosomal enzymes escape into the cytosol where they would be less active at the higher pH.

Histochemical methods can be used to demonstrate sites of enzyme activity within cells and thus act as markers for organelles which contain these enzymes. Such a method has been used in micrograph (c) to demonstrate the presence of *acid phosphatase*, a typical lysosomal enzyme; enzyme activity is represented by a very dense deposit within a lysosome **L**. Other organelles remain unstained but the outline of a mitochondrion **M** and saccules of endoplasmic reticulum **ER** can nevertheless be identified.

Fig. 1.5 Peroxisomes *(EM × 40 000)*

Peroxisomes are small, spherical, membrane-bound organelles (also known as *microbodies*) which closely resemble lysosomes in size and electron microscopic appearance. They are, however, distinguished from lysosomes by their content of an entirely different set of enzymes which can be demonstrated by histochemical techniques.

Peroxisomes contain oxidases involved in certain catabolic pathways (e.g. beta oxidation of long chain fatty acids) utilising molecular oxygen and resulting in the formation of hydrogen peroxide, a potentially cytotoxic by-product. Hydrogen peroxide is nevertheless utilised by certain phagocytic cells of the defence system to kill ingested microorganisms and also has a role in certain metabolic pathways. Peroxisomes also contain *catalase* which regulates hydrogen peroxidase concentration, utilising it in the oxidation of a variety of potentially toxic metabolites and ingested substances including phenols and alcohol.

The peroxisomes of many species have a central crystalloid structure called a *nucleoid* which contains the enzyme *urate oxidase*. This is not present in humans which thus lack the ability to metabolise urates. The peroxisomes of the liver and kidney are particularly large and abundant reflecting the functions of these organs in lipid metabolism and management of metabolic waste products.

In this micrograph, note the fine granular electron-dense contents of a peroxisome **P**, the size of which can be compared to that of adjacent mitochondria **M**.

Protein synthesis

Proteins are not only a major structural component of cells but, in the form of enzymes, mediate every metabolic process within the cell. Thus the nature and quantity of proteins present within any individual cell determines the activity of that cell. Both the structural proteins and enzymes of the cell are subject to wear and tear and are replaced continuously. Many cells also synthesise proteins for export; such proteins include glandular secretions and extracellular structural components of tissues. Protein synthesis is, therefore, an essential and continuous activity of all cells and the major function of some cells.

The principal organelles involved in protein synthesis are the *nucleus* and *ribosomes*. The nucleus of every cell contains within its complement of DNA a template for each protein that can be made by that individual as a whole. Most cells, however, only synthesise a certain defined range of proteins which are characteristic of the particular cell type and therefore only part of the DNA template is utilised. The process of protein synthesis involves *transcription* of the DNA code for a particular protein by synthesis of the specific, complementary messenger RNA (mRNA) molecule. The mRNA molecule then enters the cytoplasm to associate with ribosomes upon which protein synthesis occurs; the amino acid sequence of the resulting protein is determined by *translation* of the mRNA code.

Ribosomes are minute cytoplasmic organelles, each composed of two subunits of unequal size. Each subunit consists of a strand of RNA (ribosomal RNA) with associated ribosomal proteins; the ribosomal RNA strand and associated proteins are folded to form a condensed, globular structure. Ribosomes are highly active structures with specific receptor proteins which align mRNA strands so that transfer RNA (tRNA) molecules carrying the appropriate amino acids may be brought into position prior to the addition of their amino acids to the growing polypeptide chain. Other ribosomal proteins are involved in catalysing peptide bond formation between amino acids. Individual ribosomes are too small to be clearly resolved by electron microscopy although they are visible as small electron-dense structures at high magnification; nevertheless, the detail of ribosome structure and function are well established at the molecular level. Ribosomes may be present in the cytoplasm either alone or attached to messenger RNA molecules in small spiral-shaped aggregations called *polyribosomes* or *polysomes*. Ribosomes and polyribosomes may also be attached to the surface of the extensive intracytoplasmic membrane system known as the endoplasmic reticulum (see Fig. 1.9).

(a)

(b)

(c)

Fig. 1.6 Nucleus *(illustrations opposite) (a) EM × 15 000 (b) EM × 67 500 (c) Freeze-etched preparation × 34 000*

Micrograph (a) illustrates the typical nucleus of a highly active, protein-secreting cell, in this case a plasma cell responsible for secretion of antibody. Typical of such cells, the cytoplasm contains numerous profiles of ribosome-studded endoplasmic reticulum **ER** and considerable numbers of mitochondria **M** responsible for production of the energy required for such a metabolically active cell.

Constituents of the nucleus

The nucleus not only contains DNA, which comprises less than 20% of its mass, but also contains a large quantity of protein called *nucleoprotein* and some RNA. Most of the nucleoprotein is closely associated with DNA, these DNA-binding proteins being of two major types, *histones* and *non-histones*. Histones, which comprise the bulk of DNA-associated protein, are relatively low molecular weight proteins with a high content of positively charged amino acids which bind them readily to the negatively charged DNA strands. Histones may be involved in the folding of DNA strands and the regulation of DNA activity. The non-histone DNA-associated proteins are a heterogeneous group which may also be involved in the regulation of gene activity. The remaining nucleoproteins include enzymes responsible for DNA and RNA synthesis. All nucleoproteins are synthesised in the cytoplasm and imported into the nucleus. The nuclear RNA represents newly synthesised messenger, transfer and ribosomal RNA which has not yet passed into the cytoplasm.

Except during cell division, the chromosomes, each comprising a discrete length of the DNA complement, exist as tangled strands which extend throughout the nucleus and cannot be visualised individually by direct electron microscopy. Nuclei appear as heterogeneous structures with electron-dense and electron-lucent areas. The dense areas, called *heterochromatin*, represent that portion of the DNA complement and its associated nucleoprotein which is not active in RNA synthesis. Heterochromatin **H** tends to be clumped around the periphery of the nucleus but also forms irregular clumps throughout the nucleus. In females, the quiescent X-chromosome (equivalent to the Y-chromosome of the male) forms a small discrete mass known as a *Barr body*; Barr bodies are seen at the edge of the nucleus in a small proportion of female cells when cut in a favourable plane of section. The electron-lucent nuclear material, called *euchromatin* **E**, represents that part of the DNA which is active in RNA synthesis. Collectively, heterochromatin and euchromatin are known as *chromatin*, a name derived from the strongly coloured appearance of nuclei when stained for light microscopy.

Nucleoli

Many nuclei, especially those of cells highly active in protein synthesis, contain one or more dense structures called *nucleoli* **Nu** which are the sites of ribosomal RNA synthesis and ribosome assembly. The many different ribosomal proteins are imported from the cytoplasm and conjugated with ribosomal RNA to form the ribosomal subunits which then pass into the cytoplasm before being assembled into fully active ribosomes. Nucleoli are heterogeneous structures, the paler areas being the sites of DNA coding for ribosomal RNA and the dark areas being the sites of partially assembled ribosomes.

Each cell type has a characteristic nuclear morphology and, in general, the degree of activity of any cell may be judged by the ultrastructural appearance of its nucleus. Relatively inactive cells have small nuclei in which the chromatin is predominantly in the condensed form (heterochromatin) and in which the nucleolus is small or absent. In highly active cells, the nuclear material is dispersed (euchromatin) and nucleoli are a prominent feature.

Nuclear envelope

The nuclear envelope **NE** which encloses the nucleus is illustrated in micrograph (b). It consists of two layers of membrane (each layer of standard phospholipid bilayer structure) which represent a specialised part of the endoplasmic reticulum. The intermembranous (perinuclear) space is continuous with that of the endoplasmic reticulum **ER** and like much of the endoplasmic reticulum, the outer surface of the nuclear envelope is studded with ribosomes **R**. On the inner aspect of the nuclear envelope there is an electron-dense fibrillar layer, the nuclear lamina, consisting of polypeptides bound to membrane proteins and linked with condensed peripheral chromatin **C**. To the nuclear lamina is attached a network of filamentous proteins which provide internal support for the nuclear contents and nucleoli and thus represent the nuclear cytoskeleton.

Nuclear pores

The nuclear envelope contains numerous *nuclear pores* **NP** at the margins of which the inner and outer membranes become continuous. Each pore contains an electron-dense structure known as a *nuclear pore complex* which consists of a ring of proteins with a central channel, the whole complex being secured to and stabilised by the nuclear lamina. Nuclear pores permit and regulate the exchange of metabolites, macromolecules and ribosomal subunits between nucleus and cytoplasm.

Micrograph (c) shows an example of a technique called *freeze-etching*. Briefly, this method involves the rapid cooling of cells to subzero temperatures; the frozen cells are then fractured. Internal surfaces of the cell are thus exposed (in a somewhat random manner), the fracture lines tending to follow natural planes of weakness. Surface detail is obtained by 'etching' or subliming excess water molecules from the specimen at low temperature. A thin carbon impression is then made of the surface and this mirror image is viewed by conventional electron microscopy. Freeze-etching provides a valuable tool for studying internal cell surfaces at high resolution.

In this preparation, the plane of cleavage has included part of the nuclear envelope in which nuclear pores **NP** are clearly demonstrated. Note also the outline of the plasma membrane **PM** and mitochrondria **M**.

(a)

(b)

Fig. 1.7 Rough endoplasmic reticulum

(a) EM × 23 000 (b) EM × 50 000

The endoplasmic reticulum consists of an interconnecting network of membranous tubules, vesicles and flattened sacs (*cisternae*) which ramifies throughout the cytoplasm. Much of its surface is studded with ribosomes giving a rough or granular appearance leading to the name *rough* or *granular endoplasmic reticulum* (rER or gER). Proteins are synthesised by the ribosomes on the external surface of the rER and are then passed into the reticular lumen. Protein synthesised by rER is destined either for secretion or for incorporation in lysosomes; integral membrane proteins are also synthesised on rER. In contrast, proteins synthesised on free ribosomes are utilised within the cytosol.

These micrographs illustrate rough endoplasmic reticulum in a cell which is specialised for the synthesis and secretion of protein; in such cells rough endoplasmic reticulum tends to be profuse and to form closely packed parallel laminae of flattened cisternae.

In micrograph (a), the dimensions of the rER can be compared with that of mitochondria **M** and the nucleus **N**. The nucleus typically contains a prominent nucleolus **Nu**. Note the close association of the rER with the nuclear envelope **NE** with which it is in continuity. The chromatin in the nucleus is mainly dispersed (euchromatin) consistent with this great biosynthetic activity.

Micrograph (b) shows part of the rER at high magnification. Numerous ribosomes stud the surface of the membrane system and numerous other ribosomes lie free in the intervening cytosol.

Lipid biosynthesis

Lipids are synthesised by all cells in order to repair and replace damaged or worn membranes. Cells may also synthesise lipid as a means of storing excess energy (as cytoplasmic droplets), for lipid transport (e.g. chylomicron production by cells of the small intestine) and in the form of steroid hormones. The precursor molecules (fatty acids, triglycerides and cholesterol) are available to the cell from dietary sources, mobilisation of lipid stored in other cells or can be synthesised by most cells using simple sources of carbon such as acetyl-CoA and other intermediates of glucose catabolism. Fatty acids and triglycerides are mostly synthesised within the cytosol, whereas cholesterol and phospholipids are synthesised in areas of endoplasmic reticulum devoid of ribosomes called *smooth endoplasmic reticulum (sER)*.

Fig. 1.8 Smooth endoplasmic reticulum *(EM × 40 000)*

Smooth endoplasmic reticulum (sER) consists of an irregular network of membranous tubules and vesicles devoid of ribosomes in contrast to the flattened ribosome-studded cisternae of rough endoplasmic reticulum. It forms part of the intracellular membrane system being continuous with the rough endoplasmic reticulum and Golgi apparatus (see Fig. 1.9). The principal functions of smooth endoplasmic reticulum are lipid biosynthesis and intracellular transport; in liver cells, smooth endoplasmic reticulum also plays a major role in the metabolism of glycogen and detoxification of various noxious metabolic by-products, drugs and alcohol. In highly contractile cells (muscle), sER is involved in storage and release of calcium ions which activates the contractile mechanism (see Ch. 6). One particular enzyme, cytochrome P450, is present in large amounts in the smooth endoplasmic reticulum of liver; this enzyme hydroxylates water-insoluble hydrocarbons which

become dissolved in the lipid bilayer of the membranous vesicles.

In general, most cells do not have a prominent system of smooth endoplasmic reticulum but, rather, scattered elements can be seen amongst the other organelles. The notable exceptions are the liver and those cells specialised for lipid biosynthesis such as the steroid hormone-secreting cells of the adrenal glands and the gonads. In this micrograph from the liver, most of the membranous elements are smooth endoplasmic reticulum **sER**; however, for comparison, rough endoplasmic reticulum **rER** is included in the lower right of the field. Note the continuity of the two forms of ER. This field also includes several mitochondria **M**, a peroxisome **P**, free ribosomes and polyribosomes **R** and a whorl of membrane in a residual body **RB**.

Secretion

The export from cells of excretory (waste) products or secretory products involves the four principal mechanisms outlined earlier for the transport of materials into cells across the plasma membrane. Excretion or secretion of small molecular weight compounds or lipid-soluble materials rarely involves bulk transport, whereas secretion of proteins and protein complexes almost always involves this mode of transfer. Prior to release from the cell, proteins and other secretory products are packaged within membrane-bound vesicles. These then fuse with the surface plasma membrane thus releasing their contents by the process of exocytosis. The *Golgi apparatus* (also called *Golgi body* or *Golgi complex*) is the organelle primarily responsible for the packaging process. By a similar process, the Golgi is also responsible for lysosome formation.

The Golgi apparatus is also involved in modification of certain proteins and contains the enzymes required for the synthesis of glycoproteins; these include plasma membrane glycoproteins forming the glycocalyx. Likewise, the Golgi is also responsible for the elaboration of membrane glycolipids.

During the secretory process, large amounts of intracellular membrane become incorporated into the plasma membrane and the Golgi system recycles excess plasma membrane, returning it to an internal 'pool' of membrane. The Golgi apparatus also elaborates new membrane necessary for cell growth and formation of membrane-bound organelles such as lysosomes, as well as replacing membrane lost or damaged during normal metabolic activities.

Fig. 1.9 Golgi apparatus *(illustrations opposite) (a) Schematic diagram (b) EM × 30 000*

The diagram (a) illustrates the main structural features of the Golgi apparatus and summarises the mechanism by which secretory products are packaged within membrane-bound vesicles.

The Golgi apparatus consists of a system of stacked, saucer-shaped cisternae with the concave surface facing the nucleus. Proteins, synthesised on ribosomes of the rough endoplasmic reticulum, are transported within the endoplasmic reticulum to the vicinity of the Golgi apparatus. Small membrane-bound vesicles containing protein, known as *transfer vesicles*, bud off from the endoplasmic reticulum and then coalesce with the convex surface of the Golgi apparatus, an area of the Golgi apparatus known as the *forming face*. By a mechanism still unresolved, secretory product is passed towards the concave surface, the *maturing face*, where new vesicles containing secretory product are formed; these *secretory vesicles* are of much greater dimensions than the transfer vesicles seen at the Golgi forming face. After release from the maturing face, the contents of secretory vesicles become increasingly

condensed to form mature secretory vesicles, often termed *secretory granules*, which are then liberated at the cell surface by exocytosis.

The Golgi apparatus is a dynamically changing structure, the appearance of which varies according to the functional state of the cell; for this reason the 'classic' appearance of the Golgi apparatus is, in practice, rarely seen. Moreover, a cell may contain as many as 100 Golgi stacks or even more, all being linked by an anastomosing membrane network.

The micrograph (b) illustrates a particularly well developed Golgi apparatus; transfer vesicles **T** and elements of the rough endoplasmic reticulum **rER** are seen adjacent to the forming face. A variety of larger vesicles **V** can be seen in the concavity of the maturing face, some of which appear to be budding from the Golgi cisternae **C**; such vesicles represent both potential secretory granules and lysosomes. Note the proximity of the Golgi apparatus to the nucleus **N**; the nuclear membrane **NM** is particularly well demonstrated in this micrograph.

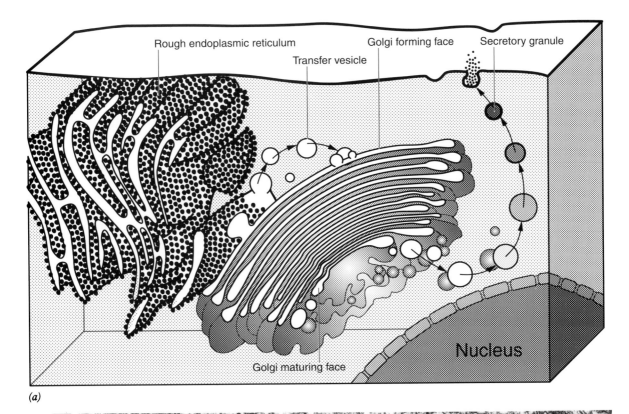

Rough endoplasmic reticulum   Golgi forming face   Secretory granule

Transfer vesicle

Nucleus

Golgi maturing face

(a)

(b)

(a)

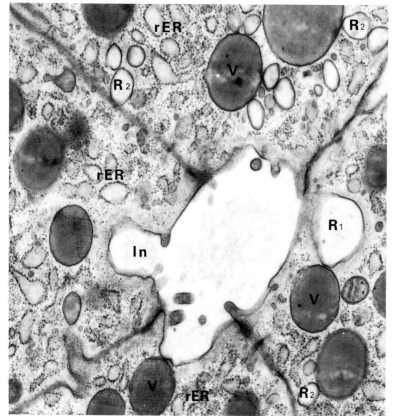

(b)

Fig. 1.10 Exocytosis

(a) EM × 14 000 (b) EM × 30 000

Micrograph (a) illustrates a typical protein-secreting cell, in this case from the pancreatic gland which produces a secretion rich in digestive enzymes. In the nucleus **N**, the chromatin is typically dispersed, and there is a prominent nucleolus **Nu**. The cytoplasm is packed with rough endoplasmic reticulum **rER**, there is a prominent Golgi apparatus **G** and scattered mitochondria **M**. Secretory vesicles **V** become increasingly electron-dense as they are concentrated towards the glandular lumen **L**.

Micrograph (b) shows the apical regions of four pancreatic secretory cells converging on a tiny central excretory duct. Large secretory vesicles **V** are seen approaching the lumen, one of which appears to be fusing with the surface plasma membrane. A deep invagination **In** in one of the plasma membranes probably represents a secretory vesicle which has just discharged its contents. A large vesicle R_1, and numerous smaller, apparently empty vesicles R_2 may represent vesicle membrane in the process of being recycled.

Energy production and storage

All cellular functions are dependent on a continuous supply of energy which is derived from the sequential breakdown of organic molecules during the process of *cellular respiration*. The energy released during this process is ultimately stored in the form of ATP molecules. In actively respiring cells, ATP forms a pool of readily available energy for all the metabolic functions of the cell. The main substrates for cellular respiration are simple sugars and lipids, particularly glucose and fatty acids. Cellular respiration of glucose (glycolysis) begins in the cytosol where it is partially degraded to form pyruvic acid, yielding a small amount of ATP. Pyruvic acid then diffuses into specialised membranous organelles called *mitochrondria* where, in the presence of oxygen, it is degraded to carbon dioxide and water; this process yields a large quantity of ATP. In contrast, fatty acids pass directly into mitochondria where they are also degraded to carbon dioxide and water; this also generates a large amount of ATP. Glycolysis may occur in the absence of oxygen and is therefore termed *anaerobic respiration*, whereas mitochondrial respiration is dependent on a continuous supply of oxygen and is therefore termed *aerobic respiration*. Mitochondria are the principal organelles involved in cellular respiration in mammals and are found in large numbers in metabolically active cells such as those in the liver and skeletal muscle.

Under favourable nutritional conditions, most cells generate and store excess glucose and fatty acids in the relatively insoluble and non-toxic forms, glycogen and triglyceride respectively. Cells vary greatly in their content of stored carbohydrate and lipid; extreme examples are nerve cells, which contain almost no intracellular glycogen or triglyceride, and fat cells, the cytoplasm of which is almost entirely filled with stored lipid.

Fig. 1.11 Mitochondria

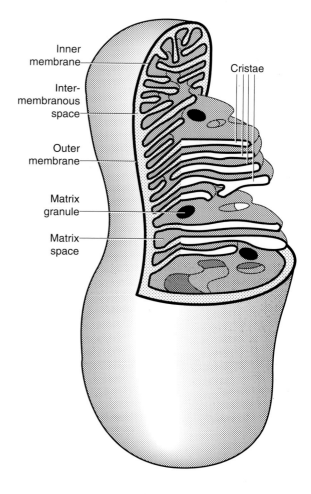

Mitochondria vary considerably in size and shape but are most often elongated, cigar-shaped organelles. They are motile and tend to localise at intracellular sites of maximum energy requirement. The number of mitochondria in cells is highly variable; liver cells contain as many as 2000 mitochondria whereas inactive cells contain very few.

Each mitochondrion consists of two layers of membrane. The outer membrane is relatively permeable and contains enzymes that convert certain lipid substrates into forms that can be metabolised within the mitochondrion. The inner membrane is thrown into folds called *cristae* projecting into the inner cavity which is filled with an amorphous substance called *matrix*. The matrix contains a number of dense *matrix granules*, the nature and function of which are unclear. The inner mitochondrial membrane is closely applied to the outer membrane leaving a narrow *intermembranous space* which extends into each crista. Aerobic respiration takes place within the matrix and inner mitochondrial membranes and this process is enhanced by the large surface area provided by the cristae. The matrix contains most of the enzymes involved in oxidation of fatty acids and the Krebs cycle. The inner membrane contains the cytochromes, the carrier molecules of the electron transport chain, and the enzymes involved in ATP production.

As organelles, mitochondria have several most unusual features. The mitochondrial matrix contains a strand of DNA arranged as a circle in a manner analogous to the chromosomes of bacteria. The matrix also contains ribosomes which have a similar structure to bacterial ribosomes.

Mitochondria synthesise at least some of their own constituent proteins, others being synthesised by the cell in which they reside. In addition, mitochondria undergo self-replication in a manner similar to bacterial cell division. It has thus been proposed that mitochondria are semi-autonomous organelles which arose during evolution as bacterial intracellular parasites of larger, more advanced cells.

Inner membrane

Cristae

Inter-membranous space

Outer membrane

Matrix granule

Matrix space

(a)

(b)

(c)

(e)

(d)

Fig. 1.12 Mitochondria, lipid droplets and glycogen *(illustrations (a) and (b) opposite)*

(a) EM × 42 000 (b) EM × 17 000 (c) EM × 25 000
(d) EM × 32 400 (e) EM × 13 000

All mitochondria conform to the same general structure but vary greatly in size, shape and arrangement of cristae; these variations often reflect the metabolic status of the cell type in which the mitochondria are found. Mitochondria move freely within the cytosol and tend to aggregate in intracellular sites with high energy demands where their shape often conforms to the available space.

Micrographs (a) and (b), both of liver cell cytoplasm, show the typical appearance of mitochondria when cut in different planes of section; note their relatively dense matrix containing a few matrix granules **G**. Glycogen is well demonstrated in micrographs (a) and (b), appearing either as irregular granules (called *α particles*) or as aggregations termed *glycogen rosettes* **GR** (also called *β particles*). As seen in micrograph (b), lipid droplets **L** are not bounded by a membrane; their size and electron density varies considerably. Note also rough and smooth endoplasmic reticulum (**rER** and **sER**), nuclei **N** and a residual body **RB**.

Mitochondria from heart muscle and steroid-secreting cells can be seen in micrographs (c) and (d) respectively. In each, the cristae are densely packed, reflecting the metabolic activity of the cell. The cristae have a characteristic shape, those of heart muscle being laminar whereas those of steroid-secreting cells are tubular. Note lipid droplets **L** in both fields.

Micrograph (e) shows the base of an absorptive cell from a kidney tubule where there is intense active transport of ions. The basal plasma membrane **PM** is deeply infolded so as to greatly increase its surface area, and elongated mitochondria are packed into the intervening spaces.

The cytoskeleton and cell movement

In order to maintain structural stability, there is within every cell a supporting framework of minute filaments and tubules known as the *cytoskeleton*. Nevertheless, the cell membrane and intracellular organelles are not rigid or static structures but are in a constant state of movement to accommodate processes such as endocytosis, phagocytosis and secretion. Some cells (e.g. white blood cells) propel themselves about by amoeboid movement, other cells have actively motile membrane specialisations such as cilia and flagella (see Ch. 5), whilst other cells (e.g. muscle cells) are highly specialised for contractility. In addition, cell division is a process which involves extensive reorganisation of cellular constituents. The cytoskeleton thus incorporates features which accommodate all these dynamic functions.

The cytoskeleton of each cell contains structural elements of three main types, *microfilaments*, *microtubules* and *intermediate filaments* as well as many accessory proteins responsible for linking these structures to one another, to the plasma membrane and to the membranes of the intracellular organelles.

- **Microfilaments.** Microfilaments are extremely fine strands (5 nm in diameter) of a protein known as *actin*. Each actin filament consists of two strings of bead-like subunits twisted together like a rope. The globular subunits are stabilised by calcium ions and associated with ATP molecules which provide energy for contractile processes.

  Actin filaments are best demonstrated histologically in skeletal muscle cells where they are arranged in bundles with another type of filamentous protein called *myosin*. Contraction occurs when the actin and myosin filaments slide relative to one another due to the rearrangement of intermolecular bonds fuelled by the release of energy from associated ATP molecules; this process is described in more detail in Chapter 6.

  Cells not considered to be overtly contractile also contain the globular subunits of various subtypes of actin which appear to assemble readily into microfilaments and then dissociate, thereby providing a dynamically changing structural framework for the cell. Membrane specialisations such as microvilli (see Fig. 5.16) also contain a skeleton of actin filaments which not only provide structural support but also cause the microvilli to shorten and elongate.

  Beneath the plasma membrane, actin in association with various transmembrane and linking proteins (predominantly *filamin*) forms a robust supporting meshwork called the *cell cortex* which protects against deformation yet can be rearranged to accommodate change in cell morphology.

- **Microtubules.** Microtubules (25 nm in diameter) are much larger than microfilaments but, like them, are made up of globular protein subunits which can readily be assembled and disassembled to provide for alterations in cell shape and position of organelles. The microtubule subunits are of two types, *alpha* and *beta tubulin*, which polymerise to form a hollow tubule; when seen in cross-section, 13 tubulin molecules make up a circle. Microtubules grow out from a specialised *microtubule organising centre* called the *centrosome* (see below) and in most cells, movement appears to be effected by the addition or subtraction of tubulin subunits from the microtubules causing them to become either lengthened or shortened. *Microtubule-associated proteins* (MAPs) stabilise the tubular structure and including *capping proteins* which stabilise the growing ends of the tubules. Two *attachment proteins*, *dynein* and *kinesin* (which can move along the tubules towards and away from the cell centre respectively), may become attached to membranous organelles (e.g. mitochondria, vesicles) providing a means by which they can be moved about within the cytoplasm. The function of the spindle during cell division is a classic example of this process on a large scale (see Fig. 2.3). In cilia, nine pairs of microtubules are disposed in a cylindrical structure, and movement occurs by rearrangement of chemical bonds between adjacent microtubule pairs (see Fig. 5.15).

- **Intermediate filaments.** Intermediate filaments (10-12 nm in diameter) are, as their name implies, intermediate in size between microfilaments and microtubules. However, in contrast, intermediate filaments have a stable fibrous structure made up of a variety of different irregular molecular strands which appear to be specific to particular cell types. For example, in epithelial cells, the intermediate filaments are composed of the protein *cytokeratin* and are known as *tonofibrils*; the filaments form a tough supporting meshwork within the cytoplasm and are anchored to the plasma membrane at strong intracellular junctions with the adjacent epithelial cells. Other tissue specific intermediate filament proteins include *vimentin* (cells of mesodermal origin), *desmin* (muscle) and *neurofilament protein* (nerve cells).

The organising centre for the cytoskeleton appears to be located near the nucleus in an area called the *centrosome* (cell centre) which contains a pair of *centrioles*. Each centriole consists of nine triplets of microtubules arranged in a cylindrical manner, the pair of centrioles being disposed at right angles to one another. The centrosome appears to act as a nucleation centre for microtubules which radiate from here towards the cell periphery. Centrioles appear to be necessary for microtubular function. For example, prior to cell division the pair of centrioles is duplicated, the pairs migrating towards opposite ends of the cell. Here they act as organising centres for the microtubules of the spindle which controls distribution of chromosomes to the daughter cells. Likewise a pair of centrioles, known as a *basal body*, is found at the base of the microtubules of cilia.

The distribution of microfilaments and intermediate filaments tends to be complementary to that of the microtubules and there is experimental evidence that, at least in some situations, microtubules may form a temporary framework around which more permanent cytoskeletal structures can be built up. The elements of the cytoskeleton are attached to one another and to the plasma membrane and the membranes of cytoplasmic organelles by a variety of linking proteins. In addition, some of the metabolic enzyme systems of the cytosol appear to be bound to various elements of the cytoskeleton. Moreover, the cytoskeleton appears to provide a mechanism whereby some molecules can be transported within the cell; such molecules are bound to microfilaments and microtubules and as these elongate and shorten, the molecules are moved from one site to another. The cytoskeletal elements may then disassemble leaving the transported molecules in new positions.

In summary, the cytoskeleton consists of three main structural elements. The microfilaments and the microtubules are relatively labile and dynamically changing structures (except where they perform highly specialised functions such as in muscle and cilia respectively), whereas the intermediate filaments serve a more static supporting function. The functions of the cytoskeleton are fourfold. Firstly, it provides the structural support for the plasma membrane, cellular organelles and some cytosol enzyme systems. Secondly, it provides the means for movement of intracellular organelles, the plasma membrane and other cytosol constituents necessary for the routine function of all cells. Thirdly, the cytoskeleton provides the locomotor mechanism for amoeboid movements and specialised motile structures such as cilia and flagella. Finally, the cytoskeleton is responsible for the property of contractility in the cells of specialised tissues such as muscle.

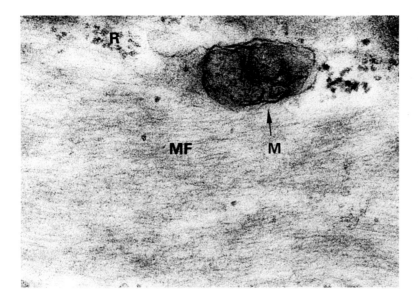

Fig. 1.13 Microfilaments
(EM × 76 500)

In general, individual microfilaments are difficult to demonstrate because of their small diameter and diffuse arrangement amongst other cytoplasmic components. In this example from a smooth muscle cell, a cell type in which cytoplasmic filaments are a predominant feature, parallel arrays of microfilaments **MF** are readily seen. The diameter of microfilaments may be compared with the diameter of a mitochondrion **M** and ribosomes **R**.

(a)

(b)

Fig. 1.14 Intermediate filaments and microtubules *(EM (a) TS × 53 000 (b) LS × 40 000)*

These micrographs are taken from nervous tissue; nerve cells contain both intermediate filaments and microtubules, allowing comparison of size and morphology. Each nerve cell has an elongated cytoplasmic extension called an axon (see Ch.7) which in the peripheral nervous system is ensheathed by a supporting Schwann cell. Micrograph (a) shows an axon in transverse section ensheathed by the cytoplasm of a Schwann cell **S**. Micrograph (b) shows part of an axon in longitudinal section. The axonal microtubules provide structural support and direct intra-axonal transport.

In longitudinal section, microtubules **MT** appear as straight, unbranched structures and in transverse section appear hollow. Their diameter can be compared with small mitochondria **M** and smooth endoplasmic reticulum **sER**.

Intermediate filaments (known as neurofilaments in nervous tissue) are a prominent feature of nerve cells, providing internal support for the cell by cross linkage with microtubules and other organelles. The neurofilaments **NF** are dispersed among and in parallel with the microtubules but are much smaller in diameter and not hollow in cross-section. Intermediate filaments **IF** are also seen in the Schwann cell cytoplasm in micrograph (a).

(a)

(b)

Fig. 1.15 Centrosome *(a) EM × 9200 (b) EM × 48 000*

The centrosome is a zone of cytoplasm usually centrally located in the cell adjacent to the nucleus **N** and often surrounded by the Golgi apparatus **G**. The centrosome, the *cell centre*, contains a pair of *centrioles* **C** together known as a *diplosome* and the surrounding cytoplasm is of increased electron density.

Centrioles are highly specialised microtubular structures and the centrosome in some way acts as the organising centre for the growth of microtubules of the cytoskeleton which radiates outwards in a star-like arrangement called an *aster*.

Each centriole is cylindrical in form, closed at one end, and consisting of nine triplets of parallel microtubules. In transverse section as seen in the lower half of micrograph (b), each triplet **T** is seen to consist of an inner microtubule which is circular in cross-section and two further microtubules which are C-shaped in cross-section. Each of the inner microtubules is connected to the outermost microtubule of the adjacent triplet by fine filaments **F**, thus forming a cylinder. The two centrioles of each diplosome are arranged with their long axes at right angles to each other as can be seen in these micrographs; the significance of this arrangement is obscure.

Structures apparently identical to centrioles form the basal bodies of cilia and flagella (see Figs. 5.15 and 18.7 and 18.8 respectively). Cilia are a cell surface specialisation, each cilium comprising a minute hair-like cytoplasmic extension containing microtubules. Cilia move in a wave-like fashion for the purpose of moving secretions across a tissue surface. Flagella are the long tails responsible for the motility of sperm but also are found in modified form at other unusual sites; microtubules also provide their means of locomotion.

Fig. 1.16 Centrosome and microtubules *(EM × 30 000)*

This micrograph shows the centrosome acting as organising centre for the microtubules of the cytoskeleton. The centrosome consists of two centrioles **C** (both cut somewhat obliquely in this specimen) typically located at the centre of the cell close to the nucleus **N**. Several microtubules **MT** are seen radiating from the centrosome towards the cell periphery.

Other features of this micrograph, which is from an antibody secreting plasma cell, include profuse rough endoplasmic reticulum **rER** distended with secretory product, several saccular profiles of an extensive Golgi complex **G** and scattered mitochondria **M**.

The integrated function of cells in tissues, organs and organ systems

As mentioned at the outset, cells are the functional units of all living organisms; indeed the most primitive organisms merely consist of single cells. In multicellular organisms, however, individual cells become specialised (differentiated) and grouped together to perform specific functions. Cells of similar morphology and function form *tissues* which are relatively homogeneous in overall structure; examples include cartilage, bone and muscle. *Organs* are anatomically discrete collections of tissues which together perform certain specific functions (e.g. liver, kidney, eye, ovary). Tissues and organs may constitute integrated functional systems which may form major anatomical entities (e.g. central nervous system, female reproductive tract, gastrointestinal tract, urinary system) or be more diffusely arranged (e.g. immune defence system, diffuse neuroendocrine system). Despite the foregoing, the terms, tissue, organ and system are not necessarily mutually exclusive and may in some cases be used interchangeably depending on the functional implications. Part 2 of this book describes five basic tissues namely blood, supporting/connective tissue, epithelia, muscle and nervous tissues as these are constituents of all organs and organ systems. Many tissues contain a mixture of functionally specialised cells and less specialised supporting tissue to which the terms *parenchyma* and *stroma* may be applied respectively.

Within tissues and organs, cells interact with one another in numerous ways during embryological development and growth, maintenance of structural integrity, response to injury (inflammation and repair), integration and control of tissue and organ functions and the maintenance of overall biochemical and metabolic integrity (homeostasis). This often involves the elaboration of structural connections between adjacent cells (various types of intercellular junctions) which in some cases may also serve as conduits for information exchange in the form of electrical excitation or chemical messengers (*cytokines*), or transfer of metabolic or other products. Some cells are indirectly bound to one another within tissues by various extracellular elements (e.g. the fibres of supporting/connective tissues). Within tissues, cellular functions are integrated by a great variety of local chemical mediators (humoral factors). At the level of systems and the body as a whole, functions are coordinated via circulating chemical messengers (hormones) and/or via the nervous system. The great pleasure to be derived from the study of histology is that all structures from the subcellular to that of organs systems always reflect these functional requirements and inter-relationships.

Light microscopical appearances of cellular organelles

Knowledge of the ultrastructure of cells has mainly been obtained from electron microscopic studies, nevertheless light microscopy still has a useful role in the demonstration of intracellular components. A major advantage of light microscopy is that a wide range of empirical and specific staining methods are available to demonstrate cellular organelles and biochemical constituents. The empirical methods, the traditional staining techniques of histology, were developed in the last century from dyes used in the textile industry.

The specific staining methods, known as *histochemical techniques*, employ reagents known to react with defined cellular constituents (e.g. lipids, glycogen and DNA) thereby staining those constituents in a characteristic manner. The activity of enzymes can similarly be demonstrated by staining for their specific substrates or end products; such methods are examples of *enzyme histochemistry*. Antibodies can be raised against specific cellular components (in this context, the 'antigen') and then conjugated with dyes or with enzymes. The antibodies are then applied to the tissue under study where they combine with the 'antigen' thus localising the dye or attached enzyme at the intracellular site of the 'antigen'; dyes can be viewed directly and the presence of enzyme can be demonstrated by an appropriate histochemical method. Such immunological methods (*immunohistochemistry*) have a high degree of specificity and are suitable for accurate localisation of cellular constituents. Histochemical, enzyme and immunological techniques have more recently been adapted for use in electron microscopy (e.g. Fig. 1.4c).

A problem common to both light and electron microscopy is the need to prevent autolytic degeneration and to preserve cellular ultrastructure; *fixatives* such as formaldehyde are therefore employed for this purpose. *Fixation* causes cross linking of macromolecules which arrests biological activity, at the same time rendering the cells more amenable to staining.

Most tissues are too thick to be examined directly in the microscope and must therefore be cut into very thin slices (*sections*). To facilitate the cutting of thin sections, the tissue is usually *embedded* in a hard medium such as paraffin wax or a plastic resin; fixed tissues generally require dehydration with organic solvents before embedding. Each stage in the fixation, dehydration, embedding, sectioning and final staining sequence may induce distortions (*artefacts*) in the cellular architecture. When biological activity of cell constituents (e.g. enzymes) must be preserved as for histochemistry, thin sections can be obtained from unfixed frozen tissue; such *frozen sections* have their own peculiar artefactual distortions. The next section illustrates examples of histological methods employed in the study of cellular ultrastructure.

(a)

(b)

Fig. 1.17 Nuclei *(a) H & E × 480 (b) Azan × 320*

Nuclei from different tissues vary greatly in morphology depending on function and level of protein synthetic activity. The nucleic acids DNA and RNA are negatively charged, thus having an affinity for basic dyes i.e. they are *basophilic*. The intensity of nuclear staining with such dyes reflects the concentration of DNA and RNA in different parts of the nucleus. The nuclei of cells active in protein synthesis are generally large and relatively lightly stained since their chromatin is widely dispersed; nucleoli are usually prominent, reflecting ribosomal RNA synthesis. In contrast, inactive cells have condensed chromatin and therefore have small, densely stained nuclei and no visible nucleoli.

The cytoplasm of highly active cells often contains much rough endoplasmic reticulum of which the ribosomal RNA is also stained by basic dyes. The intensity of cytoplasmic staining is, however, usually much less than that of the nucleus reflecting the lower concentration of nucleic acids.

The specimen shown in micrograph (a) is of brain tissue which has been stained with *haematoxylin and eosin* (H & E), the 'standard' histological staining method. Haematoxylin is

blue in colour and eosin is pink. Haematoxylin, a basic dye, is principally employed to demonstrate nuclear form whereas eosin, an acidic dye, has affinity for positively-charged structures such as mitochondria and many other cytoplasmic constituents (excluding ribosomes which are basophilic as previously described); *acidophilic* structures are therefore *eosinophilic* when stained by the H & E method. The highly active nerve cells **N** seen in micrograph (a) have huge nuclei with relatively pale-stained, dispersed nuclear chromatin and prominent nucleoli. In contrast, the surrounding relatively inactive support cells **S** have small nuclei with densely-stained, condensed chromatin and no visible nucleoli. Note the cytoplasmic basophilia of the nerve cells due to their high content of ribosomes.

The specimen in micrograph (b) also shows nervous tissue but in this case is stained by the *Azan* method which contains a red basophilic dye and a blue-green acidophilic dye. Note how the nuclear form of the neurones **N** and support cells **S** corresponds to that in micrograph (a) despite the difference in colour.

Fig. 1.18 Nucleus *(Cresyl violet × 800)*

This micrograph shows a single nerve cell at very high magnification stained by another basophilic dye, *cresyl violet*. In this cell, the dispersed chromatin and prominent nucleolus are particularly well demonstrated. Even the nuclear envelope can be distinguished, its basophilia being due to the numerous ribosomes which stud its outer surface. The basophilic clumps in the extensive nerve cell cytoplasm represent areas of prolific rough endoplasmic reticulum.

Fig. 1.19 Nucleic acids *(Acridine orange × 320)*

In this micrograph, a *fluorescent method* has been used for localising DNA and RNA. The specimen has been stained with a dye which combines with DNA and RNA. When viewed in a *fluorescent microscope*, the DNA is seen as yellow-green fluorescence and RNA as orange-red fluorescence thereby highlighting the nuclei and cytoplasm respectively. The micrograph shows plasma cells and lymphocytes in a smear of bone marrow aspirate; the plasma cells, which are very active in protein synthesis, have much cytoplasmic RNA whereas the quiescent lymphocytes have almost none.

Fig. 1.20 Golgi apparatus *(Giemsa × 300)*

This micrograph illustrates a plasma cell from a bone marrow smear; these cells are responsible for antibody production. The cytoplasm is packed with rough endoplasmic reticulum responsible for protein (antibody) synthesis and is thus strongly basophilic. There is a very well developed Golgi complex comprising numerous stacks of membrane (see Fig. 1.9) which packages the antibody prior to secretion. Since it mainly consists of lipid (membrane) which is dissolved out during preparation, the Golgi remains unstained and appears as a pale area (negative image) adjacent to the nucleus.

Fig. 1.21 Secretory granules *(Iron haematoxylin × 400)*

This staining method is used here to demonstrate the secretory granules of the pancreatic gland which secretes digestive enzymes. The secretory cells are grouped around a minute central duct **D** and the secretory granules, which are stained black, are concentrated towards the luminal aspect of the cell. Correlate this appearance with the ultrastructural appearance shown in Figure 1.10. The nuclei **N** of the secretory cells have dispersed chromatin and prominent nucleoli and are arranged around the periphery of the secretory unit.

Fig. 1.22 Secretory products

(Immunoperoxidase × 600)

In this specimen, the intracellular location of IgA antibody within plasma cells has been defined using an immunological staining technique. The reagent consists of an antibody raised against the human IgA to be demonstrated, this raised antibody being conjugated to the enzyme, *horseradish peroxidase*. The brown deposits seen in the cytoplasm of some of the cells represent the reaction product of a standard enzyme histochemical method for horseradish peroxidase, a commercially available enzyme which is frequently used in immunohistochemistry. A similar technique has been used to demonstrate glucagon secreting cells in Figure 17.21.

(a)

(b)

Fig. 1.23 Mitochondria *(a) Iron haematoxylin × 480 (b) Succinate dehydrogenase × 480*

Mitochondria are in general not seen by light microscopy. However, they are acidophilic and with the standard H & E stain are responsible for much of the eosinophilia (pink staining) of cytoplasm. In some cells, the mitochondria are profuse and may be concentrated in one region of the cell and can be demonstrated directly and indirectly by various staining methods.

Micrograph (a) shows a salivary gland duct made up of cells which are extremely active in secretion and reabsorption of a variety of inorganic ions. This takes place at the base of the cells (i.e. the surface away from the lumen **L**) and is powered by ATP produced by extremely elongated mitochondria associated with numerous basal infoldings of the plasma membrane similar to that shown in Figure

1.12(e). The cells have been stained by a modified haematoxylin method which not only stains basophilic structures (i.e. DNA and RNA) but also acidophilic structures such as mitochondria which can be seen as striations **S** in the basal aspect of the cells.

In specimen (b), which shows skeletal muscle cells in transverse section, an enzyme histochemical method for succinate dehydrogenase has been employed. Succinate dehydrogenase is an enzyme of the citric acid cycle which is exclusive to mitochondria and therefore provides a marker for mitochondria. In skeletal muscle there are three muscle types differing from each other in mitochondrial concentration. Such a staining method can be used to demonstrate their relative proportions (see also Fig. 6.13).

Fig. 1.24 Glycogen

(PAS/Haematoxylin × 600)

This histological section has been stained by a histochemical method to demonstrate the presence of glycogen which is stained magenta. The specimen is of liver, the cytoplasm of each liver cell being packed with glycogen. The section has been *counter stained* (i.e. stained with a second dye) to demonstrate the liver cell nuclei **N** (blue). It also stains the nuclei of the cells lining the blood channels **B** between the rows of liver cells; these nuclei are smaller and more condensed and hence stain more intensely.

(a)   *(b)*

Fig. 1.25 Lipid *(a) H & E × 320 (b) Osmium × 320*

Routine processing methods for microscopy generally extract lipid from tissues. Therefore lipid droplets within cells appear as unstained vacuoles as in micrograph (a). Lipids are therefore best demonstrated in frozen sections stained by specific lipid methods such as *osmium* as in micrograph (b) with which lipid is stained black. Both micrographs show brown adipose tissue at similar magnifications (see also Fig. 4.13).

Fig. 1.26 Cytoskeleton

(Silver impregnation method × 600)

Individual elements of the cytoskeleton are not easily visualised by light microscopy. However, in cells with prominent aggregations of cytoskeletal elements, e.g. nerve cells or cells undergoing division, these can be demonstrated by impregnation with silver and gold.

In this micrograph of a nerve cell body, the silver impregnated cytoskeleton which appears brown/black in colour, can be seen radiating from the vicinity of the nucleus **N** into various cytoplasmic extensions.

Fig. 1.27 Cellular pigment: melanin

(Modified azan × 600)

In general, mammalian tissues have minimal intrinsic colour when viewed in the microscope, thus the need for staining. A few tissues, however, contain intracellular pigments, the most typical being melanin which is mainly responsible for skin colour (see Fig. 9.5). This pigment which is brown in colour is also present in the nerve cells of one of the brain nuclei, the substantia nigra, shown in this micrograph. This specimen has been lightly stained by the Azan method to pick out the nuclei **N** which are stained pale blue with prominent red nucleoli.

Fig. 1.28 Cellular pigment: lipofuscin

(H & E × 320)

Lipofuscin is an intracellular pigment which probably represents an insoluble degradation product of organelle turnover (see Fig. 1.3). With increasing age, it accumulates in the cytoplasm, particularly in sympathetic ganglion cells (as seen in this micrograph), other neurones and cardiac muscle cells; it is thus sometimes referred to as 'age pigment'.

2. Cell cycle and replication

Introduction

The development of a single, fertilised egg cell to form a complex, multicellular organism involves cellular replication, growth and progressive specialisation (differentiation) for a variety of functions. The mechanism of cellular replication in all but the male and female germ cells is known as *mitosis*. Mitosis or *mitotic division* of a single cell results in the production of two *daughter cells*, each genetically identical to the parent cell. Following mitosis, the daughter cells enter a period of growth and metabolic activity prior to further mitotic division. The time interval between mitotic divisions, that is the life cycle of an individual cell, is called the *cell cycle*.

As development of the fertilised ovum progresses to produce a multicellular embryo, groups of cells and their progeny become increasingly specialised to form tissues with different specific functions. In the fully developed organism, the differentiated cells of some tissues, such as the neurones of the nervous system, lose the ability to undergo mitosis, such cells being described as *terminally differentiated*. In contrast, the cells of certain other tissues, e.g. the lining cells of gut and skin, undergo continuous cycles of mitotic division throughout the lifespan of the organism. Between these extremes are cells such as liver cells which do not normally undergo mitosis but retain the capacity to undergo mitosis should the need arise (*facultative dividers*).

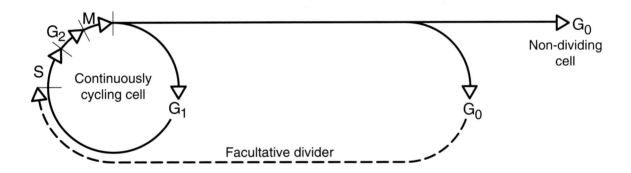

Fig. 2.1 The cell cycle

Historically, only two phases of the cell cycle were recognised: a relatively short *mitotic phase* (*M phase*) and a non-dividing phase (*interphase*), which usually occupies most of the life cycle of the cell. With the development of radio-isotopes, it was found that there is a discrete period during interphase when nuclear DNA is replicated; this phase, described as the *synthesis* or *S phase* cycle, is completed some time before the onset of mitosis. Thus interphase may be divided into three separate phases. Between the end of the M phase and the beginning of the S phase is the first gap or G_1 *phase*; this is usually much longer than the other phases of the cell cycle. During the G_1 phase, cells grow and perform their specialised functions with respect to the tissue as a *whole*. The interval between the end of the S phase and the beginning of the M phase, the *second gap* or G_2 *phase*, is relatively short and is the period in which cells prepare for mitotic division.

Some cell types progress continuously through the cell cycle to accommodate tissue growth or cell turnover whereas terminally differentiated cells leave the cell cycle after the M phase and enter a state of continuous differentiated function designated as the G_0 *phase*. Facultative dividers enter the G_0 phase but retain the capacity to re-enter the cell cycle when suitably stimulated. Some liver cells appear to enter a protracted G_2 phase in which they perform their normal differentiated functions despite the presence of a duplicated complement of DNA.

In general, the S, G_2 and M phases of the cell cycle are relatively constant in duration, each taking up to several hours to complete whereas the G_1 phase is highly variable, in some cases lasting for several days or even longer. The G_0 phase may last for the entire lifespan of the organism.

Mitosis

Somatic cell division occurs in two phases. Firstly, the chromosomes duplicated in the S phase are distributed equally and identically between the two potential daughter cells; this process is known as *mitosis*. Secondly, the dividing cell is cleaved into genetically identical daughter cells by cytoplasmic division or *cytokinesis*. Although mitosis is always equal and symmetrical, cytokinesis may, in some situations, result in the formation of two daughter cells with grossly unequal amounts of cytoplasm or cytoplasmic organelles. In other circumstances, mitosis may occur in the absence of cytokinesis as in the formation of binucleate and multinucleate cells.

Fig. 2.2 Chromosomes during mitosis *(illustrations opposite)*

(a) Diagrams (b) Chromosome spread: Giemsa × 1200

The nuclei of all cells of a species, except the germ cells of the gonads, contain the same fixed complement of DNA, a quantity called the *genome*. This is present in the form of a fixed number of *chromosomes* which is also specific to each species. DNA is a huge molecular weight polymer of many deoxyribonucleotides with a double stranded structure, each strand consisting of a backbone of alternating deoxyribose and phosphate moieties. Each deoxyribose unit is covalently bound to a purine or pyrimidine base which is in turn non-covalently linked to a complimentary base on the other strand thus linking the strands together. The bases are of four types: adenine, cytosine, thymine and guanine, with adenine only linking to thymine and cytosine only linking to guanine thus making each strand complimentary to the other (diagram 1). Linked in this way, the strands assume a double helical conformation around a common axis, the direction of the internucleotide phosphodiester bonds running in opposite directions (i.e. antiparallel) and the planes of the linked bases lying at right angles to the axis (diagram 2). The sequence of bases in either strand of the DNA molecule forms the genetic code for the individual, the bases being read in groups of three called *codons*, each codon coding for one amino acid. In human cells, there are 46 chromosomes (the diploid number) comprising 23 homologous pairs, the members of each pair having the same length of DNA and coding for the same proteins.

The extremely long DNA molecule making up each chromosome binds to a range of histone and non-histone proteins which hold the chromosome in a coiled and folded conformation, compact enough to be accommodated within the nucleus. Thus the 2 nm diameter double helix is coiled and packed through several orders of three-dimensional complexity to form an elongated structure some 300 nm in diameter and very much shorter in length than the otherwise uncoiled molecule would be. This is the form in which the chromosome is structured during the G_1 and G_0 phases of the cell cycle during which gene transcription (the prerequisite for protein synthesis) occurs.

Histologically, individual chromosomes are not visible within the nucleus of cells during interphase. During the S phase, each chromosome is duplicated (as shown in diagram 3). The resulting identical chromosomes, now known as *chromatids*, remain attached to one another at a point called the *centromere* and become even more tightly coiled and condensed; as such they may be visualised with the light microscope.

The micrograph illustrates the chromosomes of a human cell cultured in vitro and arrested at the onset of mitosis; the preparation has been treated with the enzyme *trypsin*, thus revealing a cross-banding pattern along the length of each duplicated chromosome. Each duplicated chromosome comprises two chromatids joined at the centromere **C**. Diagram 4 shows further detail of the structure of mitotic chromosomes and their supercoiled three-dimensional structure. Note the position of the kinetochore (see Fig. 2.3) which provides for attachment of certain spindle tubules during cell division.

Each member of a homologous pair of mitotic chromosomes is identical in length, centromere location and banding pattern. Micrographs such as this can be magnified and chromosomes cut out and arranged into pairs as a means of studying the normality or otherwise of an individual's chromosomal make-up. This is known as *karyotyping*.

(b)

(a)

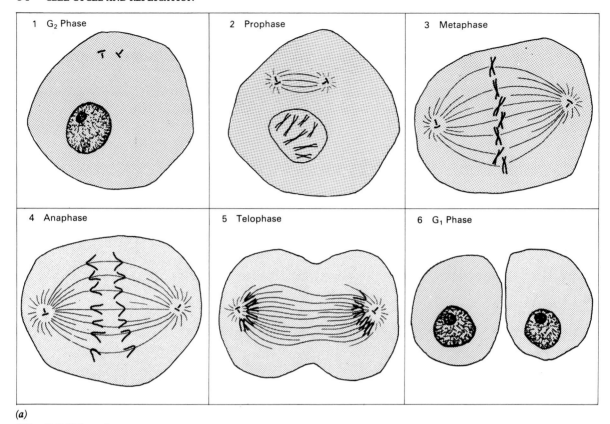

| 1 G₂ Phase | 2 Prophase | 3 Metaphase |
| 4 Anaphase | 5 Telophase | 6 G₁ Phase |

(a)

Fig. 2.3 Mitosis *(a) Schematic diagram (b) Mitotic series: Giemsa × 800 (opposite)*

The series of micrographs, shown opposite, illustrates the mitotic process in actively dividing primitive blood cells from a smear preparation of human bone marrow.

Mitosis is a continuous process which is traditionally divided into four phases: *prophase, metaphase, anaphase* and *telophase*, each stage being readily recognisable with the light microscope. Cell division requires the presence of a structure called the *mitotic apparatus* which comprises a spindle of longitudinally-arranged microtubules extending between a pair of *centrioles* (see Fig. 1.15) at each pole of the dividing cell. The mitotic apparatus is visible within the cytoplasm only during the M phase of the cell cycle since it disaggregates shortly after completion of mitosis.

Prophase. The beginning of this stage of mitosis is defined as the moment when the chromosomes (already duplicated during the preceding S phase) first become visible within the nucleus. As prophase continues, the chromosomes become increasingly condensed and shortened and the nucleoli disappear. Dissolution of the nuclear envelope marks the end of prophase.

During prophase, the microfilaments and microtubules of the cytoskeleton disaggregate into their protein subunits. During the preceding interphase, the pair of centrioles in the centrosome has duplicated and in prophase these migrate towards opposite poles of the cell whilst simultaneously a spindle of microtubules is formed between them (*interpolar microtubules*). As the centriole pairs move apart, the interpolar microtubules progressively elongate by the addition of tubulin subunits.

Metaphase. The nuclear envelope having disintegrated, the mitotic spindle moves into the nuclear area and each duplicated chromosome becomes attached, at a site called the *kinetochore*, to another group of microtubules of the mitotic spindle (*kinetochore* or *chromosome microtubules*); the

kinetochore is a plaque-like area on each duplicated chromosome and is located at the centromere, the structure which binds the duplicated chromosomes (chromatids) together (see also diagram 4, Fig. 2.2). The chromosomes then become arranged in the plane of the spindle equator, this being known as the *equatorial* or *metaphase plate*.

Anaphase. This stage of mitosis is marked by the splitting of the centromere which binds the chromatids of each duplicated chromosome. The mitotic spindle becomes lengthened by addition of tubulin subunits to its interpolar microtubules; the centrioles are thus pushed apart and the chromatids of each duplicated chromosome are drawn by the kinetochore microtubules to opposite ends of the spindle, thus achieving an exact division of the duplicated genetic material. By the end of anaphase, two groups of identical chromosomes (the former chromatids) are clustered at opposite poles of the cell.

Telophase. During the final phase of mitosis, the chromosomes begin to uncoil and to regain their interphase conformation. The nuclear envelope reforms and nucleoli again become apparent. The process of cytokinesis also takes place during telophase. The plane of cytoplasmic division is usually defined by the position of the spindle equator, thus producing two cells of equal size. The plasma membrane around the spindle equator becomes indented to form a circumferential furrow around the cell, the *cleavage furrow*, which progressively constricts the cell until it is cleaved into two daughter cells. A ring of microfilaments is present just beneath the surface of the cleavage furrow and cytokinesis occurs as a result of contraction of this filamentous ring. In the early G₁ phase, the mitotic spindle disaggregates and in many cell types the single pair of centrioles begins to duplicate in preparation for the next mitotic division.

1. Interphase

2. Early prophase

3. Late prophase

4. Metaphase

5. Early anaphase

6. Late anaphase

7. Early telophase and cytokinesis

8. Late telophase and cytokinesis

(b)

(a) *(b)* *(c)*

(d) *(e)* *(f)*

Fig. 2.4 Mitotic figures in tissue sections *(a)–(f) H & E × 400 (g) EM × 30 000 (opposite)*

This series of six light micrographs shows the appearance of mitotic figures as seen in tissue sections. In smear preparations (as shown in Fig. 2.3) an image of the whole cell is seen making the identification of mitotic cells and the stage of mitosis relatively simple. In contrast, with tissue sections, what is seen depends on the plane of section through the cell and the thickness of the section, whole cells rarely being encompassed within the section. Thus mitotic figures are more difficult to identify with certainty and the appearance is much more variable.

Specimens (a), (b) and (c) are from lymphoid tissue in which there is considerable lymphocyte proliferative activity (see Ch. 11). Cells in metaphase **M** and in cytokinesis **C** can be identified with some confidence in micrograph (a). Micrograph (b) shows another good example of a cell in metaphase **M** whilst micrograph (c) shows a dividing cell in probable late prophase **P**.

Micrograph (d) shows the proliferative basal layer of the epithelium lining the uterine cervix with a good example of a mitotic figure in late anaphase **A**. The proliferating epithelium of a duodenal crypt is illustrated in micrograph (e) and contains two dividing cells **D**; the stage of mitosis cannot be readily determined. Lastly, micrograph (f) shows a gland from the endometrium in the proliferative phase of the menstrual cycle; it contains a mitotic cell in prophase **P**.

Micrograph (g) shows an electron microscopic view of

part of a dividing cell, in this case a supporting Schwann cell in the developing nervous system. The plasma membrane **PM** can be identified but the nuclear membrane has dissolved and condensed chromatin **C** has spread out into the cytoplasm. Mitochondria **M**, smooth endoplasmic reticulum **sER** and ribosomes **R** are seen in the peripheral cytoplasm. In the centre of the nuclear material can be seen numerous microtubules **MT** in transverse section representing part of the spindle apparatus. Taken together, these features probably indicate that the cell is in anaphase, the plane of section being through one end of the dividing nuclear material and oriented at right angles to the spindle axis.

Mitotic index

The term mitotic index is used to describe the proportion of cells of a tissue which are in mitosis at a particular point in time. This can be crudely estimated by counting the number of mitotic figures per high power field and is employed in pathology as a measure of the rate of cellular proliferation in certain malignant tumours. Under experimental conditions, mitotic index can be estimated accurately by injecting the animal with thymidine which has been labelled with tritium, a radio-isotope of hydrogen. This labelled thymidine is incorporated into the replicating DNA of dividing cells which can then be identified by subjecting tissue sections to the process of autoradiography.

(g)

Meiosis

In all somatic cells, cell division (mitosis) results in the formation of two daughter cells, each one genetically identical to the mother cell. Somatic cells contain a full complement of chromosomes (the diploid number) which function as homologous pairs as described earlier. The process of sexual reproduction involves the fusion of specialised male and female cells called *gametes* to form a *zygote* which has the diploid number of chromosomes. Each gamete thus contains only half the diploid number of chromosomes; this half complement of chromosomes is known as the *haploid number* (23 in humans).

The production of haploid cells involves a unique form of cell division called *meiosis* which occurs only in the germ cells of the gonads during the formation of gametes; meiotic cell division is thus also called *gametogenesis*. Meiosis involves two cell division processes of which only the first is preceded by duplication of chromosomes.

1. First meiotic division. This results in the formation of two daughter cells, the process differing from mitosis in two important respects:

- In mitosis each duplicated chromosome divides at the centromere liberating two chromatids which migrate to opposite ends of the mitotic spindle, whereas in the first meiotic division there is no such separation of the chromatids but rather one duplicated chromosome of each homologous pair migrates to each end of the spindle. Thus at the end of the first meiotic division, each daughter cell contains a half complement of duplicated chromosomes, one chromosome being derived from each homologous pair of the mother cell.
- During the first meiotic division, and preceding the process just described, there is an exchange of alleles (alternate gene forms coding for the same characteristic) between the chromatids of homologous pairs of duplicated chromosomes. This exchange, called *chiasmata formation*, results in chromatids with a different genetic constitution from those of the mother cell.

2. Second meiotic division. This merely involves splitting of each rearranged duplicated chromosome at the centromere to liberate chromatids which migrate to opposite poles of the spindle.

Thus, meiotic cell division of a single diploid germ cell gives rise to four haploid gametes. In the male, each of the four gametes undergoes morphological development into a mature spermatozoon. In the female, unequal distribution of the cytoplasm results in one gamete gaining almost all the cytoplasm from the mother cell, whilst the other three acquire almost none; the large gamete matures to form an *ovum* and the other three, called *polar bodies*, degenerate.

During both the first and second meiotic divisions, the cell passes through stages which have many similar features to prophase, metaphase, anaphase and telophase of mitosis. Unlike mitosis, however, the process of meiotic cell division can be suspended for a considerable length of time. For example, in the development of the human female gamete, the germ cells enter prophase of the first meiotic division during the fifth month of fetal life and then remain suspended until some time after sexual maturity; the first meiotic division is thus suspended for between 12 and 45 years!

The primitive germ cells of the male, the *spermatogonia*, are present only in small numbers in the male gonads before sexual maturity. After this, spermatogonia multiply continuously by mitosis to provide a supply of cells which then undergo meiosis to form male gametes. In contrast, the germ cells of the female, called *oogonia*, multiply by mitosis only during early fetal development thereby producing a fixed complement of cells with the potential to undergo gametogenesis.

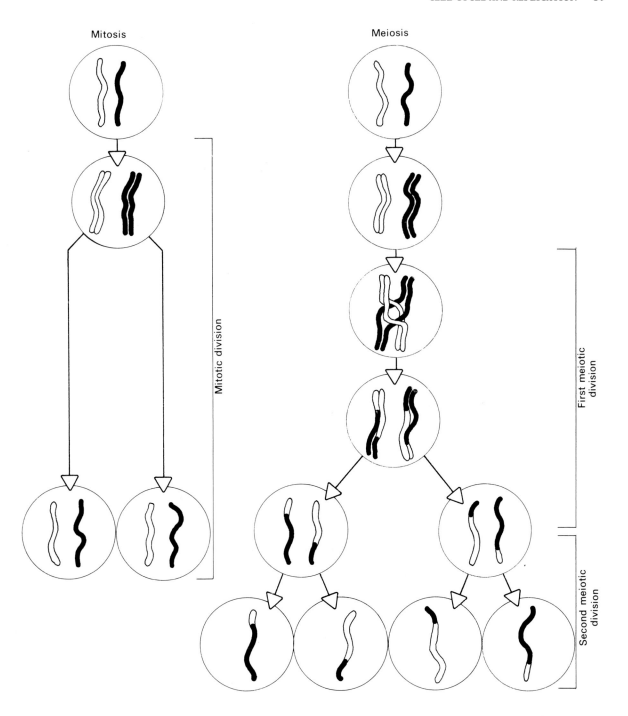

Fig. 2.5 Comparison of mitosis and meiosis

This diagram compares the behaviour of each homologous pair of chromosomes during mitosis and meiosis; the fate of only one homologous pair is represented here. The key differences between the two forms of cell division are:

- Meiosis involves two sequential cell divisions, the first meiotic cell division resulting in reduction of the chromosome complement to the diploid state and the second meiotic division resulting in the production of four haploid daughter cells, the gametes.

- Chiasmata formation occurs in meiosis only. The purpose of chiasma formation is to rearrange alleles such that every gamete is genetically different. In contrast, the products of mitosis are genetically identical.

The appearance of dead and dying cells in living tissues

Dead and dying cells are a common finding in tissues and arise as a result of normal cellular turnover, involution of tissue as part of normal development or intermittent functional requirements and finally as a result of some pathological process causing lethal cellular injury. Cell death is described as *necrosis*. The intestinal lining cells and the epidermis of skin, which are subject to regular replacement, provide the best examples of normal programmed cell death but in most normal tissues occasional necrotic cells may be encountered probably reflecting the demise of odd parenchymal or white blood cells which have outlived their usefulness. Cell necrosis on a large scale occurs in many pathological conditions when it is usually accompanied by the processes of inflammation and repair.

Nuclear changes are the most characteristic feature of necrosis. The first sign, known as *pyknosis*, results from condensation of the chromatin into a small densely staining mass. Later the nuclear material becomes fragmented (*karyorrhexis*) and ultimately breaks down with loss of the nucleus altogether (*karyolysis*).

At the same time denaturation of cytoplasmic proteins results in the formation of an amorphous cytoplasmic mass which stains intensely with eosin (bright pink). With the dissolution of the cell membrane, the cellular outline becomes increasingly difficult to distinguish (*cytolysis*).

(a)

(b)

(c)

(d)

Fig. 2.6 Necrotic cells

(a)–(d) H & E × 400

These four micrographs illustrate the typical features of necrotic cells in normal tissues. Specimens (a) and (b) are from the corpus luteum which is formed from an ovarian follicle after discharge of an ovum; it secretes the hormones involved in regulation of the menstrual cycle. Towards the end of the cycle, pituitary hormones result in involution of the corpus luteum, a process which involves progressive death of its constituent cells. In the centre of micrograph (a) is a necrotic cell **N** exhibiting pyknosis of the nucleus and amorphous cytoplasmic eosinophilia. In micrograph (b), a similar necrotic cell **N** is in a more advanced state of degeneration manifest by nuclear karyorrhexis and cytolysis.

Micrograph (c) is from a lymph node and shows two necrotic cells **N** both with markedly pyknotic nuclei. Micrograph (d) shows the tip of an intestinal villus from which degenerating cells are normally being constantly shed. Again, the necrotic cells **N** have pyknotic nuclei and amorphous eosinophilic cytoplasm.

Basic tissue types

3. Blood

Introduction

Blood is a tissue consisting of a variety of cells suspended in a fluid medium called *plasma*. It functions principally as a vehicle for the transport of gases, nutrients, metabolic waste products, cells and hormones throughout the body. Thus any sample of blood is composed not only of cells and molecules involved in transport processes but also cells and molecules in the process of being transported.

Plasma is essentially an aqueous solution of inorganic salts which is constantly exchanged with the extracellular fluid of body tissues. Plasma also contains proteins, the *plasma proteins*, of three main types: *albumins, globulins* and *fibrinogen*. Collectively, the plasma proteins exert a colloidal osmotic pressure within the circulatory system which helps to regulate the exchange of aqueous solution between plasma and extracellular fluid. The albumins, which constitute the bulk of plasma proteins, bind relatively insoluble metabolites such as fatty acids and thus serve as transport proteins. The globulins are a diverse group of proteins which include the antibodies of the immune system (see Ch.11) and certain proteins responsible for the transport of lipids and some heavy metal ions. Fibrinogen is a soluble protein which polymerises to form the insoluble protein *fibrin* during blood clotting. In general, the molecular components of plasma cannot be demonstrated by light and electron microscopy.

Blood cell types

The cells of blood are of three major functional classes: *red blood cells (erythrocytes), white blood cells (leucocytes)* and *platelets (thrombocytes)*. All are formed in the bone marrow, the process being known as *haemopoiesis*.

Erythrocytes are primarily involved in the transport of oxygen and carbon dioxide and function exclusively within the vascular system. The whole mass of red blood cells and their precursors in the bone marrow is called the *erythron*.

The leucocytes constitute an important part of the defence and immune systems of the body and, as such, act mainly outside blood vessels in the tissues; thus the leucocytes found in circulating blood are merely in transit between their various sites of activity.

Platelets play a vital role in the control of bleeding (*haemostasis*) by plugging defects in blood vessel walls and contributing to the activation of the blood clotting cascade.

Methods used to study blood and bone marrow

The standard method of examination of the blood is to make a *smear* on a glass slide. After fixation, a polychromatic *Romanowsky-type staining technique* such as the *Giemsa, Wright* or *Leishman method* is used for examination with the light microscope. Four distinctive staining characteristics can be identified according to the affinity of the various cellular organelles for the different stains employed in these methods:

- *basophilia* (deep blue)—affinity for the basic dye *methylene blue*; this is a characteristic of DNA in nuclei and RNA in the cytoplasm, i.e. ribosomes
- *azurophilia* (purple)—affinity for azure dyes; this is typical of lysosomes, one of the granule types found in leucocytes
- *eosinophilia* (pink)—affinity for the acidic dye *eosin* (thus also described as *acidophilia*); this is a particular feature of haemoglobin which fills the cytoplasm of erythrocytes
- *neutrophilia* (salmon pink/lilac)—affinity for a dye once erroneously believed to be of neutral pH; characteristic of the specific cytoplasmic granules of neutrophil leucocytes.

Bone marrow is usually studied by taking an aspirate from an active area of haemopoiesis (e.g. sternum, iliac crest). This is made into a smear, fixed and stained as for peripheral blood films. These processes induce marked artefactual alterations from that in vivo particularly in respect of cell size and morphology and this must be taken into account when comparing blood or marrow smears with tissue sections and ultrastructural preparations.

Fig. 3.1 Erythrocytes

(a) Giemsa × 1200 (b) Scanning EM × 2400

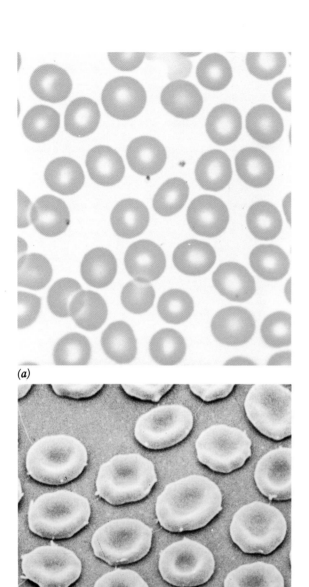

(a)

(b)

The erythrocyte is highly adapted for its principal function of oxygen and carbon dioxide transport. During differentiation, vast quantities of the iron-containing respiratory pigment *haemoglobin* are synthesised. Before release into the general circulation, the erythrocyte nucleus is extruded and, by maturity, all cytoplasmic organelles degenerate. The fully differentiated erythrocyte thus consists merely of an outer plasma membrane enclosing haemoglobin and the limited number of enzymes necessary for maintenance of plasma membrane integrity and gaseous transport functions.

Micrograph (a) demonstrates the characteristic appearance of erythrocytes in a stained smear of peripheral blood. The cells are stained pink (eosinophilia/acidophilia) due to their high content of haemoglobin, a basic protein. The pale staining of the central region of the erythrocyte is a result of its unusual biconcave disc shape.

Scanning electron microscopy reveals the biconcave disc shape of erythrocytes which provides a 20-30% greater surface area than a sphere relative to cell volume thus significantly enhancing gaseous exchange. This shape, along with the fluidity of the plasma membrane, allows the erythrocyte to deform readily, thus erythrocytes (average diameter 7.2 μm are able to pass through the smallest capillaries (3-4 μm in diameter).

The erythrocyte plasma membrane is composed of a lipid bilayer incorporating various globular proteins conforming to the standard fluid mosaic model of membrane structure (see Fig. 1.2). Immediately subjacent to the plasma membrane is a meshwork of proteins forming a cytoskeleton anchored to the membrane by one or more membrane-incorporated proteins; the main skeletal protein is the long fibre-like protein, *spectrin*. The biconcave shape of erythrocytes is determined in part by the cytoskeleton and in part by its water content, the latter being related to the concentration of inorganic ions within the cell.

The binding, transport and delivery of oxygen by haemoglobin is not dependent on erythrocyte metabolism. However, erythrocytes utilise energy in maintenance of normal electrolyte gradients across the plasma membrane, maintenance of the iron atoms of haemoglobin in the divalent form and maintenance of the sulphydryl groups of red cell enzymes and haemoglobin in the reduced, active form. The energy required for this process is derived from anaerobic metabolism of glucose. The absence of mitochondria precludes aerobic energy production and erythrocytes are thus totally dependent on glucose as an energy source.

The lifespan of an erythrocyte averages 120 days and is partly governed by its ability to maintain the biconcave shape. Without the appropriate organelles, erythrocytes are unable to replace deteriorating enzymes and membrane proteins, leading to diminished ability to pump sodium ions from the cell, uptake of water and the assumption of a spheroidal shape. Such cells are removed from the circulation by the spleen and liver (see Ch. 11).

Fig. 3.2 Erythrocytes

(EM × 6 000)

This micrograph illustrates the characteristic features of erythrocytes as seen by transmission electron microscopy. With this technique, the observed shape of the erythrocyte depends on the plane of section through the cell. The classic 'dumb-bell' shape **D** is only seen when the erythrocyte is cut through its thin central zone; more frequently, irregularly shaped erythrocytes are seen reflecting the deformation which occurs in the bloodstream. The high electron density of erythrocytes is due to the iron atoms of haemoglobin. Note the total absence of organelles. A platelet **P** is also seen in this field.

(a) *(b)*

Fig. 3.3 Reticulocytes

(a) Cresyl blue/eosin × 1200 (b) EM × 16 000

Reticulocytes are the immature form in which erythrocytes are released into the circulation from the bone marrow. They still contain sufficient mitochondria, ribosomes and Golgi elements to complete the cytoskeleton and the remaining 20% of haemoglobin synthesis. Final maturation into erythrocytes occurs within 24 to 48 hours of release. The rate of release of reticulocytes into the circulation generally equals the rate of removal of spent erythrocytes by the spleen and liver. Since the lifespan of circulating erythrocytes is about 120 days, reticulocytes constitute slightly less than 1% of circulating red blood cells.

Reticulocytes cannot be distinguished from mature erythrocytes in routinely stained blood smears, but when fresh blood is incubated with the basic dye, brilliant cresyl blue, a blue-stained *reticular* precipitate **R** is formed in the reticulocytes due to the interaction of the dye with ribosomal RNA remnants. This technique, called *supravital staining*, is illustrated in micrograph (a).

When severe erythrocyte depletion occurs, such as after haemorrhage or haemolysis, the rate of erythrocyte production in the bone marrow increases and the proportion of reticulocytes in circulating blood rises (*reticulocytosis*). Thus the reticulocyte count provides a convenient measure of the rate of red blood cell formation in the bone marrow. Note that reticulocytes are slightly larger than the surrounding mature erythrocytes. Micrograph (b) shows the ultrastructure of a reticulocyte with an adjacent mature erythrocyte for comparison. Overall the cytoplasmic density is less due to a lower concentration of haemoglobin. Scattered ribosomes can still be discerned as well as a few mitochondria **M**, a couple of degenerating mitochondria **D** and a small Golgi remnant **G**.

White cell series

Five types of leucocyte are normally present in the circulation. These are traditionally divided into two main groups based on their nuclear shape and cytoplasmic granules:

- **Granulocytes**
    Neutrophils
    Eosinophils
    Basophils
- **Mononuclear leucocytes**
    Lymphocytes
    Monocytes

Granulocytes are so named for their prominent cytoplasmic secretory granules. Each of the three different types of granulocyte has type-specific granules, the names *neutrophil*, *eosinophil* and *basophil* being derived from the staining characteristics of these *specific granules*. The granulocytes have a single multilobed nucleus which conveyed to early microscopists the erroneous impression that these cells were multinucleate and led to the confusing description of the other main group of leucocytes as mononuclear cells (see below). The multilobed nucleus may assume many morphological shapes leading to the use of the term *polymorphonuclear leucocyte* or *polymorph* as a synonym for the term granulocyte. To confuse matters further, the term polymorph is often used to refer to neutrophils since they exhibit the greatest degree of nuclear polymorphism and are by far the most prolific of the polymorphs. Granulocytes are also referred to as *myeloid cells* due to their exclusive origin from bone marrow; this should not however be taken to imply that they are the only white blood cells to be formed in the bone marrow.

Lymphocytes and monocytes have relatively non-lobulated nuclei and were described as mononuclear leucocytes by early microscopists to distinguish them from the polymorphs whose multilobed nuclei were originally believed to represent multiple nuclei. Again, to distinguish this group from the granulocytes, the term *agranulocytes* was also employed since cytoplasmic granules were not readily seen with early microscopic methods; unfortunately this may give the erroneous impression that these cells are devoid of cytoplasmic granules.

Leucocytes constitute an important part of the body's defences against foreign invaders. Neutrophils and monocytes are highly phagocytic and engulf microorganisms, cell debris and particulate matter in a non-specific manner; this activity may be enhanced and directed by immune responses to specific foreign agents (see Ch.11). Lymphocytes play the key role in all immune responses and, in contrast to the other leucocytes, their activity is always directed against specific foreign agents.

In general, all the leucocytes perform their functions in the tissues and merely use the blood as a vehicle for transit between sites of formation, storage and activity. It follows, therefore, that increased demand for particular leucocytes in various sites is reflected in increased numbers in the circulation. For example, bacterial infections attract neutrophils and this is often reflected in increased numbers of neutrophils in circulating blood (*neutrophilia*). In contrast, viral infections tend to excite a lymphocytic response and an increase in the number and proportion of lymphocytes in the peripheral circulation (*lymphocytosis*).

All leucocytes exhibit amoeboid movement which provides the means for migration in and out of the circulatory system and through the tissues.

(a) *(b)* *(c)* *(d)*

Fig. 3.4 Neutrophils

(a) and (b) Giemsa × 1200 (c) Histochemical method for alkaline phosphatase × 800 (d) Giemsa × 24 000

Neutrophils are the most common type of leucocyte in blood and constitute 40-75% of circulating leucocytes. Being highly motile and phagocytic, their principal function is in the acute inflammatory response to tissue injury where they ingest and destroy damaged tissue and invading microorganisms, particularly bacteria.

The most prominent feature of the neutrophil is the highly lobulated nucleus. When mature, there are usually five lobes connected by fine strands of nuclear material. In less mature neutrophils the nucleus is generally not as lobulated. In micrograph (a), two neutrophils in different stages of maturity are illustrated.

In neutrophils of females, the condensed, quiescent X-chromosome or Barr body (see Fig. 1.6) exists in the form of a small drumstick-shaped appendage of one of the nuclear lobes. This is known as the *drumstick chromosome* **D** and is shown in micrograph (b); it is visible in about 3% of neutrophils in peripheral blood films of females.

The cytoplasm of neutrophils is lightly stippled with purplish granules called *azurophilic granules* which represent large lysosomes; these are often referred to as *primary granules* as they are the first granules to appear during neutrophil differentiation. These granules contain the usual lysosomal acid hydrolases but also a number of microbicidal agents including *myeloperoxidase*; this can be demonstrated by the peroxidase stain and is used as a marker for the primary granules and for identification of leukaemias arising in neutrophil precursors.

The salmon-pink (neutrophilic) cytoplasmic staining of the neutrophils is a product of the specific granules of the neutrophils. These are much smaller in size than the primary granules but twice as numerous. The specific granules may also be referred to as *secondary granules*. These secretory granules are involved in many inflammatory processes including complement activation, leucocyte adhesion, collagen removal and bacterial cell wall lysis.

Recently identified *tertiary secretory granules* contain *gelatinase* (which destroys damaged collagen) as well as certain glycoproteins which appear to enhance phagocytosis.

Alkaline phosphatase activity has been traditionally used as a histochemical marker for the specific granules of neutrophils as seen in micrograph (c). Enzyme activity is indicated by a brown, granular deposit in the neutrophil cytoplasm; immature neutrophils, recognisable by their less lobulated nuclei, exhibit less enzyme activity. Recent ultracentrifugation studies have shown that alkaline phosphatase is present in a light fraction of neutrophil membranes. This may represent a fourth granule type and has been designated the *phosphasome*. Nevertheless, the function of this enzyme remains a mystery.

Micrograph (d) illustrates a neutrophil which has engulfed some coccoid bacteria; note the pseudopodium **P**, a typical feature of highly motile cells. This specimen was obtained experimentally by incubating fresh blood with bacteria. In vivo, neutrophils die after engulfing bacteria and do not re-enter the circulation.

Fig. 3.5 Neutrophil *(EM × 10 000)*

With electron microscopy, neutrophils have three distinguishing features. Firstly, the nucleus has up to five lobes which in section may appear as separate nuclei. The chromatin is highly condensed reflecting a low degree of protein synthesis. Secondly, the cytoplasm contains a considerable number of membrane-bound granules. The primary granules **P** are large, spheroidal and electron-dense, similar to the lysosomes of other cell types. The specific granules **S** are more numerous, small and often rod-like, and of variable density and shape. Tertiary granules cannot be readily identified. Thirdly, all other cytoplasmic organelles are scarce although the cytoplasm is particularly rich in dispersed glycogen.

Since the mature neutrophil has few appropriate organelles for protein synthesis, it has very limited capacity to regenerate expended lysosomal and specific enzymes which are rapidly depleted by phagocytic activity. The neutrophil is thus incapable of continuous function and degenerates after a single burst of activity. Defunct neutrophils are the main cellular constituent of *pus* and are therefore sometimes referred to as *pus cells*.

The paucity of mitochondria and the abundance of glycogen in neutrophils reflects the importance of the anaerobic mode of metabolism. Energy production via glycolysis permits neutrophils to function in the poorly oxygenated environment of damaged tissues whilst the hexose monophosphate pathway generates microbicidal oxidants.

Neutrophils are highly motile cells moving through the extracellular spaces in a crawling fashion with an undulating pseudopodium typically thrust out in the line of advance (see Fig. 3.4d). Motility and intense endocytotic activity is reflected in a large content of the contractile proteins, actin and myosin, tubulin and microtubule-associated proteins.

Neutrophil function

Neutrophils in the circulation are attracted by the presence of organisms, particularly bacteria. This process is mediated by chemotactic factors (*chemotaxins*) released from damaged tissue and generated by the interaction of antibodies with antigens on the surface of the microorganisms (see Ch. 11). The coating of organisms with antibodies and complement greatly enhances neutrophilic phagocytic activity, the phenomenon being known as *opsonisation*. Organisms which do not generate chemotaxins or become opsonised are thus relatively resistant to neutrophil phagocytosis and are thus highly pathogenic.

As the first step in phagocytosis, the organism is surrounded by pseudopodia which then fuse to completely enclose it in an endocytotic vesicle called a *phagosome*. This then fuses with cytoplasmic granules, in particular the azurophilic granules, which discharge their contents exposing the organism to a potent mixture of lysosomal enzymes. Killing is greatly enhanced by the generation of hydrogen peroxide and superoxide by enzymatic reduction of oxygen. A by-product of this powerful destructive capacity is considerable damage to the surrounding tissues in the event of leakage of the granule contents into the extracellular environment.

An important precursor to granule discharge is a phenomenon known as *neutrophil stimulation*. This involves the binding of complement fraction C5a to a significant proportion of receptors on the neutrophil plasma membrane; C5a is the most potent neutrophil chemotaxin and induces chemotaxis, degranulation and generation of hydrogen peroxide and superoxide.

(a)

0.5 µm

(b)

Fig. 3.6 Eosinophils

(a) Giemsa × 1600 (b) Human: EM × 25 000 (c) Mouse: EM × 20 000 (opposite) (d) Rat: EM × 25 000 (opposite)

Eosinophils account for 1-6% of leucocytes in circulating blood; their numbers exhibit a marked diurnal variation being greatest in the morning and least in the afternoon. Eosinophils remain in the bone marrow for several days after production, then circulate for about three to eight hours; the majority then enter the skin, pulmonary or gastrointestinal mucosae from which they may migrate into local secretions. The fate and lifespan of eosinophils are not known though few if any appear to re-enter the circulation.

Increased numbers of circulating eosinophils (*eosinophilia*) are found in many types of parasitic disease and defence against parasites appears to be one of their principal functions. Eosinophil numbers are also increased in the tissues in some allergic disorders (e.g. in the nasal and bronchial mucosae in hay fever and asthma) although their function in this context is poorly understood.

The eosinophil (12-17 µm in diameter) is larger than the neutrophil and is easily recognised by its large specific granules which stain bright red with eosin and a more brick-red with Romanowsky methods. Most cells have a bilobed nucleus but, as seen in micrograph (a), this is often partly obscured by the densely packed cytoplasmic granules.

The most characteristic ultrastructural feature of eosinophils is the large, ovoid, specific granules **S**, each containing an elongated crystalloid. In humans, as illustrated in micrograph (b), the crystalloids are relatively electron-lucent and irregular in form but in many other mammals they have a more regular, discoid shape. Micrograph (c) shows an eosinophil within the tissues of a mouse; in this species the crystalloids are also relatively electron-lucent. Micrograph (d) shows the specific granules of a rat eosinophil, the crystalloids of which are very electron-dense.

The specific granules are membrane-bound and of uniform size and the matrix contains a variety of hydrolytic enzymes including *histaminase*. The crystalloid has a cubic lattice structure and consists of an extremely alkaline (i.e. basic) protein called the *major basic protein*, other basic proteins, hydrolytic lysosomal enzymes and a peroxidase different from the myeloperoxidase of neutrophils.

Smaller granules are also present in mature eosinophils and contain *aryl sulfatase* and *acid phosphatase*; the concentration of the former is eight times greater in eosinophils than in other white cells and appears to be secreted independently of phagocytosis and degranulation.

As seen in micrograph (c), the characteristic bilobed nucleus **N** is readily seen with the electron microscope. The cytoplasm contains a fairly extensive smooth endoplasmic reticulum **sER**, clusters of ribosomes **R** and a little rough endoplasmic reticulum **rER**. Glycogen is abundant and there is a scattering of mitochondria **M**.

Eosinophil function

Eosinophils are phagocytic cells with a similar metabolism to neutrophils but with a greater oxidative capacity via the hexose monophosphate shunt; nevertheless, eosinophils appear less microbicidal than neutrophils. They have however a particular phagocytic affinity for antigen–antibody complexes.

The eosinophil plasma membrane has different immunoglobulin and complement receptors from other leucocytes. All eosinophils have receptors for IgE which may be important in the destruction of parasites; this is not present on neutrophils.

Eosinophils undergo chemotaxis in response to bacterial products and complement components; however they are preferentially attracted by substances released from basophils and mast cells, notably histamine and *eosinophil chemotactic factor of anaphylaxis (ECF-A)*, as well as activated lymphocytes.

Phagocytosis occurs in the usual manner but if the object is too large to be engulfed (e.g. a parasite), the eosinophil appears to release its granule contents into the external environment; schistosomes appear to be injured in this way. Killing is mediated by antibody and complement (see Ch. 11).

Eosinophils may have a role in ameliorating some aspects of hypersensitivity reactions as they neutralise histamine and also produce a factor called *eosinophil-derived-inhibitor* which is thought to inhibit mast cell degranulation. SRS-A, a vasoactive substance produced by basophils and mast cells (see Fig. 3.7), is inhibited by activated eosinophils. The role of aryl sulfatase (see above) is not understood; however it is not involved in the inhibition of SRS-A as once thought.

(c)

(d)

(a)

(b)

Fig. 3.7 Basophils *(a) Giemsa × 1500 (b) EM × 10 500*

Basophils are the least common leucocyte and constitute less than 1% of leucocytes in circulating blood. Characterised by large intensely basophilic cytoplasmic granules, they share many structural and functional similarities with tissue mast cells (see Fig. 4.14). It is not known whether basophils are terminally differentiated cells or the precursors of mast cells en route to peripheral tissues.

Basophils are formed in the bone marrow sharing a common precursor with the other granulocytes up to the myeloblast stage; from here, development proceeds through analogous stages as for neutrophils and eosinophils. The lifespan of basophils is unknown.

The basophil (14–16 μm in diameter) is intermediate in size between the neutrophil and eosinophil. Like the latter, it has a bilobed nucleus but this is usually obscured by numerous large, densely basophilic (deep blue) specific granules which are larger, but fewer in number, than those of eosinophils. The granules are highly soluble in water and tend to be dissolved away during common blood smear preparation, thus adding to the difficulty of identifying basophils in blood smears. Special techniques of fixation, embedding and staining may thus need to be used. When stained with the basic dye, *toluidine blue*, the granules bind the dye which changes colour to red, a phenomenon described as *metachromasia* (see Fig. 4.14).

With electron microscopy, the characteristic bilobed nucleus of the basophil is easily seen. The large specific granules **S** are membrane-bound, round or oval in shape and filled with closely packed, electron-dense material; the granules of basophils are larger and fewer in number than those of mast cells.

A small population of smaller granules is also found near the nucleus. The cytoplasm also contains free ribosomes, mitochondria and glycogen whilst the plasma membrane exhibits blunt, irregularly spaced surface projections.

Basophil function

The cytoplasmic granules of basophils and mast cells contain proteoglycans consisting of sulphated glycosaminoglycans linked to a protein core; this accounts for their metachromatic staining property. The proteoglycans are a variable mixture of *heparin* and *chondroitin sulphate*. The granules also contain *histamine* and many other mediators of inflammatory processes, e.g. *slow reacting substance of anaphylaxis (SRS-A), eosinophil chemotactic factor of anaphylaxis (ECF-A)*.

Basophil infiltration, mast cell proliferation and degranulation are features of a variety of immunological and other disorders; however the principal function of basophils and mast cells is probably in immunological responses to certain parasites.

Basophils and mast cells have membrane receptors highly specific for the Fc segment of IgE which is produced by plasma cells in response to a variety of environmental antigens (allergens). Exposure to allergen, results in the antigen forming bridges between adjacent IgE molecules which triggers rapid exocytosis of granule contents (degranulation). The release of histamine and other vasoactive mediators is thus responsible for the so-called *immediate hypersensitivity (anaphylactoid) reaction* characteristic of allergic rhinitis (hay fever), some forms of asthma, urticaria, and anaphylactic shock. Nevertheless, there are other IgE independent stimuli for mast cell degranulation.

Basophils may also account for up to 15% of infiltrating cells in allergic dermatitis and skin allograft rejection, a phenomenon known as *cutaneous basophil hypersensitivity*; this is induced by sensitised lymphocytes and is thus a type of cell mediated hypersensitivity (see Ch. 11). In this case degranulation is slow rather than rapid as in immediate hypersensitivity reactions.

(a)

(b)

Fig. 3.8 Lymphocytes

(a) Giemsa × 800 (b) EM × 15 000

Lymphocytes are the smallest cells in the white cell series, being only slightly larger than erythrocytes. They are the second most common leucocyte in circulating blood and make up 20-50% of the differential white cell count; increased numbers are commonly seen during viral infections.

Lymphocytes play the central role in all immunological defence mechanisms and are thus described in detail in Chapter 11. Blood provides the medium in which lymphocytes circulate between the various lymphoid tissues and all other tissues of the body. Most of the lymphocytes in the circulation are in a relatively inactive functional and metabolic state.

Lymphocytes are characterised by a round, densely stained nucleus and a relatively small amount of pale basophilic, non-granular cytoplasm. The amount of cytoplasm depends upon the state of activity of the lymphocyte, and in circulating blood there is a predominance of 'small' inactive lymphocytes (6–9 μm in diameter). 'Large' lymphocytes (9–15 μm in diameter) make up about 3% of lymphocytes in peripheral blood. Large lymphocytes represent activated B lymphocytes en route to the tissues where they will become antibody-secreting plasma cells; they also include *natural killer cells* (see Ch. 11).

Micrograph (a) illustrates small and large lymphocytes. In the large lymphocyte, the cytoplasm is readily visible but in the small lymphocyte the cytoplasm is almost too sparse to be seen.

Micrograph (b) shows a small lymphocyte in a pulmonary capillary. The nucleus is typically rounded but slightly indented and the chromatin is moderately condensed; nucleoli are not usually present. The sparse cytoplasm contains a few mitochondria, a rudimentary Golgi apparatus, minimal endoplasmic reticulum and a comparatively large number of free ribosomes which account for the basophilia of light microscopy. The plasma membrane exhibits small cytoplasmic projections which, with the scanning electron microscope, appear as short microvilli; these are much more numerous on B lymphocytes (see Ch. 11).

Fig. 3.9 Monocytes *(a) and (b) Giemsa × 1000 (c) EM × 20 000*

Monocytes are the largest of the white cells (up to 20 μm in diameter) and constitute from 2–10% of leucocytes in peripheral blood. They are highly motile and phagocytic cells and are the precursors of *macrophages*, large phagocytic cells of various types found in peripheral tissues and lymphoid organs.

Monocytes are characterised by a large, eccentrically placed nucleus which is stained less intensely than that of other leucocytes. As seen in these light micrographs, nuclear shape is variable but there is often a deep indentation of that aspect of the nucleus adjacent to the centre of the cell; nuclear indentation tends to become more pronounced as the cell matures, so as to give a horseshoe or even bilobed appearance. Two or more nucleoli may be visible. The extensive cytoplasm stains pale greyish blue with Romanowsky methods and contains numerous small pink-purple stained lysosomal granules and cytoplasmic vacuoles which may confer a 'frosted-glass' appearance.

With the electron microscope, the cytoplasm is seen to contain a variable number of ribosomes and polyribosomes and relatively little rough endoplasmic reticulum. The Golgi apparatus **G** is well developed and located with the centrosome in the vicinity of the nuclear indentation. Small elongated mitochondria **M** are prolific. Numerous small pseudopodia **P** extend from the cell reflecting phagocytic ability and amoeboid movement.

The cytoplasmic granules **Gr** of monocytes are electron-dense, homogeneous and membrane-bound. Histochemical studies show them to be of two types. One type represents primary lysosomes and contains acid phosphatase, aryl sulfatase and peroxidase; these are analogous to the primary (azurophilic) granules of neutrophils. The content of the other granule type is not known.

In contrast to neutrophils, monocytes are capable of continuous lysosomal activity and regeneration which utilises aerobic and anaerobic metabolic pathways depending on the availability of oxygen in the tissues.

Monocyte–macrophage system
Monocytes migrate to peripheral tissues where they assume the role of macrophages. This has lead to the concept of a single functional unit, the *monocyte-macrophage system* (*mononuclear phagocyte system*) consisting of circulating monocytes, their bone marrow precursors, and tissue macrophages both free and fixed (*histiocytes*). Included in the system are: the Kupffer cells of the liver, microglia of the CNS, Langerhans cells of the skin, antigen-presenting cells of the lymphoid organs and the osteoclasts of bone. *Multinucleate giant cells* may form by fusion of macrophages or nuclear reduplication. The system does not include vascular endothelial cells or the reticular cells and fibroblasts of lymphoid organs which may exhibit some phagocytic activity; these were included in the now obsolete concept of the *reticulo-endothelial system*.

Monocyte function
Monocytes appear to have little function in circulating blood. They respond to the presence of necrotic material (*necrotaxis*), invading microorganisms (chemotaxis) and inflammation by migration into the tissues and differentiation into macrophages; with their great capacity for phagocytosis and a large content of hydrolytic enzymes, the macrophages engulf and destroy tissue debris and foreign material as part of the process of healing and restoration of normal function.

Some of these functions form an integral part of immunological mechanisms, e.g. antigen presentation, final destruction of antigen; in this case, lymphocyte activation results in the production of factors which enhance macrophage phagocytic activity.

(a)

(b)

Fig. 3.10 Platelets *(a) Giemsa × 1600 (b) EM × 22 500*

Platelets (thrombocytes) are small, non-nucleated cells formed in the bone marrow from the cytoplasm of huge cells called *megakaryocytes*. Their numbers in circulating blood range from 150 000-400 000/ml. Platelets have a variety of functions essential to the normal process of haemostasis. Firstly, they form plugs to occlude sites of vascular damage by adhering to collagenous tissue at the margin of the wound; later the platelet plug is replaced by fibrin. Secondly, they promote clot formation by providing a surface for the assembly of coagulation protein complexes that are responsible for thrombin generation. Thirdly, platelets secrete factors that are involved in vascular repair.

Platelets are round or oval, biconvex discs varying in size from about 1.5–3.5 μm in diameter. In blood smears, as in micrograph (a), their shape is not clearly seen and they are often partially clumped together. The cytoplasm has a purple-stained, granular appearance due to their numerous organelles which are concentrated towards the centre of the cell; the peripheral cytoplasm is very poorly stained and therefore barely visible.

Platelets contain most of the cytoplasmic organelles of other cells including mitochondria, microtubules, glycogen granules, occasional Golgi elements and ribosomes as well as enzyme systems for both aerobic and anaerobic respiration. The most conspicuous organelles, as seen in micrograph (b), are the electron-dense granules which constitute about 20% of platelet volume and are of four types.

Alpha granules are variable in size and shape and contain two *platelet exclusive proteins* namely, *platelet factor 4* (regulates vascular permeability, calcium mobilisation from bone, chemotaxis of monocytes and neutrophils) and *beta thromboglobulin* (function unknown, but serum level is used to monitor platelet activation in various disease states); these granules also contain coagulation factors (fibrinogen, factor V, factor VIII/von Willebrand factor) and other proteins including *fibronectin, thrombospondin, platelet-derived growth factor* (may be involved in repair of damaged blood vessels) and other growth factors.

Dense granules are very electron-dense and appear to contain *serotonin*; serotonin is not synthesised by platelets or

their precursors but is absorbed from the plasma having been produced by enterochromaffin cells of the gut (see Ch. 17).

Lysosomes are membrane-bound vesicles distinct from the alpha granules and contain lysosomal enzymes.

Microperoxisomes are small in number and have peroxidase activity probably catalase.

The platelet plasma membrane has three unusual features relating to adherence to foreign or altered blood vessels surfaces. Firstly, it has the ability to form fibrillar bridges between one platelet and another. Secondly, a very thick, filamentous glycocalyx rich in acid mucopolysaccharides gives substance to the fibrillar bridges. Thirdly, twice as many membrane proteins are exposed to the external environment as face inwards; this is the reverse of the situation in all other cells and is as if the membrane is turned inside out.

Platelets contain a well developed cytoskeleton. Beneath the cell periphery is a *marginal band of microtubules* which depolymerise at the onset of platelet aggregation. The cytoplasm is rich in the contractile proteins actin and myosin (previously called *thrombosthenin*) and other filamentous elements, all probably involved in the functions of clot retraction and extrusion of granule contents.

Located deep to the marginal band of microtubules and also scattered throughout the cytoplasm is the *dense tubular system* (*DTS*) consisting of narrow membranous tubules which contain a homogeneous electron-opaque substance; this contains an isoenzyme of peroxidase that is specific for platelets. The function of the DTS is poorly understood but there is evidence that it may be the site of prostaglandin synthesis.

Platelets contain a system of interconnected membrane channels which are in continuity with the external environment via external pits, the cytoplasmic aspect of these membranes being associated with elements of the cytoskeleton. The function of this *canalicular membrane system* is not understood but it may be involved in the secretion of the contents of alpha granules.

Haemopoiesis

Haemopoiesis is the process by which mature blood cells develop from precursor cells. In the human adult, haemopoiesis takes place in the bone marrow mainly of the skull, ribs, sternum, vertebral column, pelvis and the proximal ends of the femurs. Before maturity, however, haemopoiesis occurs in other sites at different stages in development. In the early embryo, primitive blood cells arise in the yolk sac and, later, the liver. From the third to seventh months, the spleen is the major site of haemopoietic activity. As the bones develop during the fourth and fifth months of intra-uterine life, granulocyte and platelet formation begins in the marrow cavities with erythropoiesis becoming established by the seventh month. By birth, haemopoiesis is almost exclusive to the bone marrow although the liver and spleen may resume activity in times of need. From birth to maturity, the number of active sites of haemopoiesis in bone marrow diminishes although all bone marrow retains haemopoietic potential.

The lineage of each blood cell type has been the subject of numerous theories but only one has gained substantial experimental support, the *monophyletic theory*. This proposes that all blood cell types are derived from a single primitive stem cell type called a *multipotential (pluripotential) stem cell*. The multipotential cells replicate at a slow rate differentiating into five discrete types of *unipotential stem cells*, each committed to a different developmental lineage: erythrocytes, granulocytes, lymphocytes, monocytes and platelets. Unipotential stem cells (which are not readily distinguishable from each other histologically), divide at a rapid rate to provide histologically recognisable precursors of the mature cell types.

In vitro culture systems are used to study haemopoiesis, progenitor cells being described as *colony forming units (CFU)*. The rate of division of these cells is modulated by hormones called *poietins* (e.g. *erythropoietin*) and locally produced *colony stimulating factors* and *interleukins*.

Bone marrow

Bone marrow consists of a meshwork of vascular sinuses and highly branched fibroblasts (see Ch. 4) with the interstices packed with haemopoietic cells. The production of blood cells by the bone marrow is astronomical with an estimated daily output of about 2.5 billion erythrocytes, a comparable number of platelets, some 50–100 billion granulocytes (1.0 billion/Kg body weight/day) as well as large numbers of monocytes and immunologically naive lymphocytes. In addition to its haemopoietic function, the bone marrow, along with the spleen and liver, is one of the major sites of removal of aged and defective erythrocytes from the circulation. The bone marrow also plays a central role in the immune system being the site of B lymphocyte differentiation (the mammalian equivalent of the bursa of Fabricius of birds) as well as containing large numbers of antibody-secreting plasma cells (see Ch. 11).

Fig. 3.11 Bone marrow smear *(Giemsa × 640)*

This micrograph shows the general appearance of a smear made from an aspirate of bone marrow. Nucleate cells of developing erythrocyte and leucocyte cell lines make up a considerable proportion of the cells in contrast to smears of peripheral blood where nucleate cells (i.e. mature leucocytes) are few and far between. Cells of the same lineage are relatively easy to identify as they tend to be drawn out into trails from the various colony-forming units in the marrow; this is better seen at lower magnification than shown here.

Fig. 3.12 **Bone marrow** *(H & E × 800)*

Active bone marrow is crammed with dividing stem cells
and the precursors of mature blood cells, the predominance
of maturing erythrocytes conferring a deep red colour hence
the name *red marrow*. With increasing age, the marrow of
peripheral long bones becomes less active and is
progressively dominated by fat cells so that in mature
mammals, much of the marrow is inactive and yellow in
colour; *yellow marrow* may, however, be reactivated if the
need arises for increased haemopoiesis.

Active bone marrow consists of two main components, a
framework of reticulin (see Fig. 4.8) and specialised
fibroblasts (reticular cells) which supports the developing
blood cells and a system of interconnected blood sinusoids
which drain towards the central vein.

The bone marrow sinuses are of the continuous
endothelium type (see Ch. 8) but an unusual feature is that
the underlying basement membrane is discontinuous. The
sinus endothelial cells are active in endocytosis and probably
control passage of all materials into and out of the
haemopoietic compartment. In places, the endothelial
cytoplasm is so thin that the endothelial barrier is little more
than the inner and outer layers of plasma membrane and
such sites may provide the route of exit of mature blood cells
into the circulation.

Beyond the endothelium and its basement membrane is a
discontinuous layer of fibroblasts (reticular cells) with
extensive branched cytoplasmic processes which embrace
the outer surface of the sinus wall as well as ramifying
throughout the haemopoietic spaces. The reticular cells

synthesise reticulin fibres which, along with the cytoplasmic
processes, form a meshwork which supports the
haemopoietic cells. By the accumulation of lipid, the
reticular cells also give rise to the fat cells (adipocytes)
characteristically found in the bone marrow. Macrophages
are also present within the haemopoietic cords and are
involved in phagocytosis of cellular debris. The
haemopoietic compartment also contains typical non-
cellular supporting elements (see Ch. 4) including collagen
fibres and the large molecular weight proteins laminin and
fibronectin which bind the haemopoietic cells to the fibrous
elements of the marrow stroma. Ground substance
proteoglycans may have the function of binding growth
factors and other modulators of haemopoiesis.

This micrograph illustrates haemopoietic cords **C**
separated by broad sinusoids **S** which are filled with
erythrocytes and occasional leucocytes. Note the nuclei of
two flattened endothelial cells **E** which line the sinusoids. Of
the haemopoietic cells, only one can be reliably identified,
namely a huge megakaryocyte (responsible for platelet
formation) near the centre of the field. Note also a few
scattered adipocytes **A**.

The functional relationship between bone and bone
marrow is obscure. Bone may merely provide protection and
support for the delicate bone marrow tissue or there may be
some specific metabolic relationship between the two
tissues. In support of the latter, it has been observed that
transplanted bone marrow is unable to survive in sites other
than the medullary cavities of bone marrow.

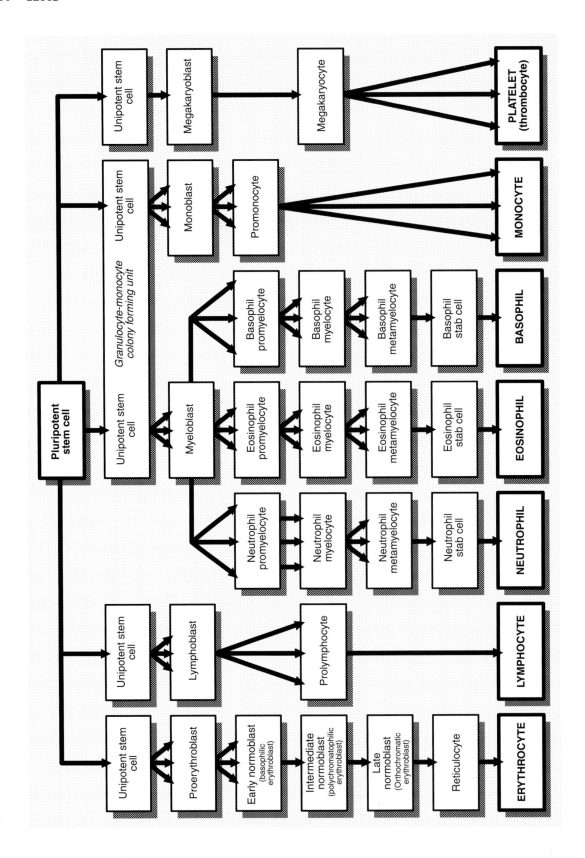

Fig. 3.13 Haemopoiesis *(illustration opposite)*

This diagram summarises the main developmental stages in blood cell formation. Such a classification is somewhat arbitrary since the process of haemopoiesis is a continuum of proliferation and progressive differentiation from stem cell to the mature form found in circulating blood.

Red cell formation (erythropoiesis). The process of erythropoiesis is directed towards producing a cell devoid of organelles but packed with haemoglobin. The first recognisable erythrocyte precursor is known as the *proerythroblast*, a large cell with numerous cytoplasmic organelles and no haemoglobin. Further stages of differentiation are characterised by three main features:

- decreasing cell size
- progressive loss of organelles; the presence of numerous ribosomes at early stages accounts for the marked cytoplasmic basophilia (blue staining) which steadily decreases as the number of ribosomes falls
- progressive increase in the cytoplasmic haemoglobin content; this accounts for the increasing eosinophilia (pink staining) of the cytoplasm towards maturity.

Haemoglobin synthesis begins during the *early normoblast (basophilic erythroblast)* stage and is complete by the end of the reticulocyte stage. Cell division ceases with the early normoblast stage, after which the nucleus progressively condenses and is finally extruded at the *late normoblast (orthochromatic erythroblast)* stage. The early normoblast stage also marks the beginning of the progressive loss of cytoplasmic organelles, only remnants of which remain by the reticulocyte stage. This process, accompanied by progressive haemoglobin synthesis, is represented morphologically by the transition from basophilia through polychromasia (intermediate normoblast) to the eosinophilia (orthochromasia) of the mature erythrocyte.

The process of erythropoiesis from stem cell to erythrocyte takes about one week. The rate of erythropoiesis is controlled by the hormone erythropoietin secreted by the kidney and by the availability of red cell components particularly iron, folic acid, vitamin B_{12} and protein precursors.

The *erythroblastic island* is the unit of erythropoiesis within the bone marrow and consists of one or two macrophages surrounded by erythrocyte progenitor cells. In bone marrow aspirates, the erythroblastic islands are broken up and ultrastructural studies of bone marrow sections are required to demonstrate their structure. The plasma membranes of the macrophages exhibit long cytoplasmic processes and deep invaginations which accommodate the dividing erythroid cells. As the erythroid cell differentiates, it migrates outwards along the cytoplasmic process of the macrophage leaving less mature cells in its wake. Approaching maturity, the erythroblast makes contact with the nearby sinusoidal endothelium and passes through its cytoplasm to enter the circulation. The nucleus is extruded prior to entry into the bloodstream and is phagocytosed by perisinusoidal macrophages. Cell culture studies indicate that endothelial cells, macrophages and fibroblasts are all essential for erythropoiesis, the fibroblasts being responsible for the production of various growth factors.

Granulocyte formation (granulopoiesis). The *myeloblast* is the earliest recognisable stage in granulopoiesis, the inappropriate name of myeloblast being derived from an outdated view that granulocytes were the only white cells formed in *myeloid tissue* (bone marrow). Myeloblasts give rise to *promyelocytes* which are characterised by the development of azurophilic granules; since the azurophilic granules develop before the specific granules, they are referred to as primary granules. As described earlier, the primary granules are merely large lysosomes.

The next stage in differentiation is the *myelocyte* which is marked by the development of specific granules, the process continuing through a further three cell divisions. The relative number and proportion of primary granules progressively decreases and the proportion of specific (secondary) granules progressively increases. From the myelocyte state through the *metamyelocyte* stage to the mature granulocyte forms, the nucleus becomes increasingly segmented. The immediate precursors of mature granulocytes tend to have an irregular horseshoe or sometimes ring-shaped nucleus and are termed *stab cells* or *band forms*.

On reaching maturity, neutrophils enter the bloodstream where some appear to circulate whilst others become adherent to the endothelial walls of small vessels (*marginated pool*) entering the circulating pool in response to exercise and stress; exit from the circulation appears to occur in a random manner. The bone marrow contains a huge pool of stored neutrophils which can be rapidly mobilised should the need arise. Corticosteroids increase the rate of release from the bone marrow and reduce the rate of exit from the circulation.

Lymphocyte formation (lymphopoiesis). Only two precursor stages, the *lymphoblast* and the *prolymphocyte*, are recognisable in the development of lymphocytes. The main feature of lymphopoiesis is a progressive diminution in cell size.

Unlike other blood cell types, lymphocytes also proliferate outside the bone marrow. This occurs in the tissues of the immune system in response to specific immunological stimulation (see Ch.11).

Monocyte formation (monopoiesis). There is considerable evidence that monocytes and granulocytes have a common progenitor, the *granulocyte-monocyte colony forming unit (CFU-GM)* and that growth of colonies requires the presence of *colony stimulating factors (CSFs)* with functions analogous to that of erythropoietin in erythropoiesis.

Two morphological precursors of monocytes are recognised, *monoblasts* and *promonocytes*, with at least three cell divisions occurring before the mature monocyte stage is reached. Monopoiesis is characterised by a reduction in cell size and progressive indentation of the nucleus. Mature monocytes leave the bone marrow soon after their formation and there is no reserve pool as for neutrophils. Monocytes spend an average of three days in the circulation before migrating by diapedesis into the tissues in an apparently random fashion after which they are unable to re-enter the circulation.

Platelet formation (thrombopoiesis). See Fig. 3.16.

In bone marrow smears, the earlier phases of haemopoiesis may be recognisable only with great difficulty, the characteristic, detailed features of each stage having been described using techniques of fixation and staining which are rarely applied in routine haematological practice. The recognition of such stages is of little practical value except in certain pathological conditions under which circumstances the classic characteristics of each cell type are often distorted.

Fig. 3.14 Erythropoiesis *(Giemsa × 1200)*

This bone marrow smear illustrates several stages in erythropoiesis. The proerythroblast **P** is the first recognisable erythrocyte precursor; the cell has a large, intensely stained, granular nucleus containing one or more paler nucleoli. The sparse cytoplasm is strongly basophilic due to its high content of RNA and lack of haemoglobin. A narrow, pale zone of cytoplasm close to the nucleus represents the Golgi apparatus.

Three increasingly differentiated normoblast forms can also be recognised. An early normoblast (basophilic erythroblast) **N₁** can be distinguished from the proerythroblast stage by its smaller size and smaller nucleus which has more condensed chromatin. More advanced in the maturation sequence is an intermediate normoblast (polychromatophilic erythroblast) **N₂**, the cytoplasm of which exhibits both basophilia and eosinophilia (i.e. polychromasia), the latter due to increasing haemoglobin content. The nucleus is also condensed and is accompanied by several small fragments called *Howell-Jolly bodies*, an unusual finding in normal erythropoiesis. With further haemoglobin synthesis and degeneration of cytoplasmic ribosomes, the late normoblast (orthochromatic erythroblast) stage **N₃** is reached and by this time the nucleus is extremely condensed prior to being extruded from the cell.

Fig. 3.15 Granulocyte precursors *(Giemsa × 1600)*

This micrograph illustrates three phases of neutrophil granulocyte development. A neutrophil myelocyte **M₁** is recognised by its large, eccentrically located nucleus, a prominent Golgi apparatus (negative image) and cytoplasm containing many azurophilic (primary) granules. The next stage towards maturity, the metamyelocyte **M₂**, is a smaller cell characterised by indentation of the nucleus and loss of prominence of the azurophilic granules. The final stage before maturity, the stab cell **M₃**, has a more highly segmented nucleus approaching that of the mature neutrophil.

(a)

Fig. 3.16 Megakaryocytes and platelet
formation *(a) EM × 22 500 (b) Giemsa × 800*

Megakaryocytes are responsible for platelet production and
are the largest cells seen in bone marrow aspirates
(30–100 μm in diameter).

These huge polyploid cells have a large irregular,
multilobular nucleus containing clumped dispersed
chromatin and devoid of nucleoli. The extensive cytoplasm
is filled with fine basophilic granules reflecting the profusion
of cytoplasmic organelles. With light microscopy, the
margin of the cell is often difficult to define clearly due to
numerous disaggregating platelets, **P**, cytoplasmic
processes, ruffles and blebs.

The precursor of the megakaryocyte in the bone marrow
is the *megakaryoblast* which undergoes as many as seven
reduplications of nuclear and cytoplasmic constituents
without cell division (*endomitosis*), each associated with
increasing ploidy, nuclear lobulation and cell size.

Cytoplasmic maturation involves the elaboration of
granules, vesicles and *demarcation membranes* and
progressive loss of free ribosomes and rough endoplasmic
reticulum.

The megakaryocyte cytoplasm is divided into three zones.

A *perinuclear zone* contains the Golgi apparatus and
associated vesicles, rough and smooth endoplasmic
reticulum, developing granules, centrioles and spindle
tubules; the zone remains attached to the nucleus after
platelet shedding.

The *intermediate zone* contains an extensive system of
interconnected vesicles and tubules known as the
demarcation membrane system (*DMS*) which is in continuity

(b)

with the plasma membrane and has the function of
delineating developing platelet fields (i.e. potential
platelets); at least some of the DMS appears to be derived
from the Golgi.

The outer *marginal zone* is filled with cytoskeletal
filaments and is traversed by membranes connecting with
the demarcation membrane system.

Platelets are formed not by budding, as often described,
but rather by fragmentation of the megakaryocyte cytoplasm
with the release of demarcated platelet fields; like platelets,
they are very uneven in size. Platelets appear to be released
in at least two different ways. In the bone marrow,
megakaryocytes exude pseudopodia called *proplatelets* into
the sinusoidal lumens, each representing a string of platelet
fields which then fragment in the circulation.
Mature megakaryocytes also appear to enter the bone
marrow sinusoids intact and pass to the pulmonary vascular
bed where they fragment into platelets.

Cell type	Erythrocyte	Neutrophil	Eosinophil	Basophil	Lymphocyte	Monocyte	Platelets
Size	6.7-7.7 μm	12-14 μm	12–17 μm	14-16 μm	6–15 μm	16-20 μm	1.5–3.5 μm
Number per litre	$3.9 - 6.5 \times 10^{12}$	$2.0 - 7.5 \times 10^9$	$1.3 - 3.5 \times 10^9$	$0 - 0.44 \times 10^9$	$0 - 0.1 \times 10^9$	$0.2 - 0.8 \times 10^9$	$150 - 400 \times 10^9$
Differential leucocyte count	—	40–75%	1–6%	<1%	20–50%	2–10%	—
Duration of development	5–7 days	6–9 days	6–9 days	3–7 days	1–2 days	2–3 days	4–5 days
Lifespan of mature cell	120 days	6 hours to a few days	8–12 days	?	?	months to years	8–12 days

Fig. 3.17 Mature cell types in circulating blood

4. Supporting/connective tissues

Introduction

Connective tissue is the term traditionally applied to a basic type of tissue of mesodermal origin which provides structural and metabolic support for other tissues and organs throughout the body. Connective tissues usually contain blood vessels and mediate the exchange of nutrients, metabolites and waste products between tissues and the circulatory system. The traditional term 'connective tissue' thus hardly does justice to the wide range of functions of this type of tissue and it is now probably more appropriate to use the term *supporting tissue*.

Supporting tissues occur in many different forms with diverse physical properties. In most organs, loose supporting tissues act as a biological packing material between cells and other tissues with more specific functions. Dense forms of supporting tissue provide tough physical support in the dermis of the skin, comprise the robust capsules of organs such as the liver and spleen, and are the source of great tensile strength in ligaments and tendons. Cartilage and bone, the major skeletal components, are merely rigid forms of supporting tissue. The function of the skeletal tissues is however so specialised that they are considered separately in Chapter 10. Supporting tissues have important metabolic roles such as the storage of fat (white adipose tissue) and the regulation of body temperature in the newborn (brown adipose tissue). Some of the cells of supporting tissue constitute a major part of the body's defences against pathogenic microorganisms. The processes of tissue repair are largely a function of supporting tissues.

All supporting/connective tissues have two major constituents, *cells* and *extracellular material*. The extracellular material determines the physical properties of each type of supporting tissue. Extracellular material consists of a matrix of organic material called *ground substance* within which are embedded a variety of *fibres*. A group of *structural glycoproteins* are the third constituent of the extracellular matrix and mediate the interaction of cells with the other constituents.

The cells of supporting/connective tissue

The cells of supporting tissue may be divided into three types according to their basic function:

- Cells responsible for synthesis and maintenance of the extracellular material. These cells are termed *fibroblasts*, and are derived from precursor cells in primitive supporting tissue (*mesenchyme*). Fibroblasts with additional contractile function are found in some tissues and are known as *myofibroblasts*. It is customary to describe a precursor or immature cell by the suffix 'blast' as in erythroblast (see Fig. 3.17) and the mature form by the suffix 'cyte' as in erythrocyte. This convention, however, is not commonly used in respect of supporting tissues, where the term 'fibrocyte' would be a more appropriate term than fibroblast for the mature cell form.
- Cells responsible for the storage and metabolism of fat. These cells are known as *adipocytes* and may collectively form *adipose tissue*.
- Cells with defence and immune functions. This group of cells includes the mast cells and tissue macrophages as well as all types of white blood cells.

Ground substance

Ground substance derived its name from being an amorphous transparent material which has the properties of a semi-fluid gel. Tissue fluid is loosely associated with ground substance, thereby forming the medium for passage of molecules throughout supporting tissues and for the exchange of metabolites with the circulatory system.

Ground substance consists of a mixture of long, unbranched polysaccharide chains of seven different types, each composed of repeating disaccharide units. One of the disaccharide units is usually a uronic acid and the other an amino sugar (either N-acetyl glucosamine or N-acetyl galactosamine) thus giving rise to the modern term *glycosaminoglycans (GAGs)*; these were formerly called *mucopolysaccharides*. The glycosaminoglycans are acidic (negatively-charged) due to the presence of hydroxyl, carboxyl and sulphate side groups on the disaccharide units.

Hyaluronic acid is the predominant GAG in the loose supporting tissues and is the only one without sulphate side groups; the other GAGs (*chondroitin-4-sulphate, chondroitin-6-sulphate, dermatan sulphate, heparan sulphate, heparin sulphate* and *keratan sulphate*) differ from hyaluronic acid in that they are covalently linked to a variety of protein molecules to form proteoglycans (formerly known as mucoproteins); these proteoglycans are huge molecules consisting of 90–95% carbohydrate. Further, the proteoglycans may form non-covalent links with hyaluronic acid chains to form even larger molecular complexes.

Unlike many proteins, GAG molecules are not flexible enough to form globular aggregates but remain in an expanded form, thus occupying a huge volume for relatively small mass. In addition, their highly charged side groups render them extremely hydrophilic thus attracting a large volume of water and positive ions, particularly sodium, which constitute *extracellular fluid*. The extracellular fluid imparts the characteristic turgor of supporting tissue.

In summary, ground substance is basically composed of glycosaminoglycans in the form of hyaluronic acid and proteoglycans. These huge molecules are entangled and electrostatically linked to one another and their water of hydration, to form a flexible gel through which metabolites may diffuse. The size of the spaces between the GAG molecules and the nature of electrostatic changes determine the permeability characteristics of any particular supporting tissue, a fact of particular significance in the structure of basement membranes (see later). The mechanical properties of ground substance are reinforced by the fibrous proteins of the extracellular tissue to which the components of ground substance are also bound.

The fibres of supporting/connective tissue

The fibrous components of supporting tissue are of two main types: *collagen* (including *reticulin* which was formerly considered a separate fibre type) and *elastin*.

Collagen is the main fibre type found in most supporting tissues and is the most abundant protein in the human body. Its most notable function is the provision of tensile strength. Collagen is secreted into the extracellular matrix in the form of *tropocollagen* which consists of three polypeptide chains (alpha chains) bound together to form a helical structure 300 nm long and 1.5 nm in diameter. In the extracellular matrix, the tropocollagen molecules polymerise to form collagen. Eleven different types of collagen (designated I to XI) have now been delineated on the basis of morphology, amino acid composition and physical properties.

- *Type* I *collagen* is found in fibrous supporting tissue, the dermis of the skin, tendon, ligaments and bone, in a variable arrangement from loose to dense according to the mechanical support required. The tropocollagen molecules are aggregated to form fibrils strengthened by numerous intermolecular bonds. Parallel collagen fibrils are further arranged into strong bundles 2–10 μm in diameter which confer great tensile strength to the tissue; these bundles are visible with the light microscope.

- *Type* II *collagen* is found in hyaline cartilage and consists of fine fibrils which are dispersed in the ground substance. *Type* III *collagen* makes up the fibre type known as reticulin which was previously thought to represent a separate species of fibre because of its affinity for silver salts. Reticulin fibres form the delicate branched 'reticular' supporting meshwork in highly cellular tissues such as the liver, bone marrow and lymphoid organs. *Collagen type* IV does not form fibrils but rather a mesh-like structure and is an important constituent of basement membranes. The remaining collagen types are present in various specialised situations where their fibrillar structure has yet to be fully elucidated.

Elastin is a rubber-like material which is arranged as fibres and/or discontinuous sheets in the extracellular matrix particularly of skin, lung and blood vessels where it confers the properties of stretching and elastic recoil. Elastin is synthesised by fibroblasts in a precursor form known as *tropoelastin* which undergoes polymerisation in the extracellular tissues. Deposition of elastin in the form of fibres requires the presence of microfibrils of the structural glycoprotein *fibrillin* (see below) which become incorporated around and within the elastic fibres.

The structural glycoproteins

The structural glycoproteins are a group of molecules composed principally of protein chains bound to branched polysaccharides; much has yet to be learned about their role in the function of extracellular material. The structural glycoproteins include two fibril-forming molecules, *fibrillin* and *fibronectin*, and a number of non-filamentous proteins including *laminin*, *entactin* and *tenascin* which function as links between cells and extracellular matrix.

Fibrillin forms microfibrils 8-12 nm in diameter which, in certain specialised situations e.g. the mesangium of the kidney (see Ch. 16), appear to enhance adhesion between other extracellular constituents. As mentioned earlier, fibrillin is a constituent of elastic fibres where it appears to play a role in the orderly deposition of the fibres.

Fibronectin plays a part in controlling the deposition and orientation of collagen in extracellular matrix and the binding of the cell to the extracellular material. Cell membranes incorporate a group of transmembrane protein complexes called *integrins* which act as *cell adhesion molecules*. One of these, the *fibronectin receptor*, establishes bonds within the cell to the actin filaments of the cytoskeleton and binds with fibronectin externally. The fibronectin in turn binds with collagen and the glycosaminoglycan, heparin sulphate, thus establishing structural continuity between the cytoskeleton and the extracellular matrix.

Laminin is a major component of basement membranes binding with specific cell adhesion molecules so as to form links between cell membranes and other constituents of the basement membrane. Entactin, another non-fibrillary protein, has the function of binding laminin to type IV collagen in basement membranes. Tenascin also binds to integrins, and is important in the embryo where it appears to be involved in control of nerve cell growth.

Basement membranes

The epithelial, muscle and nervous tissues, of which all specialised composite tissues and organs are comprised, derive mechanical and nutritional support from supporting/connective tissue, the boundary being invariably marked by a condensed layer of extracellular material traditionally known as the *basement membrane*. The term derives from the fact that the first basement membranes to be recognised were those lying beneath the basal cells of surface epithelia. In the context of muscle and nervous tissue, the term *external lamina* may also be applied.

Epithelia in particular are almost entirely composed of closely packed cells with minimal intercellular material between them. The basement membrane provides structural support as well as binding the epithelium to the underlying supporting tissue. Basement membrane is also involved in the control of epithelial growth and differentiation forming an impenetrable barrier to downward epithelial growth; this is only breached if epithelia undergo malignant transformation. Epithelium is devoid of blood vessels and the basement membrane must therefore permit the flow of nutrients, metabolites and other molecules to and from the epithelium. Where an epithelium acts as a selective barrier to the passage of molecules from one compartment to another (e.g. between the lumen of blood vessels and surrounding tissues), the basement membrane assumes a critical role in regulating permeability. This reaches an extreme of sophistication in the kidney where the glomerular basement membrane is part of the highly selective filter for molecules passing from the blood stream into the urine. Critical association of basement membranes with epithelial structure and function was thus responsible for the basement membrane being traditionally discussed as if it were a uniquely epithelial structure. Increasing understanding demands that it be considered as one of the supporting tissues.

The main constituents of basement membranes and external laminae are the glycosaminoglycan *heparan sulphate*, the fibrous protein *collagen type IV*, and the structural glycoproteins *fibronectin*, *laminin* and *entactin*. Fibronectin appears to be produced by fibroblasts of the supporting tissue but the remainder are at least partly, if not exclusively, elaborated by the tissues being supported.

With the electron microscope, the basement membrane is seen to consist of three layers. A relatively electron-lucent layer, the *lamina lucida* (ranging from 10–50 nm in width), abuts the basal cell membrane of the parenchymal tissue. The intermediate layer is electron dense and is thus known as the *lamina densa*; depending on the tissue, this varies from 20–300 µm in thickness. Beyond the lamina densa is a broad, relatively electron-lucent layer known as the *lamina fibroreticularis* which merges with the underlying supporting tissue.

The electron-dense material of both lamina lucida and lamina densa represents a fine meshwork of collagen type IV which is exclusive to basement membranes. Another major constituent of these layers is laminin which binds the type IV collagen to the other basement membrane constituents and to laminin receptors in the parenchymal basal plasma membranes. Entactin mediates the binding of laminin to type IV collagen. The fibroreticular layer probably represents a condensation of the underlying supporting tissue. Its collagen content is mainly of type III (reticulin) which, via the fibrillar glycoprotein fibronectin, is also bound to integrins in the parenchymal basal plasma membrane.

Fig. 4.1 Basement membrane

(a) PAS/Haematoxylin × 400 (b) Jones' methenamine silver × 100 (c) EM × 5 000 (d) EM × 45 000

With the light microscope, basement membranes can be seen beneath certain epithelial tissues where they happen to be relatively thick or where histochemical or other methods have been employed which are specific for particular basement membrane constituents. Micrograph (a) shows a duodenal crypt lined by mucus-secreting cells and is stained by the PAS method. This has affinity for the complex carbohydrates of the proteoglycans in the basement membrane **BM** as well as the mucus **M** at the luminal aspect of the crypt lining cells. In micrograph (b), a silver impregnation method which has affinity for reticulin demonstrates the basement membrane **BM** of the tubules.

Micrograph (c) shows the epithelial lining of mouse trachea. A basement membrane **BM** can be clearly seen separating it from the underlying supporting tissue which contains the cell body and nucleus of a fibroblast **F**, numerous fine fibroblastic cytoplasmic processes **Fc**, bundles of collagen fibrils **C** (cut in transverse section) and elastin fibres **E**.

At higher magnification in micrograph (d), the three

layers of the basement membrane can be seen. The relatively electron-lucent *lamina lucida* **LL** abuts the basal epithelial cell membrane. The intermediate layer is electron-dense and represents the *lamina densa* **LD**. Beyond the lamina densa is the broad, relatively electron-lucent *lamina fibroreticularis* **LF** which merges with the fibrous and fibrillary (reticular) components of the underlying supporting tissue. In this field, note collagen fibrils **C**, part of a fibroblast **F** and elastin **E**. The basement membrane typically passes uninterrupted beneath the intercellular space **IS** between two epithelial cells **Ep** and beneath a basal invagination **In** of one of these cells.

The lamina densa was formerly known as the *basal lamina*. The terms *basal lamina* and *basement membrane* were often used interchangeably until it was realised that all three layers seen with the electron microscope represent the single layer seen with the light microscope. This has led to considerable terminological confusion and, if used, the term basal lamina should be confined to its meaning as lamina densa.

(a)

(b)

Fig. 4.2 Collagen *(EMs × 124 000 (a) Section (b) Teased preparation)*

The typical appearance of Type I collagen, the most common variety, is shown in these specimens. The characteristic feature is a pattern of cross-banding with a periodicity of approximately 64 nm which results from the polymerisation of tropocollagen molecules (300 nm in length) such that each molecule overlaps the next by approximately one-quarter of its length.

Fig. 4.3 Primitive mesenchyme *(H & E × 400)*

Primitive mesenchyme is the embryological tissue from which all types of supporting/connective tissue, including that of the skeleton, are derived. Mesenchymal cells are relatively unspecialised and are capable of differentiation into all the cell types found in mature supporting tissue. Some mesenchymal cells remain in fully mature supporting tissue and provide a pluripotential source of cells as the need arises for replacement or repair.

Mesenchymal cells **M** have an irregular, star (stellate) or spindle (fusiform) shape with delicate branching cytoplasmic extensions which form an interlacing network throughout the tissue. The oval nuclei have dispersed chromatin and visible nucleoli. The extracellular material consists almost exclusively of ground substance and does not contain mature fibres. Thus, mesenchyme represents a very loose variant of supporting tissue; in the well developed fetus, it is often referred to as *mucous tissue*. The circulatory system of the embryo is poorly developed until a late stage and mesenchyme permits free diffusion of metabolites to and from developing tissues.

Fig. 4.4 Mature fibroblasts *(H & E × 320)*

This micrograph demonstrates the typical histological appearance of mature fibroblasts in a relatively loose type of supporting tissue; collagen fibres are stained pink in this preparation. The fibroblast nuclei **F** are condensed and elongated in the direction of the collagen fibres. The cytoplasm is greatly reduced in volume, the cell being long and thin with fine cytoplasmic processes extending into the matrix to meet up with those of other fibroblasts; these are usually very difficult to see with the light microscope. The main function of fibroblasts is to maintain the integrity of supporting tissues by continuous slow turnover of the extracellular matrix constituents.

Fig. 4.5 Fibroblasts *(EM × 12 000)*

This micrograph illustrates the body of a mature fibroblast within loose collagenous supporting tissue. The nucleus **N** is moderately condensed, and nucleoli are not a prominent feature. The small quantity of cytoplasm contains a relatively sparse network of rough endoplasmic reticulum **rER**; the Golgi apparatus **G** is poorly developed and few mitochondria are present.

Fine tapering cytoplasmic extensions **E** of adjacent fibroblasts can be seen on either side of the central fibroblast. Bundles of collagen fibres are seen in transverse **Ct** and longitudinal section **Cl** in the extracellular matrix.

During active synthesis of extracellular fibres, the fibroblast cytoplasm becomes much expanded and the rough endoplasmic reticulum and Golgi apparatus become prominent features. Fibroblasts synthesise and secrete the precursors of the glycosaminoglycans, collagen, elastin and all other extracellular constituents; however, in the mature, relatively inactive fibroblast, few secretory vesicles are found.

Fig. 4.6 Active fibroblasts: healing wound
(H & E × 400)

Active fibroblasts **F** are readily demonstrated in healing wounds, as in this micrograph. The nuclei are large and rounded in shape with prominent nucleoli reflecting active protein synthesis. The cytoplasm is extensive and its strongly stained, granular appearance is evidence of an extensive system of rough endoplasmic reticulum involved in protein synthesis. The relative absence of formed fibres in the extracellular matrix permits the meshwork of cytoplasmic extensions between fibroblasts to be visualised somewhat more easily than in less active supporting tissues.

Fibroblasts with a contractile function (myofibroblasts) play an important role in contraction and shrinkage of the resultant scar tissue.

Fig. 4.7 Common forms of supporting tissue

(a) H & E × 320 (b) Masson's trichrome × 320 (c) Azan × 320 (d) H & E × 100 (e) H & E × 320

These micrographs illustrate a variety of common forms of supporting tissue. In the past, rather rigid descriptive classifications have been employed, e.g. 'dense regular connective tissue', 'dense irregular connective tissue', 'loose (areolar) connective tissue' etc. but in reality supporting tissues exhibit a great diversity of density and regularity and such rigid descriptions have outlived their usefulness.

The first three micrographs show collagen fibres stained by three common histological methods. Collagen is acidophilic due to its positively-charged side groups, thus in standard H & E preparations, collagen is eosinophilic (i.e. pink-stained). With the trichrome stain, collagen stains green or blue (depending on the variant of the stain used) and with the Azan staining method, collagen is deep blue. These three specimens are of the dense supporting tissue of the skin (dermis) where the collagen fibres are arranged in coarse irregular interwoven bundles which confer great tensile strength. Fibroblasts are recognised by their highly condensed nuclei (stained red with Azan).

Micrograph (d) shows the capsule **C** of the adrenal gland

A demonstrating again the typical dense arrangement of collagen fibres where mechanical support is the primary function. The collagen fibres are elongated and arranged in a regular manner to provide a well organised and robust enveloping capsule. Similar capsules invest the liver, spleen, lymph nodes, salivary glands, gonads and other encapsulated organs. Fibroblast nuclei are elongated in the direction of the collagen fibres.

Loose collagenous tissue supports the epithelial linings of the gastrointestinal, respiratory and urinary tracts, forms the deeper layers of the skin and occurs as a loose interstitial packing in many other organs. Such supporting tissue is illustrated in micrograph (e). The collagen fibres are loosely arranged and pursue a wave-like course in unstretched preparations. The open (*areolar*) spaces between collagen fibres are filled with ground substance which is not stained in this type of preparation since it is dissolved away during tissue processing. Several small blood vessels **BV** are seen. This type of tissue is traditionally referred to as *areolar tissue*.

Fig. 4.8 Reticulin fibres

(Silver impregnation method/Haematoxylin × 800)

Reticular tissue forms a delicate supporting framework for many highly cellular organs such as endocrine glands, lymph nodes and the liver. In such organs, a fine network of branching fibres ramifies throughout the parenchyma usually anchored to a dense, collagenous capsule and septae which traverse the tissue. Reticulin is a non-banded form of collagen designated collagen Type III.

Reticulin fibres are usually poorly stained in common preparations but are able to absorb metallic silver by which they are stained black. This phenomenon led early histologists to believe that reticulin had a completely different chemical composition from that of collagen. Reticulin is the earliest type of collagen fibre to be produced during the development of all supporting tissues and is also present in varying quantities in most mature supporting tissues.

This micrograph shows the fine reticular architecture of part of a lymph node; the framework provides loose support for lymphoid cells, the nuclei of which have been counterstained blue. Reticulin is also a major component of the walls of small blood vessels **BV** as seen at the top of the field.

(a)

(b)

(c)

Fig. 4.9 Elastin fibres

(a) Spread preparation: Elastin/H & E × 320 (b) Elastic van Gieson × 100 (c) H & E × 400

Elastin is found in varying proportions in most supporting tissues conferring elasticity to enable recovery of tissue shape following normal physiological deformation. Elastin is thus present in large amounts in tissues such as lung, skin and urinary bladder.

In most tissues, elastin occurs as short branching fibres which form an irregular network throughout the tissue. This is not easily seen in tissue sections but is better demonstrated in *spread preparations* such as in micrograph (a) in which elastin fibres **E** are stained black, collagen fibres **C** are stained pink and nuclei are stained blue. A branched capillary **Cap** crosses the field and two densely stained plasma cells **P** are also seen (see Ch. 11).

Micrograph (b) shows a histological section stained specifically for elastin; with this method, elastin is stained black and collagen is stained red. The specimen is of the dermis of the skin. The dominant feature is the coarse, closely packed, interwoven bundles of collagen between which are dispersed numerous finer elastic fibres. Most of the elastic fibres are cut in transverse or oblique section but some are cut in longitudinal section making them readily identifiable.

Micrograph (c) shows the wall of a large artery, this being made up mainly of smooth muscle cells, collagen and thick sheets of elastin (see Ch. 8). Like the collagen and smooth muscle cytoplasm, the elastin **E** is eosinophilic; it is only recognisable in this situation because the elastin sheets are very thick and because the elastin has a relaxed wave-like conformation due to collapse of the vessel wall.

Fig. 4.10 Elastin *(EM × 50 000)*

This micrograph shows elastin **E** in the delicate supporting tissue underlying the epithelium of mouse trachea. The field also contains collagen fibrils **C** (cut in transverse section) and the fine cytoplasmic extensions of fibroblasts **F** responsible for elaboration of the extracellular constituents.

The elastin is not made up of fibrils but rather is an amorphous mass of polymerised tropoelastin. Microfibrils **M** of the structural glycoprotein fibrillin which is involved in the process of elastin deposition can just be discerned at this magnification (in transverse section) lying within and around the elastin. Microfibrils can also be seen in the lower part of the field cut in longitudinal section **L** in association with small amounts of elastin.

Adipose tissue

Most supporting tissues contain cells which are adapted for the storage of fat; these cells, called *adipocytes*, are derived from primitive mesenchyme. Adipocytes are found in isolation or in clumps throughout loose supporting tissues or may constitute the main cell type as in adipose tissue.

Stored fat within adipocytes is derived from three main sources: dietary fat circulating in the bloodstream as chylomicrons, triglycerides synthesised in the liver and transported in blood, and triglycerides synthesised from glucose within adipocytes. Adipose tissue is often regarded as an inactive energy store, however it is an extremely important participant in general metabolic processes in that it acts as a temporary store of substrate for the energy-deriving processes of almost all tissues. Adipose tissue, therefore, generally has a rich blood supply. The rate of fat deposition and utilisation within adipose tissue is largely determined by dietary intake and energy expenditure, but a number of hormones and the sympathetic nervous system profoundly influence the fat metabolism of adipocytes.

There are two main types of adipose tissue:

- **White adipose tissue:** this type of adipose tissue comprises up to 20% of total body weight in normal, well-nourished male adults and up to 25% in females. It is distributed throughout the body particularly in the deep layers of the skin (see Ch.9). In addition to being an important energy store, white adipose tissue acts as a thermal insulator under the skin and functions as a cushion against mechanical shock in such sites as around the kidneys.

- **Brown adipose tissue:** this highly specialised type of adipose tissue is found in newborn mammals and some hibernating animals, where it plays an important part in body temperature regulation. Only small amounts of brown adipose tissue are found in human adults and, although previously thought to contribute little to thermoregulation, there is now increasing evidence that (at least in some individuals) brown adipose tissue may play a role in burning off excess energy thus preventing obesity.

(a)

(b)

Fig. 4.11 White adipose tissue

(a) Masson's trichrome × 480
(b) EM × 6 000

The typical appearance of white adipose tissue is illustrated in micrograph (a). Fat stored in adipocytes accumulates as lipid droplets which fuse to form a single large droplet which distends and occupies most of the cytoplasm. The adipocyte nucleus **N** is compressed and displaced to one side of the stored lipid droplet and the cytoplasm is reduced to a small rim around the periphery. In routine histological sections, the lipid content of adipocytes is extracted during tissue processing leaving a large, unstained space within each cell. Note the minute dimensions of blood capillaries **C** compared with the size of the surrounding adipocytes.

The electron micrograph (b) shows the periphery of two adjacent adipocytes. Contrary to the impression given by light microscopy, the main lipid droplet **L** in each cell has an irregular outline with numerous tiny droplets **D** at the periphery in the process of fusion with the main droplet. The lipid is not bounded by a membrane. The thin rim of cytoplasm contains the usual organelles most notably mitochondria **M**. In the adjacent extracellular tissue can be seen a fibroblastic cytoplasmic process **F** and collagen fibrils **C**.

(c)

Fig. 4.12 Fibrofatty tissue

(H & E × 200)

This micrograph demonstrates the typical appearance of adipocytes **A** scattered within loose, collagenous supporting tissue. Adipocytes occur either singly or in groups, particularly in the tissues supporting the lining of the gastrointestinal tract as shown here. Like the adipocytes of white adipose tissue, the size of adipocytes in loose supporting tissue depends on the equilibrium between dietary fat intake and energy expenditure.

(a)　(b)　(c)

Fig. 4.13 Brown adipose tissue

(a) H & E × 100 (b) H & E × 200 (c) H & E × 320
(d) Rabbit: EM × 4070

These micrographs demonstrate the typical histological appearance of brown adipose tissue. As seen in micrographs (a) and (b), brown adipose tissue is arranged in lobules separated by fibrous septae **S** which convey blood vessels and sympathetic nerve fibres. Within the cytoplasm, lipid is stored in the form of multiple small droplets, giving the cytoplasm a vaculated appearance. The cytoplasm is relatively copious and stains strongly due to the presence of numerous mitochondria.

At high magnification in micrograph (c), the nuclei of brown adipocytes are seen to be eccentrically located within the cell but, unlike those of white adipocytes, the nuclei are plump and surrounded by a significant quantity of strongly eosinophilic cytoplasm. The stored lipid is contained within multiple droplets, all of which have been dissolved away during tissue processing. A frozen section of brown adipose tissue stained for lipid is shown in Figure 1.25(b). Note the rich network of capillaries **C** between the brown adipocytes.

The electron micrograph (d) shows brown adipose tissue taken from a newborn rabbit and readily demonstrates the multilocular nature of stored lipid **L**. The cytoplasm of brown adipocytes is crammed with mitochondria **M** which have numerous, closely packed cristae. These mitochondria are extremely rich in cytochromes, molecules involved in oxidative energy production; this accounts for the brown colour of brown adipose tissue when examined macroscopically.

Unlike the metabolism of other tissues, in brown adipose cells the process of electron transport is readily uncoupled from the phosphorylation of ADP to form ATP. The energy derived from oxidation of lipids, and energy released by electron transport in the uncoupled state, is dissipated as heat which is rapidly conducted to the rest of the body by the rich vascular network of brown adipose tissue. Note the intimate association of capillaries **C** with the brown adipocyte in this micrograph.

Using these metabolic processes, neonatal humans and

(d)

other mammals utilise brown adipose tissue to generate body heat during the vulnerable period after birth. Brown adipose tissue undergoes involution in early infancy and in adult humans is found only in odd sites such as around the adrenal gland and great vessels. The production of heat by brown adipose tissue is controlled directly by the sympathetic nervous system.

The defence cells of supporting tissue

The supporting tissues not only contain cells responsible for their synthesis, maintenance and metabolic activity, but also a variety of cells with defence and immune functions. Traditionally, these cells have been divided into two categories: fixed (intrinsic) cells and wandering (extrinsic) cells.

The intrinsic defence cells of supporting tissue are the *tissue-fixed macrophages* (*histiocytes*) and *mast cells*. Tissue-fixed macrophages are now generally believed to be derived from circulating monocytes (see Fig. 3.9) which have become at least temporarily resident in supporting tissues. Mast cells are functionally analogous to basophils (see Fig. 3.7) but there are structural differences which suggest that mast cells are not merely basophils resident in the tissues.

The wandering category of defence and immune cells includes all the remaining members of the white blood cells series (see Ch.3). Although leucocytes are usually considered as a constituent of blood, their principal site of activity is outside the blood circulation, particularly within loose supporting tissues. Leucocytes are normally found only in relatively small numbers but in response to tissue injury and other disease processes their numbers increase greatly. The supporting tissues of those regions of the body which are subject to the constant threat of pathogenic invasion, such as the gastrointestinal and respiratory tracts, contain a large population of leucocytes, even in the absence of overt disease.

The reticulo-endothelial concept

The term *reticulo-endothelial system* has long been used to describe a diverse group of cells found in many tissues but in particular the bone marrow, liver, spleen, lymph nodes and thymus. The principal functional characteristic of such cells is their ability to phagocytise particulate matter and effete (worn out or dead) cells, e.g. old blood cells. Such phagocytic cells are found lining certain blood and lymph-filled spaces, such as the sinusoids of the liver (see Fig. 15.8), bone marrow (see Fig. 3.12) and spleen (see Fig. 11.25), and in this context they have some features in common with the *endothelial cells* which line all blood and lymphatic vessels (see Ch. 8).

Certain highly cellular tissues, such as lymph nodes and the haemopoietic cords of bone marrow, have a supporting framework of reticulin fibres (see Fig. 4.8) upon which are draped cells with long cytoplasmic processes morphologically similar to primitive mesenchymal cells (see Fig. 4.3); these cells are traditionally described as *reticulum* or *reticular cells*. Some if not all of these cells are probably responsible for synthesis of the reticulin framework, being thus analogous to fibroblasts; many of these cells, if not all, may also exhibit considerable phagocytic activity.

Because of the close structural and functional association of these cell types with the haemopoietic, macrophage-monocyte (see Fig. 3.9) and immune systems, they were thought to represent some common functional denominator. Consequently, 'reticulo-endothelial' and related terms became widely and often indiscriminately applied to tissues and cells within these systems. Scientific advances have rendered the concept so imprecise as to serve little purpose and it should now be considered of historical interest only.

(a)

Fig. 4.14 Mast cells

(a) Thin section, toluidine blue × 1200 (b) EM × 12 000

Mast cells are found in all supporting tissues but are particularly prevalent beneath the skin, gastrointestinal lining, the serosal lining of the peritoneal cavity and around blood vessels. Their major constituents and functions are very similar to those of basophils which are described in detail with Figure 3.7. Whether or not they are derived from circulating basophils is in dispute, but mast cells are long lived with the ability to proliferate within the tissues. Mast cell degranulation results in the release of histamine and other vasoactive mediators which induce the immediate hypersensitivity (anaphylactoid) response (characteristic of urticaria, allergic rhinitis and asthma) and anaphylactic shock.

Mast cells are not readily identified in routine histological sections due to the water solubility of their densely basophilic granules which tend to be lost during preparation. Thus special techniques of fixation, embedding and staining must be employed. With suitable staining, however, the characteristic feature of mast cells is an extensive cytoplasm packed with large granules which are nevertheless smaller in size, though more numerous, than those of basophils. When stained with certain blue basic dyes such as *toluidine blue*, the granules bind to the dye changing its colour to red. This property is known as *metachromasia*.

The light micrograph demonstrates two mast cells **M** in the supporting tissue underlying the tracheal surface. A pale nucleus can be seen in one cell but the plane of section is outside the nucleus of the other. Note the large, densely packed granules which exhibit metachromasia.

In the electron micrograph (b), mast cell granules **G** are seen to be membrane-bound and to contain a dense amorphous material. The granules are liberated from the cell by exocytosis when stimulated during an inflammatory or allergic response. The cytoplasm contains a few rounded mitochondria **Mi** and a little rough endoplasmic reticulum. The non-segmented nucleus has less condensed chromatin than that of basophils. Other differences from basophils include a more uniform distribution of their thin surface processes, a greater number of cytoplasmic filaments and a lack of glycogen granules.

2.0 µm

(b)

Fig. 4.15 Leucocytes in loose supporting tissue *(H & E × 640)*

The appearance of leucocytes within tissue sections differs greatly from the appearance seen in blood smears (see Ch. 3). In this micrograph, a variety of leucocytes are seen in the loose supporting tissue beneath the lining of the large intestine, a site which is normally rich in such cells even in the absence of inflammation.

Fibroblasts **F**, are identified by their relatively large, elongated nuclei. Erythrocytes **Er** within small blood vessels are intensely eosinophilic (red stained); the presence of erythrocytes (approximate diameter 7 µm) provides a reference for the size of other cells of the granulocyte series (see Ch. 3).

Of the granulocytes, neutrophils are only rarely seen in the tissues except in acute or chronic inflammation. Neutrophils **N** are recognised by their multilobed nuclei and poorly stained cytoplasm. Eosinophils **Eo** are present in large numbers in normal supporting tissues and are recognised by their bilobed nuclei and strongly eosinophilic cytoplasmic granules. Basophils, and their analogues mast cells, are poorly stained in H & E preparations and are therefore difficult to recognise.

Lymphocytes **L** are easily recognised by their small, densely-stained nuclei and a thin halo of poorly stained cytoplasm. Plasma cells **P**, immunologically activated lymphocytes responsible for antibody synthesis (see Ch. 11),

are recognised by their large granular nuclei and extensive basophilic (blue-stained) cytoplasm containing a pale stained peri-nuclear area which represents a well developed and active Golgi apparatus. The basophilia of plasma cells is largely attributable to profuse rough endoplasmic reticulum involved in the synthesis of antibody molecules.

Large mononuclear phagocytes, analogous to the monocytes of blood, are distributed throughout all supporting tissues where they may exhibit intense phagocytic activity; these cells are also known as macrophages, tissue-fixed macrophages, and histiocytes when present in supporting tissue. Inactive macrophages are small and drape themselves on the fibres of the extracellular matrix and may be difficult to distinguish from fibroblasts. In contrast, actively phagocytic macrophages are plump and may move in an amoeboid manner through the ground substance. When actively phagocytic, macrophages may be easily recognised by their large size and content of engulfed material; note, however, that active macrophages have an extremely variable appearance, depending on the nature of their phagocytic activity. Most of the cytoplasmic detail of the macrophages **M** shown in this preparation is obscured by engulfed material which appears brown. For comparison, a different example of the appearance of active macrophages is seen in Figure 11.12(b).

Fig. 4.16 Macrophage *(EM × 11 600)*

The ultrastructural features of macrophages vary widely according to their state of activity and tissue location. This micrograph shows an active macrophage obtained from the peritoneum of a rat which had previously been injected intra-peritoneally with latex particles; a number of particles **P** have been engulfed by the macrophage.

The macrophage nucleus is irregular with heterochromatin typically clumped around the nuclear envelope. The cytoplasm contains a few mitochondria **M** and a variable amount of free ribosomes and rough endoplasmic reticulum **rER**. In quiescent macrophages, lysosomes **L** are abundant but their number is much reduced in actively phagocytic cells; lysosomes are later regenerated by the Golgi apparatus. The macrophage cytoplasm contains an assortment of phagosomes and residual bodies **R**. Residual material may be released from the macrophage by exocytosis. Such material may remain sequestered in the tissues, as occurs with the dyes used in tattooing of the skin, or the material may be returned to the circulation for excretion or re-use in biosynthetic processes. Actively

phagocytic cells exhibit irregular cytoplasmic projections or pseudopodia **Pp** which are involved in amoeboid movement and phagocytosis.

In addition to their role as tissue scavengers, macrophages play an important role in immune mechanisms (see Ch. 11) since they are often the first cells to make contact with antigens. Macrophages process antigenic material in some way before presenting it to lymphocytes; lymphocytes are then stimulated to undergo specific immune responses. Macrophages involved in this way are described as *antigen presenting cells*. As a result of various immune mechanisms, antigenic material may become combined or coated with substances such as antibodies and complement which are then collectively known as *opsonins*. Opsonins greatly enhance the phagocytic ability of macrophages and other phagocytes such as neutrophils (see Ch. 3), a process which is known as *opsonisation*. Other substances such as lymphokines, which are released during the immune response, act directly upon macrophages to increase greatly their metabolic and phagocytic activity.

5. Epithelial tissues

Introduction

The epithelia are a diverse group of tissues which, with rare exceptions, cover or line all body surfaces, cavities and tubes. Epithelia thus function as interfaces between different biological compartments. As such, epithelia mediate a wide range of activities such as selective diffusion, absorption and/or secretion, physical protection and containment; all these major functions may be exhibited at a single epithelial surface. For example, the epithelial lining of the small intestine is primarily involved in absorption of the products of digestion, but the epithelium also protects itself from noxious intestinal contents by the secretion of a surface coating of mucus.

Surface epithelia form continuous sheets comprising one or more layers of cells. The cells are separated by a minute quantity of intercellular material which may represent the fused glycocalyces of adjacent cells (see Ch.1). Epithelial cells are closely bound to one another by a variety of membrane specialisations called *cell junctions* which provide physical strength and mediate exchange of 'information' and metabolites.

All epithelia are supported by a *basement membrane* of variable thickness. Basement membranes separate epithelia from underlying supporting tissues and are never penetrated by blood vessels; epithelia are thus dependent on the diffusion of oxygen and metabolites from adjacent supporting tissues. The structure of basement membranes is described in detail in Chapter 4.

Classification of epithelia

Epithelia are traditionally classified according to three morphological characteristics:

- The number of cell layers: a single layer of epithelial cells is termed *simple epithelium*, whereas epithelia composed of several layers are termed *stratified epithelia*.
- The shape of the component cells: this is based on the appearance in sections taken at right angles to the epithelial surface. In stratified epithelia the shape of the outermost layer of cells determines the descriptive classification. Cellular outlines are often difficult to distinguish, but the shape of epithelial cells is usually reflected in the shape of their nuclei.
- The presence of surface specialisations such as cilia and keratin: an example is the epithelial surface of skin which is classified as 'stratified squamous keratinising epithelium' since it consists of many layers of cells, the surface cells of which are flattened (squamous) in shape and covered by an outer layer of the proteinaceous material, keratin (see Fig. 5.7).

Epithelia may be derived from ectoderm, mesoderm or endoderm although in the past it was thought that true epithelia were only of ectodermal or endodermal origin. Two types of epithelia derived from mesoderm, i.e. the lining of blood and lymphatic vessels and the linings of the serous body cavities, were not considered to be epithelia and were termed *endothelium* and *mesothelium* respectively. By both morphological and functional criteria, such distinction has little practical value; nevertheless, the terms endothelium and mesothelium are still used to describe these types of epithelium.

Glandular epithelia

Epithelium which is primarily involved in secretion is often arranged into structures called *glands*. Glands are merely invaginations of epithelial surfaces which are formed during embryonic development by proliferation of epithelium into the underlying tissues. Glands which maintain their continuity with the epithelial surface, discharging their secretions onto the free surface via a duct, are called *exocrine glands*.

In some cases, the duct degenerates during development leaving isolated islands of epithelial secretory tissue deep within other tissues. The secretory products of such glands, known as *endocrine* or *ductless glands*, pass into the bloodstream; their secretions are known as *hormones* (see Ch. 17). Nevertheless some endocrine glands develop by migration of epithelial cells without the formation of a duct.

Simple epithelia

Simple epithelia are defined as surface epithelia consisting of a single layer of cells. Simple epithelia are almost always found at interfaces involved in selective diffusion, absorption or secretion. They provide little protection against mechanical abrasion and thus are not found on surfaces subject to such stresses. The cells comprising simple epithelia range in shape from extremely flattened to tall columnar, depending on their function. For example, flattened simple epithelia are ideally suited to diffusion and are therefore found in the air sacs of the lung (alveoli), the lining of blood vessels (endothelium) and lining body cavities (mesothelium). In contrast, highly active epithelial cells, such as the cells lining the small intestine, are generally tall since they must accommodate the appropriate organelles. Simple epithelia may exhibit a variety of surface specialisations, such as microvilli and cilia, which facilitate their specific surface functions.

(a)

(b)

(c)

Fig. 5.1 Simple squamous epithelium

(a) Diagram (b) H & E × 800
(c) Spread preparation, silver method/neutral red × 320

Simple squamous epithelium is composed of flattened, irregularly shaped cells forming a continuous surface which may be referred to as *pavemented epithelium*; the term 'squamous' derives from the comparison of the cells to the scales of a fish. Like all epithelia, this delicate lining is supported by an underlying basement membrane **BM** as shown diagrammatically, although this is rarely thick enough to be seen with routine light microscopy.

Simple squamous epithelium is found lining surfaces involved in passive transport (diffusion) of either gases (as in the lungs), or fluids (as in the walls of blood capillaries). Simple squamous epithelium also forms the delicate lining of the pleural, pericardial and peritoneal cavities where it permits passage of tissue fluid into and out of these cavities. Reflecting the minimal metabolic activity of these cells, the nuclear chromatin is condensed and the cytoplasm is sparse and contains few organelles.

Micrograph (b) shows a small blood vessel and illustrates the typical appearance of simple squamous epithelium in section. The epithelial lining cells **E** (known as endothelium in the circulatory system) are so flattened that they can only be recognised by their nuclei which bulge into the vessel lumen. The supporting basement membrane is thin and, in haematoxylin and eosin stained preparations, has similar staining properties to the endothelial cell cytoplasm; hence it cannot be seen in this micrograph.

In the preparation used in micrograph (c), the mesothelial lining of the peritoneal cavity has been stripped from the underlying tissues and spread onto a slide thus permitting a surface view of simple squamous epithelium. The intercellular substance has been stained with silver thereby outlining the closely interdigitating and highly irregular cell boundaries. The nuclei **N** are stained red.

(a)

(b)

Fig. 5.2 Simple cuboidal epithelium *(a) Diagram (b) Azan × 400*

Simple cuboidal epithelium represents an intermediate form between simple squamous and simple columnar epithelium; the distinction between tall cuboidal and low columnar is often arbitrary and is of descriptive value only. In section perpendicular to the basement membrane, the epithelial cells appear square, leading to its traditional description as cuboidal epithelium; on surface view, however, the cells are actually polygonal in shape. The nucleus is usually round and located in the centre of the cell.

Simple cuboidal epithelium usually lines small ducts and tubules which may have excretory, secretory or absorptive functions; examples are the small collecting ducts of the kidney, salivary glands and pancreas.

The micrograph shows the cells lining a small collecting tubule in the kidney. Although the boundaries between individual cells are indistinct, the nuclear shape provides an approximate indication of the cell size and shape. Reflecting the considerable metabolic activity of these cells, the nuclear chromatin is relatively dispersed and nucleoli are prominent. The underlying basement membrane appears as a prominent blue line with the Azan staining method.

(a)

(b)

Fig. 5.3 Simple columnar epithelium *(a) Diagram (b) H & E × 800*

Simple columnar epithelium is similar to simple cuboidal epithelium except that the cells are taller and appear columnar in sections at right angles to the basement membrane. The height of the cells may vary from low to tall columnar depending on the site and/or degree of functional activity. The nuclei are elongated and may be located towards the base, the centre or occasionally the apex of the cytoplasm; this is known as *polarity*. Simple columnar epithelium is most often found on highly absorptive surfaces such as in the small intestine, although it may constitute the lining of highly secretory surfaces such as that of the stomach.

The micrograph illustrates an unusually tall example of simple columnar epithelium and is taken from the lining of the gall bladder where it has the function of absorbing water, thus concentrating bile. Note the typically elongated nuclei which in this location exhibit basal polarity.

The luminal plasma membranes of highly absorptive epithelial cells are often arranged into numerous, minute, finger-like projections called *microvilli* which greatly increase the surface area of the absorptive interface. Microvilli are far too small to be resolved individually by light microscopy although they may collectively give the appearance of a *striated* or *brush border* at the luminal surface (see Fig. 5.16).

(a)   *(b)*

Fig. 5.4 Simple columnar ciliated epithelium *(a) Diagram (b) Azan × 320*

This type of simple columnar epithelium is traditionally described as a separate entity because of the presence of surface specialisations called cilia **C** on the majority of the cells. Among the ciliated cells are scattered non-ciliated cells which usually have a secretory function.

Cilia are much larger than microvilli and are readily visible with the light microscope. Each cilium consists of a finger-like projection of the plasma membrane, its cytoplasm containing a motile specialisation of the cytoskeleton (see Fig. 5.15). Each cell may have up to 300 cilia which, along with those of other cells, beat in a wavelike manner, generating a current which propels fluid or minute particles over the epithelial surface. Simple columnar ciliated epithelium is not common in humans except in the female reproductive tract.

This micrograph taken from the Fallopian tube (oviduct) shows one of its numerous folds covered by simple columnar ciliated epithelium. The predominant cell type in this epithelium is tall columnar and ciliated, the nuclei being located towards the luminal aspect of the cells. The less numerous, blue-stained cells with basally located nuclei are not ciliated and have a secretory function. Ciliary action facilitates transport of the ovum from the ovary towards the uterus. As in this preparation, cilia are often stuck together in clumps by surface secretions or they may become flattened during tissue processing and therefore difficult to distinguish.

(a)   *(b)*

Fig. 5.5 Pseudostratified columnar ciliated epithelium *(a) Diagram (b) H & E × 600*

Another variant of simple columnar epithelium is described in which the majority of cells are also usually ciliated. The term *pseudostratified* is derived from the appearance of this epithelium in section which conveys the erroneous impression that there is more than one layer of cells. In fact, this is a true simple epithelium since all the cells rest on the basement membrane. The nuclei of these cells however are disposed at different levels, thus creating the illusion of cellular stratification. Not all the ciliated cells extend to the luminal surface; such cells are capable of cell division providing replacements for cells lost or damaged.

Pseudostratified columnar ciliated epithelium may be distinguished from true stratified epithelia by two characteristics. Firstly, the individual cells of the pseudostratified epithelium exhibit polarity, with nuclei being mainly confined to the basal two thirds of the epithelium. Secondly, cilia are never present on stratified epithelia.

Pseudostratified epithelium is almost exclusively confined to the larger airways of the respiratory system in mammals and is therefore often referred to as *respiratory epithelium*. Micrograph (b) illustrates the lining of a bronchus. In the respiratory tract, the cilia propel a surface layer of mucus containing entrapped particles towards the pharynx in what is often described as the *mucociliary escalator*.

Stratified epithelia

Stratified epithelia are defined as epithelia consisting of two or more layers of cells. Stratified epithelia have mainly a protective function and the degree and nature of the stratification is related to the kinds of physical stresses to which the surface is exposed. In general, stratified epithelia are poorly suited for the functions of absorption and secretion by virtue of their thickness, although some stratified surfaces are moderately permeable to water and other small molecules. The classification of stratified epithelia is based on the shape and structure of the surface cells since cells of the basal layer are usually cuboidal in shape.

(a) (b) (c) (d)

Fig. 5.6 Stratified squamous epithelium *(a) Diagram (b) H & E × 100 (c) H & E × 400 (d) Papanicolou × 400*

Stratified squamous epithelium consists of a variable number of cell layers which exhibit transition from a cuboidal basal layer to a flattened surface layer. The basal cells divide continuously, their offspring being progressively pushed towards the free surface where they are ultimately shed. During the process, the cells undergo first maturation, then degeneration, the surface cells showing overt signs of degeneration; this is particularly evident in the nuclei which become progressively condensed (pyknotic) and flattened, before ultimately disintegrating.

Stratified squamous epithelium is well adapted to withstand abrasion since loss of surface cells does not compromise the underlying tissue; it is poorly adapted to withstand desiccation. This type of epithelium lines the oral cavity, pharynx, oesophagus, anal canal, uterine cervix and vagina, sites which are subject to mechanical abrasion but which are kept moist by glandular secretions.

The epithelium demonstrated in micrograph (b) is from the uterine cervix. Note the highly cellular basal layer and the transformation through the large polygonal cells of the intermediate layers to the degenerate superficial squamous cells. The junction between epithelium and underlying supporting tissue is irregular, enhancing the adhesion of the epithelium to the underlying tissues.

Micrograph (c) shows the deep layers at high magnification; a few lymphocytes **L** are scattered at this level. The basement membrane **BM** is quite thick and, as in all epithelia, blood vessels **BV** do not extend beyond the basement membrane.

Micrograph (d) shows a smear made from cells scraped from the uterine cervix as it projects into the vagina. The degenerate, scaly superficial cells stain pink with this staining method, the living cells from deeper layers staining blue.

Fig. 5.7 Stratified squamous keratinising epithelium *(H & E × 320)*

This specialised form of stratified squamous epithelium constitutes the epithelial surface of the skin (epidermis) and is adapted to withstand the constant abrasion and desiccation to which the body surface is exposed. During maturation, the epithelial cells undergo a process called *keratinisation* resulting in the formation of a tough, non-cellular surface layer consisting of the protein, *keratin* **K** (see Ch. 9). Keratinisation may be induced in normally non-keratinising stratified squamous epithelium such as that of the oral cavity when exposed to excessive abrasion or desiccation.

Fig. 5.8 Stratified cuboidal epithelium
(H & E × 320)

Stratified cuboidal epithelium is a thin, stratified epithelium which usually consists of only two or three layers of cuboidal or low columnar cells. This type of epithelium is usually confined to the lining of the larger excretory ducts of exocrine glands such as the salivary glands. Stratified cuboidal epithelium is probably not involved in significant absorptive or secretory activity but merely provides a more robust lining than would be afforded by a simple epithelium.

(a)

(b)

Fig. 5.9 Transitional epithelium *(a) Diagram (b) H & E × 320*

Transitional epithelium is a form of stratified epithelium almost exclusively confined to the urinary tract in mammals where it is highly specialised to accommodate a great degree of stretch and to withstand the toxicity of urine. This epithelial type is so named because it has some features which are intermediate (transitional) between stratified cuboidal and stratified squamous epithelia. In the relaxed (contracted) state, transitional epithelium appears to be about four to five cell layers thick. The basal cells are roughly cuboidal, the intermediate cells are polygonal and the surface cells are large and rounded and may contain two nuclei. In the stretched state, transitional epithelium often appears only two or three cells thick (although the actual

number of layers remains constant) and the intermediate and surface layers are extremely flattened.

The micrograph shows the appearance of transitional epithelium from the lining of a contracted bladder. The shape and apparent size of the basal and intermediate cells vary considerably depending on the degree of distension, but the cells of the surface layer usually retain several characteristic features. Firstly, the surface cells are large and pale-stained and present a scalloped surface outline. Secondly, the luminal surface of the cells appears thickened and more densely stained. Thirdly, the nuclei of the surface cells are large and round, and often exhibit prominent nucleoli; some surface cells are binucleate **B**.

Membrane specialisations of epithelia

The intercellular, luminal and basal surfaces of epithelial cells exhibit a variety of specialisations.

Intercellular surfaces. The apposed surfaces of epithelial cells are linked by several different types of membrane and cytoskeletal specialisations. These *cell junctions* permit epithelia to form a continuous cohesive layer in which all of the cells 'communicate' and co-operate to achieve the particular functional requirements of the epithelium.

Cell junctions are of three functional types:

- *Occluding junctions*, also known as *tight junctions*, are located immediately beneath the luminal surface of simple columnar epithelium (e.g. intestinal lining) where they seal the intercellular spaces so that luminal contents cannot penetrate between the lining cells. Each tight junction forms a continuous circumferential band or zonule around the cell and is thus also known as a *zonula occludens*.

- *Adhering junctions* tightly bind the constituent cells of the epithelium together and act as anchorage sites for the cytoskeleton of each cell so that the cytoskeletons of all cells are effectively linked into a single functional unit. Adhering junctions are of two morphological types. Deep to the tight junctions of columnar epithelial cells, an adhering junction forms a continuous band (*zonula adherens*) around the cell providing structural reinforcement to the occluding junction. Secondly, adhering junctions in the form of small circular patches or spots called *desmosomes (macula adherens)* are circumferentially arranged around columnar cells deep to the continuous adhering junction. The combination of zonula occludens, zonula adherens and circumferentially arranged desmosomes is known as a *junctional complex*. Desmosomes (spot adhering junctions) are also widely scattered elsewhere in epithelial intercellular interfaces binding the whole epithelial mass into a structurally coherent whole.

- *Communicating junctions*, also known as *gap* or *nexus junctions* due to their ultrastructural appearance, are circular intercellular contact areas containing hundreds of tiny pores which permit passage of small molecules between adjacent cells. Molecules involved in such cytoplasmic interchange include ions responsible for electrical excitation of cell membranes, nutrients and chemical signalling agents.

Adhering junctions and communicating junctions are not exclusive to epithelia and are also present in cardiac and visceral muscle where they appear to serve similar functions.

Luminal surfaces. The luminal surfaces of epithelial cells may incorporate three main types of specialisation, *cilia*, *microvilli* and *stereocilia*. Cilia are relatively long, motile structures which are easily resolved by light microscopy. In contrast, microvilli are short, often extremely numerous projections of the plasma membrane which cannot be individually resolved with the light microscope. Stereocilia are merely extremely long microvilli usually found only singly or in small numbers in odd sites such as the male reproductive tract; stereocilia are not motile and are thus quite inappropriately named.

Basal surfaces. The interface between all epithelia and underlying supporting tissues is marked by a non-cellular structure known as the *basement membrane* which provides structural support for epithelia and constitutes a selective barrier to the passage of materials between epithelium and supporting tissue. Details of basement membrane structure are provided in the introduction to Chapter 4 and illustrated in Figure 4.1. The basal plasma membranes of some simple epithelia which are very active in ion transport (e.g. the cells of the kidney tubules) exhibit deep basal folds. These greatly enhance surface area and provide an arrangement by which the energy-providing mitochondria can be situated in intimate association with the plasma membrane; an example is shown in Figure 1.12(e). *Hemidesmosomes*, a variant of the desmosome, are present on the inner aspect of the basal plasma membrane adjacent to the basement membrane and provide a means of anchorage of the cytoskeleton to the basement membrane and underlying supporting tissue.

(a)

(b)

Fig. 5.10 Intercellular junctions

(a) Schematic diagram (b) Junctional complex: EM × 125 000

The illustration demonstrates, in a highly schematic manner, the three-dimensional (circumferential) arrangement of the junctional complex with respect to the cell surface and the detailed structure of the various types of intercellular junction of which it is comprised.

Between the cells of simple cuboidal and simple columnar epithelia, a junctional complex encircles each cell preventing access of luminal contents to the intercellular spaces and strengthening the luminal surface against cellular disaggregation.

As seen in the micrograph of intestinal columnar epithelium, the junctional complex begins immediately below the luminal surface and is made up of three components, a *tight junction* **TJ** *(zonula occludens), a continuous adhering junction* or *zonula adherens* **ZA** and a row of *spot-adhering junctions* or *desmosomes* **D**.

In this field, the bases of microvilli **Mv** which cover the surface of small intestinal lining cells can be identified. As described in Figure 5.16, each microvillus contains a core of cytoskeletal microfilaments **Mf** which insert into a zone of condensed intermediate and microfilaments lying just beneath the cell surface, the *terminal web* **TW**; this finds anchorage in the zonula adherens. The desmosome **D** is the anchorage point for intermediate filaments **IF** of the cytoskeleton.

0.1 μm

Fig. 5.11 Occluding (tight) junctions *(EM × 190 000)*

The occluding or tight junction (zonula occludens) forms a collar around each cell immediately beneath the cell surface sealing the intercellular space from ingress of luminal contents. As seen in this electron micrograph, the outer electron-dense layers of opposing cell membranes are seen to come extremely close together with minimal intercellular material between them. In places, the plasma membranes appear to fuse completely, these sites being represented at the molecular level by the opposed membranes exhibiting a system of fine matching ridges known as *sealing strands* which 'stitch' the membranes together in the manner of two pieces of cloth, haphazardly stitched together on a sewing machine (see Fig. 5.10(a)). Continuing this analogy, each 'stitch' comprises a pair of membrane proteins, one an integral part of each opposing plasma membrane, linked tightly together.

As well as sealing the intercellular space from the luminal environment, tight junctions may prevent migration of 'floating' membrane proteins from their appropriate domains on the cell surface (e.g. luminal surface proteins are confined to that surface).

Structurally similar but discontinuous strips of tight junction called *fascia occludens* are found between the endothelial cells lining blood vessels except in the vessels of the brain where they are of the continuous (zonula occludens) type.

TJ

ZA

TW

TW

D

IF

D₂

IF

0.2 μm

Fig. 5.12 Adhering junctions *(EM × 95 000)*

As previously described, adhering junctions provide anchorage points for cytoskeletal elements, in effect linking the cytoskeletons of individual cells into a strong transcellular network. These junctions are of two forms, the continuous belt (zonula adherens) and the spot or patch type (macula adherens or desmosome). The zonula adherens (also known as a belt desmosome) forms a single continuous band lying deep to the zonula occludens (tight junction) beneath the cell surface of certain columnar lining epithelia. A row of desmosomes is also disposed circumferentially around the apical aspect of columnar epithelium, forming the third component of the junctional complex. Larger desmosomes are also scattered over the intercellular surfaces of all epithelial cells. This micrograph from the intestinal lining illustrates a junctional complex comprising tight junction **TJ**, zonula adherens **ZA** and desmosome **D**. At a deeper level, a large desmosome **D₂** represents one of the scattered intercellular adhering junctions.

At the zonula adherens, opposing plasma membranes diverge and the intercellular space contains a relatively electron-lucent material of unknown composition which forms a strong bond between the opposing membrane surfaces. The cytoplasmic aspect of the membrane provides anchorage for the fine meshwork of microfilaments making up the terminal web **TW**. Contraction of the terminal web probably regulates tension at the epithelial surface. It may also provide for small lateral movements thus keeping the microvilli in a state of gentle agitation maximising contact of microvilli with molecules in the luminal contents and preventing clogging.

Desmosomes have a somewhat different structure. The widened space between opposed plasma membranes contains numerous fine transverse filaments called *transmembrane linkers* which appear to form an electron-dense line where they link up midway across the intercellular space. Within the cells, intermediate filaments **IF** insert into an electron-dense plaque on the inner aspect of the desmosome (see also Fig. 5.10(a)). Desmosome numbers are greatest in stratified squamous epithelia reflecting their role in providing structural integrity at surfaces subject to considerable mechanical stress, e.g. friction.

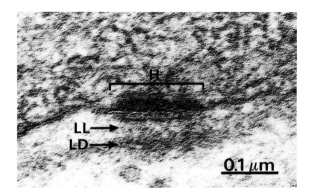

Fig. 5.13 Hemidesmosome *(EM × 150 000)*

Hemidesmosomes **H** are found along the basal plasma membranes of certain epithelia providing anchorage of the cytoskeleton to the plasma membrane at the base of the cell and to the underlying basement membrane.

On the cytoplasmic aspect of the plasma membrane is a structure akin to half a desmosome into which insert intermediate filaments. The underlying lamina densa **LD** is thickened and more electron-dense as is the lamina lucida **LL** which contains an electron-dense line like that of an intercellular desmosome.

(a)

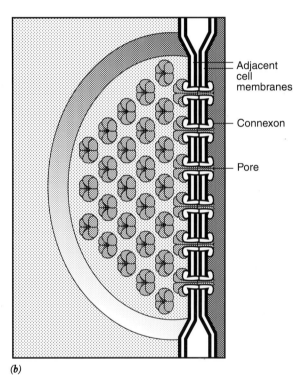

Adjacent
cell
membranes

Connexon

Pore

(b)

Fig. 5.14 Communicating (gap, nexus) junctions *(a) EM × 80 000 (b) Diagram*

Communicating junctions are broad patches where adjacent plasma membranes are closely opposed leaving a narrow intervening gap (hence the name gap junction). A gap junction **G** is demonstrated in the electron micrograph which is taken from intestinal epithelium.

As seen in the diagram, each gap junction contains numerous pores which permit the passage of positively charged ions and other small molecules (less than 2 nm in diameter) from the cytoplasm of one cell to another. Large molecules and negatively charged ions are denied access. Thus they serve as sites for exchange of metabolites, control molecules for growth, development, cell recognition and differentiation. Gap junctions also provide the means of electrical coupling of visceral and cardiac muscle cells permitting synchronous contraction.

Each pore consists of a minute tubular structure called a *connexon* which traverses the intercellular gap. The connexon comprises a pair of grommet-like cylinders, one penetrating each of the opposing cell membranes. Each cylinder is made up of six transmembrane protein molecules as indicated in the diagram. Tubal patency is maintained by the proteins being arranged in a slightly twisted conformation. This is highly sensitive to the intracellular concentration of calcium ions which, if increased, results in closure of the pores. A rise in intracellular calcium concentration is a feature of cell death and this mechanism appears to provide a means of sealing off necrotic cells and their potentially noxious contents from adjacent viable cells.

Communicating junctions are more numerous in embryonic epithelia where they appear to be involved in exchange of chemical messengers, in cell recognition, differentiation and control of cell position. They are also probably involved in the passage of nutrients from cells deep in the epithelium (adjacent to supporting tissues and blood vessels) to cells more remote from the nutritional supply.

(a)

Fig. 5.15 Cilia

(a) Thin section, toluidine blue × 800 (b) EM × 20 000
(c) Schematic diagram

Cilia are motile structures which project in parallel rows from certain epithelial surfaces, notably in the respiratory and female reproductive tracts. Cilia beat with a wave-like synchronous rhythm propelling surface films of mucus or fluid in a consistent direction over the epithelial surface. In the airways, mucus traps debris from inspired air, the cilia moving the mucus upwards towards the throat where it is swallowed thus keeping the airways clean. In the oviducts, ciliary action helps to transport the ovum from the ovary towards the uterus.

Cilia measure from about 7–10 μm in length and may therefore be around half the length of the cell (depending on cell size). A single epithelial cell may have up to 300 cilia usually of similar length.

Micrographs (a) and (b) show ciliated cells from the respiratory tract. Cilia **C** are readily visible with light microscopy although during processing they often become matted together and flattened making them less conspicuous. In micrograph (b), the proximal parts of three cilia **C** are seen in longitudinal section and, more superficially, the tips of a number of others otherwise lying outside the plane of section. Note the internal microtubular contents. Small surface microvilli **Mv** are seen between the cilia providing a useful size comparison.

Each cilium is bounded by an evagination of the luminal plasma membrane and, as shown diagrammatically, contains a central core called the *axoneme* consisting of 20 microtubules arranged as a central pair surrounded by nine peripheral doublets. At its base, the axoneme inserts into a structure called a *basal body* which has a microtubular arrangement identical to that of a centriole, i.e. nine triplets of microtubules forming a short cylinder (see Fig. 1.15). Each peripheral doublet of the cilium axoneme is continuous with the two inner microtubules of the corresponding triplet of the basal body. Basal bodies **BB** can be readily identified in micrograph (b).

Each axoneme doublet consists of one tubule of circular cross-section closely applied to another incomplete tubule which is C-shaped in cross-section. From each complete tubule, pairs of 'arms' consisting of the protein *dynein*, which has ATPase activity, extend towards the incomplete tubule of the adjacent doublet as well as towards the central microtubule pair. Ciliary action results from longitudinal movement of the doublets relative to one another, energy for the process being provided in the form of ATP by mitochondria **M** in the subjacent cytoplasm as in micrograph (b).

(b)

(c)

(a)

Fig. 5.16 Microvilli

(a) H & E × 320 (b) EM × 4 000 (c) EM × 30 000

Microvilli are minute finger-like projections of the luminal plasma membrane found in many epithelia particularly those specialised for absorption where their presence may increase the surface area as much as 30-fold. Microvilli are only 0.5–1.0 μm in length and are thus very short in relation to the size of the cell, a feature contrasting markedly with cilia (see Fig. 5.15). Furthermore, individual microvilli are too small to be resolved by light microscopy.

Some epithelia have only a small number of irregular microvilli. However, epithelia in such highly absorptive sites as in the small intestine and proximal renal tubules have up to 3000 regular microvilli per cell; collectively these can be seen with the light microscope as so-called *striated* and *brush borders* respectively. Micrographs (a) and (b) illustrate the typical features of microvilli constituting the striated border **SB** of cells lining the small intestine.

As seen at very high magnification in micrograph (c), the cytoplasmic core of each microvillus contains fine protein filaments **F** which insert into the terminal web, a specialisation of the cytoskeleton lying immediately beneath the cell surface; at the periphery of the cell the terminal web is anchored to the zonula adherens (see Fig. 5.12) enhancing the surface stability of the epithelium. At the tip of the microvillus, the filaments attach to an electron-dense part of the plasma membrane. The filaments, of which the principal constituent is actin, maintain stability of microvilli and may also mediate some contraction and elongation of the microvilli, thus preventing clogging.

(b)

(c)

Fig. 5.17 Stereocilia *(H & E × 320)*

Extremely long microvilli, readily visible with light microscopy, are found in small numbers in parts of the male reproductive tract such as the epididymis (shown in this micrograph) and other odd sites. Originally, these structures were thought to be an unusual form of cilia and were termed stereocilia; however, electron microscopy has shown that they do not have the internal structure of cilia but merely a filamentous skeleton like that of microvilli. Stereocilia **S** are thought to facilitate absorptive processes in the epididymis but the reason for their unusual form is not known.

Fig. 5.18 Goblet cell *(PAS/Haematoxylin × 800)*

Goblet cells are modified columnar epithelial cells which synthesise and secrete mucus. Goblet cells are scattered amongst the cells of many simple epithelial linings, particularly those of the respiratory and gastrointestinal tracts, and are named for their resemblance to drinking goblets.

The distended apical cytoplasm contains a dense aggregation of *mucigen granules* which, when released by exocytosis, combine with water to form the viscid secretion called mucus. Mucigen is composed of a mixture of neutral and acidic proteoglycans (mucopolysaccharides) and therefore can be readily demonstrated by the PAS method which stains carbohydrates magenta. The 'stem' of the goblet cell is occupied by a condensed, basal nucleus and is crammed with other organelles involved in mucigen synthesis.

In this example from the lining of the small intestine, note the tall columnar nature of the surrounding absorptive cells. The PAS-positive surface coating is not only due to secreted mucus but also to the presence of a thick glycocalyx (see Ch. 1) on the numerous microvilli which characterise small intestine absorptive cells.

Fig. 5.19 Goblet cell

(EM × 5 000)

This micrograph shows two goblet cells amongst columnar absorptive cells **A** of the small intestine; the nucleus of the goblet cell on the right is outside the plane of section, the nucleus **N** of the other being typically highly condensed. The cytoplasm is packed with rough endoplasmic reticulum **rER**; a few mitochondria **M** are present. A prominent Golgi apparatus **G** is found in the supranuclear region.

The protein component of mucigen is synthesised by the rough endoplasmic reticulum and passed to the Golgi apparatus where it is combined with carbohydrate and packaged into membrane-bound, secretory vacuoles containing mucigen **Mu**. Goblet cells secrete at a steady basal rate and may be stimulated by local irritation to release their entire mucigen contents. Sparse microvilli **Mv** are seen at the surface of the goblet cell and may be associated with the secretory process. Note the microvilli forming the brush border **BB** of the absorptive cells.

Mucus has a variety of functions. In the upper gastrointestinal tract it protects the intestinal lining cells from autodigestion whilst in the lower tract it lubricates the passage of faeces. In the respiratory tract it protects the lining from drying, contributes to the humidification of inspired air and acts as a sticky surface trap for fine dust particles and microorganisms.

Exocrine glands

Exocrine glands discharge their secretory product via a duct onto an epithelial surface. The cells of which they are composed are highly specialised epithelial cells, the internal structure of the cells reflecting the nature of the secretory product and the mode of secretion (see Ch. 1).

Endocrine glands may be classified according to two major characteristics, which are described below.

The morphology of the gland. Exocrine glands may be broadly divided into simple and compound glands. *Simple glands* are defined as those with a single, unbranched duct. The secretory portions of simple glands have two main forms, tubular or acinar (spherical), which may be coiled and/or branched. *Compound glands* have a branched duct system and their secretory portions have similar morphological forms to those of simple glands.

The means of discharge of secretory products from the cells. This occurs in three ways:

- *Merocrine secretion* (also called *eccrine* secretion) involves the process of exocytosis and is the most common form of secretion; proteins are usually the major secretory product.
- *Apocrine secretion* involves the discharge of free, unbroken, membrane-bound vesicles containing secretory product; this is an unusual mode of secretion and applies to lipid secretory products in the breasts and some sweat glands.
- *Holocrine secretion* involves the discharge of whole secretory cells with subsequent disintegration of the cells to release the secretory product. Holocrine secretion occurs principally in sebaceous glands.

In general, all glands have a continuous basal rate of secretion which is modulated by nervous and hormonal influences. The secretory portions of some exocrine glands are embraced by contractile cells which lie between the secretory cells and the basement membrane. The contractile mechanism of these cells is thought to be similar to that of muscle cells and has given rise to the term *myoepithelial cells*.

Fig. 5.20 Exocrine gland types

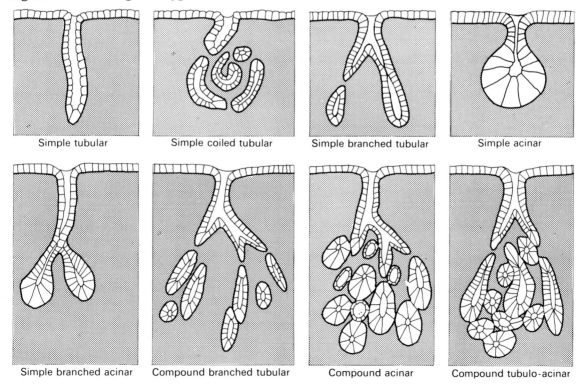

Simple tubular   Simple coiled tubular   Simple branched tubular   Simple acinar

Simple branched acinar   Compound branched tubular   Compound acinar   Compound tubulo-acinar

Fig. 5.21 Simple tubular glands

(H & E × 50)

This example of simple tubular glands is taken from the large intestine. This type of gland has a single, straight tubular lumen into which the secretory products are discharged. In this example, the entire duct is lined by secretory cells; the secretory cells are goblet cells. In other sites mucus is secreted by columnar cells which do not have the classic goblet shape but nonetheless function in a similar manner.

Fig. 5.22 Simple coiled tubular glands

(H & E × 80)

Sweat glands are almost the only example of simple coiled tubular glands. Each consists of a single tube which is tightly coiled in three dimensions; portions of the gland are thus seen in various planes of section. Sweat glands have a terminal secretory portion **S** lined by simple cuboidal epithelium which gives way to a non-secretory (excretory) duct **D** lined by stratified cuboidal epithelium.

Fig. 5.23 Simple branched tubular glands

(H & E x 60)

Simple branched tubular glands are found mainly in the stomach. The mucus-secreting glands of the pyloric part of the stomach are shown in this example. Each gland consists of several tubular secretory portions **T** which converge onto a single, unbranched duct **D** of wider diameter; this is also lined by mucus-secreting cells. Unlike those of the large intestine (see Fig. 5.21), these mucous cells do not have a goblet shape.

Fig. 5.24 Simple acinar glands

(H & E × 128)

Simple acinar glands occur in the form of pockets in epithelial surfaces and are lined by secretory cells. In this example of the mucus-secreting glands of the penile urethra, the secretory cells are pale stained compared to the non-secretory cells lining the urethra **U**. Note that the term *acinus* can be used to describe any rounded exocrine secretory unit.

Fig. 5.25 Simple branched acinar gland

(Masson's trichrome × 80)

Sebaceous glands provide a good example of simple branched acinar glands. Each gland consists of several secretory acini **A** which empty into a single excretory duct; the excretory duct **E** is formed by the stratified epithelium surrounding the hair shaft. The mode of secretion of sebaceous glands is holocrine, i.e. the secretory product, sebum, accumulates within the secretory cells and is discharged by degeneration of the cells.

Fig. 5.26 Compound branched tubular gland

(H & E × 20)

Brunner's glands of the duodenum, as shown in this example, are described as compound branched tubular glands. Although difficult to visualise here, the duct system **D** is branched, thus defining the glands as compound glands; the secretory portions **S** have a tubular form which is branched and coiled.

Fig. 5.27 Compound acinar gland

(Chrome alum haematoxylin/ Phloxine × 320)

Compound acinar glands are those in which the secretory units are acinar in form and drain into a branched duct system. The pancreas shown in this micrograph consists of numerous acini, each of which drains into a minute duct. These minute ducts **D**, which are just discernible in the centre of some acini, drain into a system of branched excretory ducts **E** of increasing diameter and lined by simple cuboidal epithelium.

Fig. 5.28 Compound tubulo-acinar gland

(H & E × 200)

Compound tubulo-acinar glands have three types of secretory units namely branched tubular, branched acinar and branched tubular with acinar end-pieces called *demilunes*. The submandibular salivary gland shown here is the classic example. It contains two types of secretory cells, mucus-secreting cells and serous cells; the former are poorly stained but the latter, which have a protein-rich secretion (digestive enzymes), stain strongly due to their large content of rough endoplasmic reticulum. Generally, the mucous cells form tubular components **T** whereas the serous cells form acinar components **A** and demilunes **D**. Two excretory ducts **E** are also seen.

Endocrine glands

Endocrine glands are ductless glands, the secretory products diffusing directly into the bloodstream. The secretory products are known as hormones and control the activity of cells and tissues usually far removed from the site of secretion.

Fig 5.29 Endocrine gland *(a) Diagram (b) Isamine blue Eosin × 128*

Most endocrine glands consist of clumps or cords of secretory cells surrounded by a rich network of small blood vessels. Each clump of endocrine cells is surrounded by a basement membrane, reflecting its epithelial origin. Endocrine cells release hormones into the intercellular spaces from which they diffuse rapidly into surrounding blood vessels.

The micrograph of the pituitary gland shows the typical features of endocrine glands. The secretory cells **S** are arranged in cords and clumps and are surrounded by delicate supporting tissue containing a rich network of broad capillaries **C**. The basement membrane surrounding each clump of endocrine cells is not visible at this magnification. Like many other endocrine glands, the secretory cells of the pituitary are of several different types; in this case, the majority are eosinophilic (red stained), some stain blue and some stain very little.

Fig. 5.30 Follicular endocrine gland *(a) Diagram (b) H & E × 150*

The thyroid gland is an unusual endocrine gland which stores hormone within spheroidal cavities enclosed by the secretory cells; these spheroidal units are called *follicles*. Secretion of stored hormone involves reabsorption of hormone from the follicular lumen, release into the surrounding interstitial spaces, and then diffusion into the rich capillary network which embraces each follicle.

The micrograph shows typical thyroid follicles **F** of variable size. The secretory cells lining the follicles are of flattened cuboidal shape. Stored thyroid hormone is bound to a glycoprotein which is strongly eosinophilic. The relatively sparse interfollicular supporting tissue is mainly occupied by capillaries **C** which can be identified by the strongly eosinophilic (pink stained) erythrocytes within them.

6. Muscle

Introduction

Contractility is an inherent property of all cells and is necessary for the performance of basic functions involving movement such as phagocytosis and cell division, and more specialised functions such as motility as in white blood cells.

In multicellular organisms, some cells are specialised to enable movement of tissues or organs. These cells may function as single contractile units, namely the myoepithelial cells surrounding the acini of some exocrine glands (see Ch. 5) and the pericytes which invest very small blood vessels (see Ch. 8). Alternatively, contractile cells may be aggregated to form muscles for the movement of large structures such as the skeleton or the viscera. Recent evidence, partly based on the study of the contractile mechanisms of some unicellular organisms, suggests that there is a similar contractile mechanism in all cells. This mechanism consists of fibrillar proteins arranged in an organised manner in the cytoplasm and linked by intermolecular bonds. Contraction results from the rearrangement of the intermolecular bonds with the utilisation of chemical energy.

There are three types of muscle tissue:

- **Skeletal muscle.** This is responsible for the movement of the skeleton and organs such as the globe of the eye and the tongue. Skeletal muscle is often referred to as *voluntary muscle* since it is capable of voluntary (conscious) control. The arrangement of the contractile proteins gives rise to the appearance of prominent cross-striations in some histological preparations and hence the name *striated muscle* is often applied to skeletal muscle.

- **Visceral muscle.** This type of muscle forms the muscular component of visceral structures such as blood vessels, the gastrointestinal tract, the uterus and the urinary bladder. Since visceral muscle is under inherent autonomic and hormonal control, it is described as *involuntary muscle*. As the arrangement of contractile proteins does not give the histological appearance of cross-striations, the name *smooth muscle* is also commonly applied.

- **Cardiac muscle.** Cardiac muscle has many structural and functional characteristics intermediate between those of skeletal and visceral muscle and provides for the continuous, rhythmic contractility of the heart. Although striated in appearance, cardiac muscle is readily distinguishable from skeletal muscle and should not be referred to by the term 'striated muscle'.

The highly specialised functions of the cytoplasmic organelles of muscle cells has led to the use of a special terminology for some muscle cell components: plasma membrane or plasmalemma = *sarcolemma*; cytoplasm = *sarcoplasm*; endoplasmic reticulum = *sarcoplasmic reticulum*; mitochondria = *sarcosomes*.

Muscle cells of all three types are surrounded by a thin basement membrane or external lamina (see Ch. 4) which binds the cells to adjacent cells and supporting tissue.

Skeletal muscle

Skeletal muscles have a wide variety of morphological forms and modes of action, nevertheless all have the same basic structure. Skeletal muscle is composed of extremely elongated, multinucleate contractile cells, often described as *muscle fibres*, bound together by collagenous supporting tissue. Individual muscle fibres vary considerably in diameter from 10–100 μm and may extend throughout the whole length of a muscle reaching up to 35 cm in length.

Skeletal muscle contraction is controlled by large motor nerves, individual nerve fibres branching within the muscle to supply a group of muscle fibres, collectively described as a *motor unit*. Excitation of any one motor nerve results in simultaneous contraction of all the muscle fibres of the corresponding motor unit. The structure of neuromuscular junctions is described in Figure 7.12. The vitality of skeletal muscle fibres is dependent on the maintenance of their nerve supply which, if damaged, results in atrophy of the fibres. Skeletal muscle contains highly specialised stretch receptors known as neuromuscular spindles which are shown in Figure 7.30.

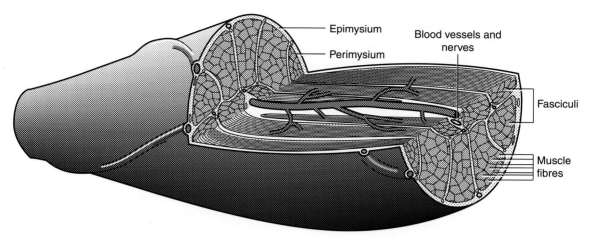

Fig. 6.1 Skeletal muscle

This diagram illustrates the arrangement of the basic components which make up a typical skeletal muscle.

The individual muscle cells (muscle fibres) are grouped together into elongated bundles called *fasciculi* with delicate supporting tissue called *endomysium* occupying the spaces between individual muscle fibres.

Each fascicle is surrounded by loose collagenous tissue called *perimysium*. Most muscles are made up of many fasciculi and the whole muscle mass is invested in a dense collagenous sheath called the *epimysium*. Large blood vessels and nerves enter the epimysium and divide to ramify throughout the muscle in the perimysium and endomysium.

The size of the fasciculi reflects the function of the particular muscle concerned. Muscles responsible for fine, highly controlled movements, e.g. the external muscles of the eye, have small fasciculi and a relatively greater proportion of perimysial supporting tissue. In contrast, muscles responsible for gross movements only, e.g. the muscle of the buttocks, have large fasciculi and relatively little perimysial tissue. Within each muscle, the supporting tissue component contains both collagen and elastic fibres acting as a flexible skeleton to which individual muscle fibres and fasciculi are anchored. This connective tissue becomes continuous with that of the tendons and muscle attachments (see Ch. 10) which distribute and direct the motive forces of the muscle to bone, skin etc. as appropriate.

Fig. 6.2 Skeletal muscle

(Trichrome stain × 150)

This micrograph shows part of a fasciculus of a skeletal muscle at high magnification. The individual purple-stained muscle cells (fibres) are highly elongated and arranged in parallel, the spaces between them being occupied by small amounts of endomysial supporting tissue. The endomysium, which consists mainly of reticulin fibres (unstained) and a small amount of collagen (stained blue in this preparation), conveys numerous small blood vessels, lymphatics and nerves throughout the muscle. In this micrograph, a small nerve bundle **N** is seen; tiny blood vessels **V** can be identified by the rows of erythrocytes contained within them.

Fig. 6.3 Skeletal muscle *(Masson's trichrome × 300)*

This micrograph shows the skeletal muscle of the tongue which is made up of numerous small fasciculi oriented in various different directions. This staining method clearly distinguishes skeletal muscle cells, stained red, from supporting tissue, the collagen of which is stained blue.

In the centre and at the upper right of the field are fasciculi cut in transverse section **TS**, the remaining fasciculi being cut longitudinally. The spaces between the fasciculi are filled with loose collagenous tissue, the perimysium **P**, which is continuous with the delicate endomysium, separating individual muscle fibres in each fasciculus. The supporting tissue of skeletal muscle also contains elastin fibres (not distinguishable in this preparation) which are most numerous in muscles attached to soft tissues as in the tongue and face. Note the rich network of capillaries **C** in the endomysium and perimysium.

Fig. 6.4 Skeletal muscle blood supply

(Perfusion method × 128)

This specimen was prepared by perfusing the blood supply of a skeletal muscle with a red dye; the muscle fibres were then teased apart to reveal the endomysial capillary bed.

Large blood vessels enter the epimysium and divide to ramify throughout the muscle in the perimysium. Fine branches arise from the perimysial arteries and pass between the muscle fibres transversely to their long axes. These give rise to numerous capillaries which run longitudinally through the endomysium. Frequent transverse anastomoses between the capillaries result in a fine, elongated capillary network surrounding each muscle fibre.

(a)

(b)

(c)

Fig. 6.5 Skeletal muscle and its embryogenesis

(H & E (a) Mature skeletal muscle × 320 (b) Myoblasts × 150 (c) Myotubes × 150)

Micrograph (a) demonstrates the characteristic histological features of skeletal muscle fibres in longitudinal section. Skeletal muscle fibres are extremely elongated, unbranched cylindrical cells with numerous flattened nuclei located at fairly regular intervals just beneath the sarcolemma (plasma membrane).

During embryological development, certain mesenchymal cells in each myotome differentiate into long, mononuclear skeletal muscle precursors called *myoblasts* which then proliferate by mitosis; this is shown in micrograph (b). Subsequently, the myoblasts fuse end to end forming progressively elongated multinucleate cells called *myotubes*, seen in micrograph (c), which may eventually contain up to 100 nuclei.

Synthesis of the contractile proteins begins after myoblast fusion, the proteins being laid down initially in the central axis of the myotube, the nuclei being displaced peripherally as more contractile protein is formed. Most of the process of muscle development is completed by the time of birth along with the process of innervation. Thereafter, growth occurs by increase in bulk of the muscle cell cytoplasm.

Mature muscle cells are highly differentiated and, if damaged, have very limited capacity for repair and regeneration. Nevertheless, a few myoblasts (*satellite cells*) persist after maturity; they are capable of mitosis and appear to play some part in repair of muscle after injury.

Regular cross-striations are the characteristic feature of skeletal muscle fibres and can be seen in longitudinal sections as in micrograph (a). The cross-striations result from the arrangement of the contractile proteins as described later.

Fig. 6.6 Skeletal muscle *(TS: H & E × 320)*

This micrograph of skeletal muscle cut in transverse section shows the extreme peripheral location of the nuclei of skeletal muscle fibres. In unfixed tissue, the fibres appear oval or round; however, in the more commonly used fixed tissue preparations such as this, the fibres appear artefactually irregular and polyhedral. Similarly, the wide endomysial spaces are a shrinkage artefact.

In the endomysial spaces, note the numerous minute capillaries **C** recognisable by the eosinophilic erythrocytes contained within them. Compare the huge diameter of the muscle fibres which may be as great as 0.1 mm in diameter with that of the capillaries, the latter being approximately 7 μm across. Note also a strand of perimysial tissue **P** cutting across the field separating two fasciculi from one another.

Fig. 6.7 Skeletal muscle

(a) TS: Iron haematoxylin × 1200
(b) Schematic diagram

Micrograph (a) shows a transverse section through several skeletal muscle fibres at very high magnification. The plane of section includes only one skeletal muscle nucleus **N**. Note the presence of erythrocytes in endomysial capillaries **C**.

In some preparations such as this, the transversely-sectioned muscle fibres are seen to be packed with numerous dark dots. These represent the cut ends of *myofibrils*, elongated cylindrical structures which lie parallel to one another in the sarcoplasm.

As shown diagrammatically in (b), each myofibril exhibits a repeating pattern of cross-striations which is a product of the highly ordered arrangement of the contractile proteins within it; this can only be seen with electron microscopy (see Fig. 6.8). Furthermore, the parallel myofibrils are arranged with their cross-striations in register giving rise to the regular striations seen with light microscopy in longitudinal sections of skeletal muscle as in Fig. 6.5.

(a)

(b)

Muscle fibre   Myofibrils

(a)

(b)

(c)

Fig. 6.8 Skeletal muscle

*(a) Heidenhain's haematoxylin ×
1200 (b) EM × 2860
(c) EM × 18 700*

This series of micrographs shows the
arrangement of the contractile proteins
within skeletal muscle and explains the
striations seen with light microscopy.

Micrograph (a) shows the striations
of a skeletal muscle fibre at a
magnification close to the limit of
resolution. They are composed of
alternating broad light **I** bands
(isotropic in polarised light) and dark
(anisotropic) **A** bands. Fine dark lines
called **Z** bands (Zwischenscheiben) can
be seen bisecting the light I bands.
Note the nucleus **N** at the extreme
periphery of the cell.

Micrograph (b) shows the electron
microscopic appearance of muscle cell
at the same magnification and with a
nucleus **N** situated in a similar
position. The sarcoplasm is filled with myofibrils
M oriented parallel to the long axis of
the cell. These are separated by a small
amount of sarcoplasm containing rows
of mitochondria **Mt** in a similar
orientation.

Each myofibril has prominent
regular cross-striations arranged in
register with those of the other
myofibrils and corresponding to the I,
A and Z bands seen in light
microscopy. The Z bands are the most
electron-dense and divide each
myofibril into numerous contractile
units, called *sarcomeres*, arranged end to
end.

With further magnification in (c),
the arrangement of the contractile proteins
(*myofilaments*) may be seen in each
sarcomere. The dark **A** band is bisected
by the lighter **H** (heller) band, which is
further bisected by a more dense **M**
(Mittelscheibe) band. Irrespective of
the degree of contraction of the muscle
fibre, the A band remains constant in
width. In contrast, the I and H bands
narrow during contraction and the Z
bands are drawn closer together. These
findings are explained by the *sliding
filament theory* (Fig. 6.9).

Mitochondria **Mi** and numerous
glycogen granules **G** provide a rich
energy source in the scanty cytoplasm
between the myofibrils. The mature
muscle cell contains little rough
endoplasmic reticulum; it contains,
however, a smooth membranous system
S which is involved in activation of the
contractile mechanism (see Figs.
6.10–6.12).

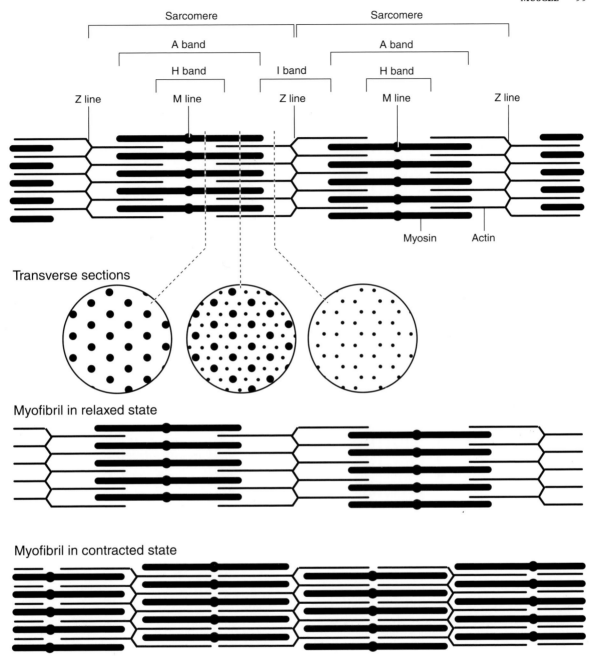

Fig. 6.9 The arrangement of myofilaments in the sarcomere

The sarcomere consists of two types of myofilaments, *thick filaments* and *thin filaments*. Each type remains constant in length irrespective of the state of contraction of the muscle. The thick filaments, which are composed mainly of the protein myosin, are maintained in register by their attachment to a disc-like zone represented by the M line. Similarly the thin filaments, which are composed mainly of the protein *actin*, are attached to a disc-like zone represented by the Z line. The I and H bands, both areas of low electron-density, represent areas where the thick and thin filaments do not overlap one another.

The widely accepted sliding filament theory proposes that under the influence of energy released from ATP, the thick and thin filaments slide over one another, thus causing shortening of the sarcomere.

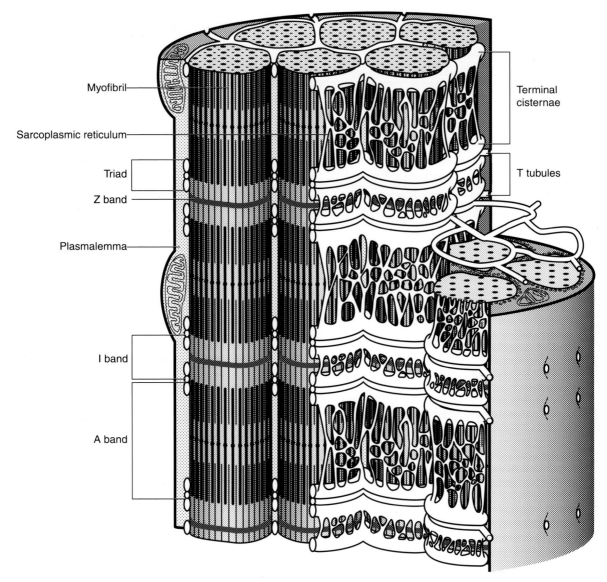

Myofibril

Sarcoplasmic reticulum

Triad

Z band

Plasmalemma

I band

A band

Terminal cisternae

T tubules

Fig. 6.10 The conducting system for contractile stimuli

To permit the synchronous contraction of all sarcomeres in the muscle fibre, a system of tubular extensions of the muscle cell plasma membrane (sarcolemma) extends transversely into the muscle cell to surround each myofibril at the region of the junction of the A and I bands. Known as the *T system*, its lumen is continuous with the extracellular space. (In amphibian skeletal muscle, which was the first to be studied, the T tubules are disposed at the Z bands; the same applies in cardiac muscle).

Between the T tubules, a second membrane system derived from smooth endoplasmic reticulum, the *sarcoplasmic reticulum*, forms a membranous network which embraces each myofibril. On either side of each T tubule,

the sarcoplasmic reticulum exhibits a flattened cisternal arrangement, each pair of *terminal cisternae* and a T tubule forming a *triad* near the junction of the I and A bands of each sarcomere.

Calcium ions are concentrated within the lumen of the *sarcoplasmic reticulum*. Depolarisation of the sarcolemma of the muscle fibre is rapidly disseminated throughout the sarcoplasm by the T tubule system. This promotes the release of calcium ions from the sarcoplasmic reticulum into the sarcoplasm surrounding the myofilaments. Calcium ions activate the sliding filament mechanism resulting in muscle contraction.

Fig. 6.11 Skeletal muscle *(EM × 33 000)*

This electron micrograph of mammalian skeletal muscle cut in longitudinal section demonstrates the main elements of the conducting system. In the vicinity of the junction of the **A** and **I bands** (and depending on the state of contraction) are tubular triads **Td** each comprising a central flattened tubule of the T system **T** and a pair of terminal cisternae **TC** of the sarcoplasmic reticulum. Within the A bands can be seen tubular elements of the sarcoplasmic reticulum **SR** connecting the terminal cisternae. Likewise within the I bands, similar though less regular longitudinal tubular profiles of sarcoplasmic reticulum are seen. The conducting system of 'slow-twitch' (red) fibres as shown here (see Fig. 6.13) is more regular than that of 'fast-twitch' (white) fibres where this pattern is more difficult to discern. Note the distribution of mitochondria **M**, regularly arranged between the sarcomeres within the I bands in immediate association with that part of the actin and myosin filaments which interact during the process of contraction. The reason for this appearance is evident in the following micrograph.

Fig. 6.12 Skeletal muscle *(EM × 44 000)*

This micrograph shows parts of two skeletal muscle cells cut in transverse section in the vicinity of the junction of A and I bands; the intercellular space **ICS** bisects the field. Note the external lamina **L** adjacent to the plasmalemma. Sarcomeres at the upper right and lower left of this field have been sectioned through the end part of the A band and thus show both actin and myosin filaments. The remaining sarcomeres are cut through the I band and contain only actin filaments. This results from the fact that the bands of all sarcomeres within any one muscle cell are not exactly in register with one another.

Each sarcomere is ensheathed by a network of tubules of the sarcoplasmic reticulum **SR**. The plane of section has also included a part of a broader diameter T tubule system **T** which branches to encompass several different sarcomeres. Direct communication of T tubules with the intercellular space is difficult to visualise as the tubules appear to ramify into a complex tubular system just beneath the plasmalemma; the continuity of T tubule lumen and the intercellular space has been convincingly demonstrated however by experimental techniques. Note the extraordinary serpentine branched mitochondria **M** which lie between the sarcomeres within the I bands, giving rise to the mitochondrial appearance seen in longitudinal section in the previous micrograph.

(a)

(b)

Fig. 6.13 Skeletal muscle *(TS: Histochemical techniques (a) Succinate dehydrogenase × 200 (b) ATP-ase × 600)*

The mode of activity of skeletal muscle varies from one part of the body to another. Some muscles, such as those involved in the maintenance of posture, are required to contract almost continuously whilst others, such as the extra-ocular muscles, make rapid short-lived movements. In humans, distinction between these types cannot be made on gross examination of the muscle. In domestic poultry, however, the extremes are easily identified by a difference in colours; for example, leg muscles are red and flight (breast) muscles are white.

Correspondingly, 'slow-twitch' and 'fast-twitch' muscle fibre types can be demonstrated by nerve stimulation studies. The metabolic requirements of each fibre type differ markedly, the slow red fibres mainly relying on aerobic metabolism and the fast white fibres using predominantly anaerobic pathways. Most muscles actually contain a mixture of these extreme fibre types as well as an intermediate type.

Aerobic (*type I*) muscle fibres are small in cross section and contain abundant mitochondria. They also contain a large content of *myoglobin*, an oxygen-storage molecule analogous to haemoglobin, which accounts for the red colour of such fibres. In addition these fibres have a rich blood supply.

In contrast, anaerobic (*type II*) muscle fibres are large in cross-section, contain few mitochondria and relatively little myoglobin; they also have a relatively poor blood supply. These muscle fibres are, however, rich in glycogen and glycolytic enzymes. These characteristics account for the 'white' colour of such fibres. Anaerobic fibres predominate in muscles responsible for intense but sporadic contraction such as the biceps and triceps of the arms.

The activity of the specific mitochondrial enzyme *succinate dehydrogenase*, which catalyses one of the stages of Krebs' cycle, demonstrates the relative proportions of mitochondria within the muscle fibres. In micrograph (a), note the presence of intensely stained small-diameter aerobic fibres **A**, poorly stained large-diameter anaerobic fibres **An** and intermediate fibres **I**.

Similarly, the amount of ATP-ase activity can be used to determine the relative proportions of different fibre types as in micrograph (b). The small aerobic fibres **A** have the greatest activity and stain strongly, whilst the anaerobic fibres **An** show little ATP-ase activity; intermediate fibres **I** predominate in this specimen. The type of metabolism of each fibre is determined by the frequency of impulses in its motor nerve supply. Any one motor nerve supplies fibres of one type only and all the fibres of a particular motor unit are of the same metabolic type. Indeed, if the motor nerve supply to one type of fibre is experimentally transplanted to supply another fibre type, this fibre type will become converted to the metabolic pattern of the former.

Visceral muscle

In contrast to skeletal muscle, which is specialised for relatively forceful contractions of short duration and under fine voluntary control, visceral muscle is specialised for continuous contractions of relatively low force producing diffuse movements resulting in contraction of the whole muscle mass rather than contraction of individual motor units. Contractility is an inherent property of visceral muscle, occurring independently of neurological innervation often in a rhythmic or wave-like fashion. Superimposed on this inherent contractility are the influences of the autonomic nervous system, hormones and local metabolites which modulate contractility to accommodate changing functional demands. For example, the smooth muscle of the intestinal wall undergoes continuous rhythmic contractions which result in waves of constriction passing along the bowel, propelling the luminal contents distally. This activity is enhanced by parasympathetic stimulation and influenced by a variety of hormones released in response to changes in the nature and volume of the gut contents. The structure of autonomic neuromuscular junctions is described in Chapter 7.

The cells of visceral muscle are relatively small with only a single nucleus. The fibres are bound together in irregular branching fasciculi, the arrangement varying considerably from one organ to another according to functional requirements.

(a)

(b)

Fig. 6.14 Visceral muscle

(LS (a) H & E × 480
(b) Masson's trichrome × 480)

As seen in these micrographs, visceral muscle fibres are elongated, spindle-shaped cells with tapered ends which may occasionally be bifurcated. Visceral muscle fibres are generally much shorter than skeletal muscle fibres and contain only one nucleus which is elongated and centrally located in the cytoplasm at the widest part of the cell; however, depending on the contractile state of the fibres at fixation, the nuclei may sometimes appear to be spiral-shaped.

Visceral muscle fibres are bound together in irregular, branching fasciculi and these fasciculi, rather than individual fibres, are the functional contractile units. Within the fasciculi, individual muscle fibres are arranged roughly parallel to one another with the thickest part of one cell lying against the thin parts of adjacent cells.

The contractile proteins of visceral muscle are not arranged in myofibrils as in skeletal and cardiac muscle, thus visceral muscle cells are not striated, giving rise to the common name of smooth muscle.

Between individual muscle fibres and between fasciculi is a network of supporting collagenous tissue which is well demonstrated in micrograph (b) in which the collagen is stained blue.

Fig. 6.15 Visceral muscle *(LS: H & E × 320)*

This micrograph illustrates smooth muscle from the bowel wall cut in longitudinal section. In this case, the fibres are arranged in a highly regular manner and packed so closely that it is difficult to identify individual cell outlines although cell shape can be deduced from that of the nuclei.

Fig. 6.16 Visceral muscle

(TS: H & E × 600)

This micrograph shows smooth muscle in transverse section at very high magnification. The spindle-shaped cells are sectioned at various different points along their length which gives the erroneous impression that they are of differing diameters. Nuclei are only included in the plane of section where fibres have been cut through their widest diameter. Note the plump nuclear shape and central location of nuclei within the cytoplasm.

Fig. 6.17 Visceral muscle

(Masson's trichrome × 150)

In many tubular visceral structures such as the ileum seen in this micrograph, smooth muscle is disposed in layers with the cells of one layer arranged at right angles to those of the adjacent layer. This arrangement permits a wave of contraction to pass down the tube propelling the contents forward; this action is called *peristalsis*.

Typically, the longitudinal smooth outer muscle layer **L** is closely applied to the inner circular layer **C** with only a minimal amount of supporting tissue between; in this specimen the collagen is stained blue. The supporting tissue contains clumps of large cells with pale nuclei which represent parasympathetic ganglia **G** (see Fig. 7.19).

(a)

(b)

Fig. 6.18 Visceral muscle *(EM (a) ×8 000 (b) ×21 000)*

At low magnification, micrograph (a) demonstrates the spindle shape and elongated, central nuclei **N** of visceral muscle cells. The cells at the lower right are cut longitudinally and those at the upper left transversely. Between them is a band of supporting tissue **S** containing the cytoplasmic processes of fibroblasts **F**. Note the relative sparsity of mitochondria **M** and other intracellular organelles.

At high magnification in micrograph (b), details of the plasma membrane and endomembrane system can be seen. The plasma membrane contains numerous flask-shaped invaginations. In some areas these are irregular in shape and size and may be involved in pinocytosis. In other areas, the invaginations are regular in shape and distribution and are called *caveolae* **C**.

The endomembrane system contains some elements which represent a poorly developed Golgi and endoplasmic reticulum **ER**. Other vesicular and tubular structures **S** are seen near the plasma membrane, often in association with caveolae; these probably constitute a system analogous to the sarcoplasmic reticulum of skeletal muscle with the caveolae being analogous to the T tubule system.

Parallel myofilaments occupy most of the cytoplasm analogous to the thin (actin) filaments of skeletal muscle. Thick (myosin) filaments have also been demonstrated using special techniques. The mechanism of smooth muscle contractility is therefore believed to be basically similar to that of skeletal muscle. *Dense bodies* **D** (best seen at low magnification) are a feature of visceral muscle and are involved in maintaining the longitudinal orientation of the contractile filaments.

The narrow intercellular spaces are of almost uniform width but at numerous sites the plasma membranes of adjacent cells form specialised cell junctions. Nexus (gap) junctions **N** mediate spread of excitation throughout visceral muscle (see Fig. 5.14). Junctions **J** resembling the desmosomes of epithelia provide anchorage points for contractile proteins and *desmin*, the intermediate filament of smooth muscle.

Cardiac muscle

Cardiac muscle exhibits many structural and functional characteristics intermediate between those of skeletal and visceral muscle. Like the former, its contractions are strong and utilise a great deal of energy, and like the latter the contractions are continuous and initiated by inherent mechanisms though modulated by external autonomic and hormonal stimuli.

Cardiac muscle fibres are essentially long, cylindrical cells with one or at most two nuclei, centrally located within the cell. The ends of the fibres are split longitudinally into a small number of branches the ends of which abut onto similar branches of adjacent cells giving the impression of a continuous three-dimensional cytoplasmic network; this was formerly described as a *syncytium* before the discrete intercellular boundaries were recognised.

Between the muscle fibres, delicate collagenous tissue analogous to the endomysium of skeletal muscle supports the extremely rich capillary network necessary to meet the high metabolic demands of strong continuous activity.

Cardiac muscle fibres have an arrangement of contractile proteins similar to that of skeletal muscle and are consequently striated in a similar manner. However, this is often difficult to visualise with light microscopy due to the irregular branching shape of the cells and their myofibrils. Cardiac muscle fibres also have a system of T tubules and sarcoplasmic reticulum analogous to that of skeletal muscles. In the case of cardiac muscle, however, there is a slow leak of calcium ions into the cytoplasm from the sarcoplasmic reticulum after recovery from the preceding contraction; this causes a succession of automatic contractions independent of external stimuli. The rate of this inherent rhythm is then modulated by external autonomic and hormonal stimuli.

Between the ends of adjacent cardiac muscle cells are specialised intercellular junctions called *intercalated discs* which not only provide points of anchorage for the myofibrils but permit extremely rapid spread of contractile stimuli from one cell to another. Thus, adjacent fibres are caused to contract almost simultaneously, thereby acting as a functional syncytium. In addition, a system of highly modified cardiac muscle cells constitute the pacemaker regions of the heart and ramify throughout the organ as the Purkinje system thus co-ordinating contraction of the myocardium as a whole in each cardiac cycle; this is illustrated and described in more detail in Chapter 8.

Muscle fibre

Cross striations

Capillary

Intercalated disc

Nucleus

Fig. 6.19 Cardiac muscle

(a)

(b)

Fig. 6.20 Cardiac muscle

(a) LS: H & E × 198
(b) TS: H & E × 480
(c) Thin section, toluidine blue × 640

In longitudinal section in micrograph
(a), cardiac muscle cells are seen to
contain one or two nuclei and an
extensive cytoplasm which branches to
give the appearance of a continuous
three-dimensional network. In routine
H & E preparation such as this, the
cross-striations are not readily visible.
The elongated nuclei are mainly
centrally located, a characteristic well
demonstrated in transverse section as in
micrograph (b).

Micrograph (c) illustrates an
extremely thin resin-embedded section
at very high magnification. The
branching cytoplasmic network is
readily seen with prominent
intercalated discs **D** marking the
intercellular boundaries.
Note the typical cross-striations.

In each of these specimens, note the
delicate supporting tissue filling the
intercellular spaces and containing an
extensive network of blood capillaries
C.

(c)

(a)

Fig. 6.21 Cardiac muscle

(EM (a) ×5 000 (b) ×38 000)

Micrograph (a) illustrates portions of six cardiac muscle cells labelled C_1 to C_6. None of their nuclei are included in the plane of section. Cells C_1 and C_2 abut one another end to end and are demarcated by an intercalated disc **D**. Cells C_3 and C_4 are demarcated in a similar fashion. The intercellular space contains a capillary **Cap** and a fibroblast **F**.

The sarcomeres of cardiac muscle have an identical banding pattern to that of skeletal muscle. The sarcomeres are not, however, arranged into single columns making up cylindrical myofibrils as in skeletal muscle, but form a branching myofibrillar network continuous in three dimensions throughout the cytoplasm. The branching columns of sarcomeres are separated by sarcoplasm containing rows of mitochondria and sarcoplasmic reticulum. The great abundance of mitochondria in cardiac muscle reflects the enormous metabolic demands of continuous cardiac muscle activity.

Conduction of excitatory stimuli to the sarcomeres of cardiac muscle is mediated by a system of T tubules and sarcoplasmic reticulum essentially similar in arrangement to that of skeletal muscle. The T tubules, however, ramify throughout the cardiac muscle cytoplasm at the Z lines and their origins are seen as indentations in the sarcolemma which thus has a somewhat scalloped outline.

The conducting system can be seen at high magnification in micrograph (b). T tubules **T** and sarcoplasmic reticulum **SR** form poorly defined triads compared to those of skeletal muscle. Note the typical closely packed cristae of the mitochondria **M**, a lipid droplet **L** and glycogen granules **G**.

(b)

Fig. 6.22 Cardiac muscle: intercalated disc *(EM × 31 000)*

Intercalated discs are specialised transverse junctions between cardiac muscle cells at sites where they meet end to end; they always coincide with the Z lines. Intercalated discs bind the cells, transmit forces of contraction and provide areas of low electrical resistance for the rapid spread of excitation throughout the myocardium.

The intercalated disc is an interdigitating junction and consists of three types of membrane to membrane contact. The predominant type of contact, the *fascia adherens* **FA**, resembles the zonula adherens of epithelial junctional complexes (see Fig. 5.12) but is more extensive and less regular. The actin filaments at the ends of terminal sarcomeres insert into the fasciae adherentes and thereby transmit contractile forces from cell to cell. *Desmosomes* **D**

occur less frequently and provide anchorage for intermediate filaments of the cytoskeleton. Gap (nexus) junctions **N** (see Fig. 5.14) are present mainly in the longitudinal portions of the interdigitations and are sites of low electrical resistance through which excitation passes from cell to cell.

Note the similarity of the sarcomeres of cardiac and skeletal muscle (see Fig. 6.8). The mitochondria **M** are elongated or spheroidal and have abundant closely packed cristae rich in oxidative enzyme systems. The sarcoplasm within and between the sarcomeres is rich in glycogen granules **G**. Lace-like profiles of sarcoplasmic reticulum **SR** and parts of T tubules **T** can be identified.

Fig. 6.23 Cardiac muscle: intercalated disc *(EM × 27 000)*

This micrograph shows a transverse section through cardiac muscle in the vicinity of a Z line incorporating an intercalated disc. The tortuous course of the intercellular junction as well as circles of apparently isolated paired cell membranes (arrowed) reflect the manner in which the ends of the cardiac muscle fibres interdigitate with one another. Most of the intercellular junction comprises fasciae adherentes with interspersed desmosomes **D** and some nexus junctions **N**.

Beneath the plasmalemma are dilated tubules **T** representing part of the T tubule system. Elements of the sarcoplasmic reticulum **SR** can be seen surrounding the sarcomeres. Beyond the plasma membrane lies the external lamina **EL**. A fibroblast cytoplasmic extension **F** is present in the extracellular space at the right of the field. At the upper right is an endomysial capillary, its endothelium **E** containing numerous pinocytotic vesicles; the lumen contains a lymphocyte **L**.

7. Nervous tissues

Introduction

The function of the nervous system is to receive stimuli from both the internal and external environments which are then analysed and integrated to produce appropriate, co-ordinated responses in various effector organs. The nervous system is composed of an intercommunicating network of specialised cells called *neurones* which constitute most sensory receptors, the conducting pathways, and the sites of integration and analysis.

The functions of the nervous system depend on a fundamental property of neurones called *excitability*. As in all cells, the resting neurone maintains an ionic gradient across its plasma membrane thereby creating an electrical potential. Excitability involves a change in membrane permeability in response to appropriate stimuli such that the ionic gradient is reversed and the plasma membrane becomes *depolarised*; a wave of depolarisation, known as an *action potential*, then spreads along the plasma membrane. This is followed by the process of *repolarisation* in which the membrane rapidly re-establishes its resting potential. At *synapses*, the sites of intercommunication between adjacent neurones, depolarisation of one neurone causes it to release chemical transmitter substances, *neurotransmitters*, which initiate an action potential in the adjacent neurone.

Within the nervous system, neurones are arranged to form pathways for the conduction of action potentials from receptors to effector organs via integrating neurones. Neurotransmitters not only mediate neurone-to-neurone transmission but also act as chemical intermediates between the nervous system and effector organs which also exhibit the property of excitability. The effector organs of voluntary nervous pathways are generally skeletal muscle whilst those of involuntary pathways are usually smooth muscle, cardiac muscle and muscle-like epithelial cells (myoepithelial cells) within some exocrine glands.

The nervous system is divided anatomically into the *central nervous system* (CNS) comprising the brain and spinal cord, and the *peripheral nervous system* (PNS) which constitutes all nervous tissue outside the CNS. Functionally, the nervous system is divided into the *somatic nervous system* which is involved in voluntary functions, and the *autonomic nervous system* which exerts control over many involuntary functions. Histologically, however, the entire nervous system merely consists of variations in the arrangement of neurones and their supporting tissues.

This chapter encompasses the cell and tissue types found in the nervous system and includes the structure of the peripheral nervous system and relatively simple types of sensory receptor. Details of the arrangement of nervous tissue in the central nervous system are the subject of Chapter 20 whilst the structure of the highly specialised organs of sensory reception associated with the cranial nerves, e.g. eye and ear, is presented in Chapter 21.

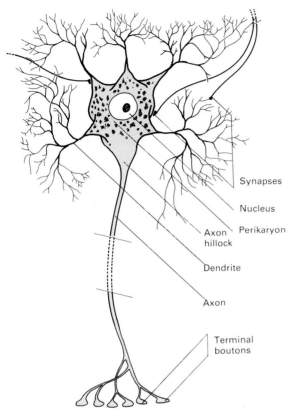

Synapses

Nucleus

Axon hillock

Perikaryon

Dendrite

Axon

Terminal boutons

Fig. 7.1 The neurone

Despite great variation in size and shape in different parts of the nervous system, all neurones have the same basic structure as shown in this idealised diagram. The neurone consists of a large *cell body* containing the nucleus surrounded by cytoplasm known as the *perikaryon*. Processes of two types extend from the cell body, namely a single *axon* and one or more *dendrites*.

Dendrites are highly branched, tapering processes which either end in specialised sensory receptors (as in primary sensory neurones), or form synapses with neighbouring neurones from which they receive stimuli. In general, dendrites function as the major sites of information input into the neurone.

Each neurone has a single axon arising from a cone-shaped portion of the cell body called the *axon hillock*. The axon is a cylindrical process up to one metre in length terminating on other neurones or effector organs by way of a variable number of small branches which end in small swellings called *terminal boutons*.

Action potentials arise in the cell body as a result of integration of afferent (incoming) stimuli; action potentials are then conducted along the axon to influence other neurones or effector organs. Axons are commonly referred to as *nerve fibres*.

In general, the cell bodies of all neurones are located in the central nervous system; exceptions are the cell bodies of most primary sensory neurones and the terminal effector neurones of the autonomic nervous system where in both cases the cell bodies lie in aggregations called *ganglia* in peripheral sites.

Multipolar neurone

Bipolar neurone

Pseudo-unipolar neurone

Fig. 7.2 Basic neurone types

Throughout the nervous system, neurones have a wide variety of shapes which fall into three main patterns according to the arrangement of the axon and dendrites with respect to the cell body.

The most common form is the *multipolar neurone* in which numerous dendrites project from the cell body; the dendrites may all arise from one pole of the cell body or may extend from all parts of the cell body. In general, intermediate, integratory and motor neurones conform to this pattern.

Bipolar neurones have only a single dendrite which arises from the pole of the cell body opposite to the origin of the axon. These unusual neurones act as receptor neurones for the senses of smell, sight and balance.

Most other primary sensory neurones are described as *pseudo-unipolar neurones* since a single dendrite and the axon arise from a common stem of the cell body; this stem is formed by the fusion of the first part of the dendrite and axon of a bipolar type of neurone during embryological development.

As a general rule, neurone impulses are conveyed along dendrites towards the nerve cell body (afferent) whilst axons usually convey impulses away from the nerve cell body (efferent).

Neurones are terminally differentiated cells and are completely incapable of cell division and replacement in the event of cell death. However, regeneration of axons and dendrites can occur in the event of damage, provided the neurone cell body remains viable.

Dendrite

Synapse

Nucleolus

Rough
endoplasmic
reticulum
(Nissl body)

Golgi

Mitochondrion

Nucleus

Neurofilament

Microtubule

Axon hillock

Axon

Smooth endoplasmic reticulum

(a)

Fig. 7.3 Ultrastructure of the neurone (a) Schematic diagram (b) EM × 19 000 (opposite)

The diagram (a) illustrates the main ultrastructural features of the neurone, in this case a multipolar neurone with an axon and two dendrites. The nucleus is large, round or ovoid and usually centrally located within the perikaryon. Reflecting the intense metabolic activity of the neurone (and consequent need to replace damaged enzymes), the chromatin is completely dispersed and the nucleolus is a conspicuous feature.

The cytoplasm of the cell body contains large aggregations of rough endoplasmic reticulum which correspond to the *Nissl substance* of light microscopy (see Fig. 7.4); the rough endoplasmic reticulum extends into the dendrites but not into the axon hillock or axon. Rough endoplasmic reticulum is a much more prominent feature in large neurones, such as somatic motor neurones, than in smaller neurones such as those of the autonomic nervous system. A diffuse Golgi apparatus is found adjacent to the nucleus. Smooth endoplasmic reticulum is not a prominent feature of the perikaryon but tubules, cisternae and vesicles are prominent in the axon and dendrites. The mitochondria of the perikaryon are numerous and have the usual rod-like appearances; those of the axon are extremely slender and elongated.

Neurones are very metabolically active and expend much energy in maintaining ionic gradients across the plasma membrane. Neurones synthesise neurotransmitter substances or their precursors in the perikaryon from where they are transported along the axon to the synapse to be released when appropriately stimulated.

Numerous intermediate filaments (neurofilaments) and microtubules are arranged in parallel bundles throughout the perikaryon and along the length of the axon and dendrites. The intermediate filaments provide structural support and the microtubules are involved in axonal transport of neurotransmitter substances, enzymes, membrane and other cellular constituents.

The electron micrograph (b) shows part of the cell body of a neurone and includes a portion of the nucleus **N**. At the lower right, part of the neuronal plasma membrane **PM** is seen including a synapse **S** with the terminal bouton **TB** of an adjacent neurone. Features of the cytoplasm of the perikaryon are areas of rough endoplasmic reticulum **rER**, free ribosomes **R** and scattered mitochondria **M**. An extensive Golgi complex **G** is represented by several stacks of flattened membranous cisternae. Associated with the Golgi are several multivesicular bodies **MB** involved in transport to other organelles including lysosomes **L**. Microtubules **T** can be identified in oblique section but neurofilaments are not readily identifiable.

(b)

1.0 μm

(a)

(b)

(c)

(d)

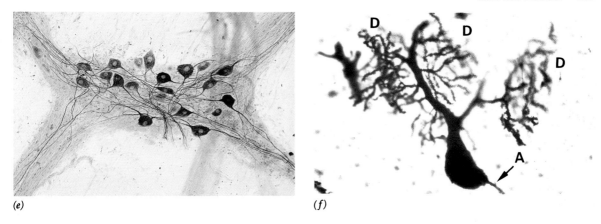

(e) *(f)*

Fig. 7.4 Neurones and methods of study with light microscopy *(micrographs (a) to (d) opposite)*

(a) H & E × 480 (b) Nissl method × 1200 (c) Gold method × 1200 (d) Gold/toluidine blue × 600
(e) Spread preparation, Gold method × 320 (f) Golgi–Cox × 320

The large size and complex morphology of neurones, the extreme elongation of axons, and the need to study neuronal interconnections has resulted in an extensive range of techniques being employed in neurohistology.

Methods which demonstrate nuclei, cell bodies and their cytoplasmic contents include routine stains such as H & E and more specific techniques for demonstrating particular cytoplasmic elements such as the Nissl method for RNA; however, these methods are of limited use in the study of axons and dendrites.

Heavy metal impregnation techniques with gold and silver are valuable in the study of neurone morphology including axons and dendrites and were widely employed by the pioneers of neuro-anatomy such as Cajal and Golgi from whom they take their names. Thick sections are often used with such methods as there is then a much greater chance of whole cells being included in the plane of section. Likewise, *spread preparations* often permit the examination of complete neurones and their cytoplasmic processes. Heavy metals are also deposited in the neuronal microtubules thus permitting study of the cytoskeleton.

Micrograph (a), stained with H & E, shows neurones **N** in the brain; the nuclei are huge in comparison with those of surrounding support cells; dispersed chromatin and prominent nucleoli reflect a high level of protein (enzyme) synthesis. The extensive cytoplasm is basophilic (blue-stained) due to extensive ribosomal RNA. No detail can be seen of cytoplasmic processes.

In micrograph (b), the Nissl method stains ribosomes

(Nissl substance) dark blue giving the neuronal cytoplasm a granular appearance; DNA in the nucleus and nucleoli has similar staining properties. In this specimen, note the axon **A** which is devoid of Nissl substance beyond the axon hillock.

A very similar neurone is shown in micrograph (c) using a heavy metal impregnation technique. Virtually the only intracellular detail that can be seen is the cytoskeleton and a negative image of the nucleus. Note the numerous axons with tiny terminal boutons **B** making synapses with the cell body.

Micrograph (d) employs another gold method which provides excellent detail of neuronal shape and shows the presence of the cytoskeleton in the dendrites and axons; the blue counter-stain demonstrates the nuclei of surrounding support cells. Note that detail of neuronal processes is lost when these pass out of the plane of section.

Spread preparations, as shown in micrograph (e), overcome this problem to a certain extent. This example shows neurones in a small peripheral ganglion, their main cytoplasmic processes being very clearly delineated.

Finally, micrograph (f) illustrates a very thick section stained by a silver impregnation method and shows a Purkinje cell in the cerebellar cortex. These cells have a single small axon **A** at one pole and an extraordinary, finely branching dendritic tree **D** at the other pole. Note that the base of the dendritic system (arrowed) is in this case much larger than that of the axon.

Myelinated and non-myelinated nerve fibres

In the peripheral nervous system, all axons are enveloped by highly specialised cells called *Schwann cells* which provide both structural and metabolic support. In general, small diameter axons (e.g. those of the autonomic nervous system and small pain fibres) are simply enveloped by the cytoplasm of Schwann cells; these nerve fibres are said to be *non-myelinated*. Large diameter fibres are wrapped by a variable number of concentric layers of the Schwann cell plasma membrane forming a *myelin sheath*; such nerve fibres are said to be *myelinated*. Within the central nervous system, myelination is similar to that in the peripheral nervous system except that the myelin sheaths are formed by cells called *oligodendrocytes* (see Fig. 7.22). In the CNS, non-myelinated fibres have no specific cellular support but are indirectly supported by the mass of surrounding nerve cell processes and support cells called *astrocytes* (see Fig. 7.21).

In all nerve fibres, the rate of conduction of action potentials is proportional to the diameter of the axon; myelination greatly increases axon conduction velocity compared with that of a non-myelinated fibre of the same diameter.

(a)

(c)

(b)

Fig. 7.5 Non-myelinated nerve fibres *(a) Diagram (b) EM × 15 000 (c) EM × 36 000*

The relationship of non-myelinated axons with their supporting Schwann cell is illustrated in diagram (a). One or more axons become longitudinally invaginated into the Schwann cell so that each axon is embedded in a channel, invested by the Schwann cell plasma membrane and cytoplasm. The Schwann cell plasma membrane becomes apposed to itself along the opening of the channel, thus effectively sealing the axon within an extracellular compartment bounded by the Schwann cell. The zone of apposition of the Schwann cell membrane is called the *mesaxon*. Note that more than one axon may occupy a single channel within the Schwann cell. Each Schwann cell extends for only a short distance along the nerve tract and at its termination the ensheathment is continued by another Schwann cell with which it interdigitates closely end to end.

At low magnification in micrograph (b), non-myelinated axons **A** of various sizes are seen ensheathed by Schwann cells; one of the Schwann cells has been sectioned transversely through its nucleus **S**. Note the variable number of axons enclosed by each Schwann cell. Delicate cytoplasmic extensions of fibroblasts **F** and collagen fibrils **C** cut in cross-section can be seen in the endoneurium.

At high magnification in micrograph (c), part of the cytoplasm of a Schwann cell **S** is shown ensheathing several axons **A**; axons are readily identified by their content of smooth endoplasmic reticulum and microtubules, seen in cross-section. Several mesaxons **M** can be seen. The external surface of the Schwann cell is bounded by an external lamina **L** equivalent to basement membrane in epithelia.

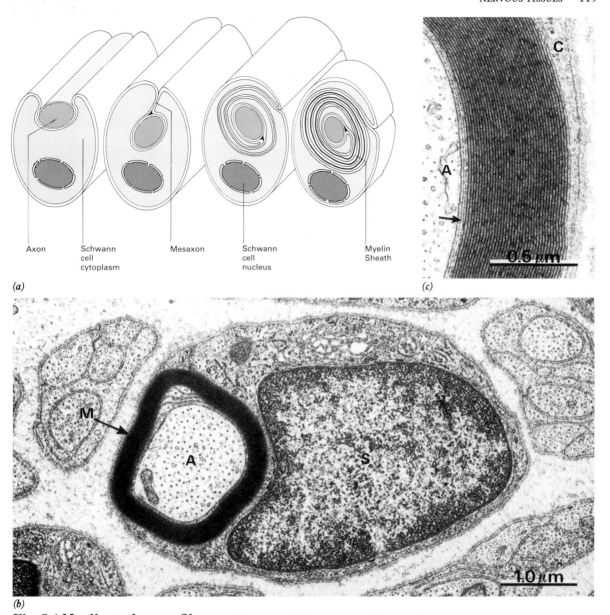

Axon   Schwann   Mesaxon   Schwann   Myelin
        cell   cell   Sheath
        cytoplasm   nucleus

(a)   *(c)*

(b)

Fig. 7.6 Myelinated nerve fibre *(a) Diagram (b) EM × 20 000 (c) EM × 46 000*

In peripheral nerves, myelination begins with the invagination of a single nerve axon into a Schwann cell; a mesaxon is then formed. As myelination proceeds, the mesaxon rotates around the axon thereby enveloping the axon in concentric layers of Schwann cell cytoplasm and plasma membrane. The cytoplasm is then excluded so that the inner leaflets of plasma membrane fuse with each other and the axon becomes surrounded by multiple layers of membrane which together constitute the myelin sheath. The single segment of myelin produced by each Schwann cell is termed an *internode*; this ensheaths the axon between one node of Ranvier and the next (see Fig. 7.7).

In the CNS, oligodendrocytes are responsible for the process of myelination which follows a similar pattern; a single oligodendrocyte, however, forms multiple myelin internodes, which contribute to the ensheathment of as many as 50 individual axons (see Fig. 7.22). In micrograph

(b), a myelinated nerve fibre from the PNS is sectioned transversely at the level of the nucleus of an ensheathing Schwann cell **S**. The single axon **A** is enveloped by many layers of fused Schwann cell plasma membrane forming the myelin sheath **M**.

Micrograph (c) shows that Schwann cell cytoplasm is absent within the compact myelin sheath which consists of many regular layers of membrane. The darker lines, termed the *major dense lines*, arise by fusion of cytoplasmic leaflets. The intervening *intraperiod* lines represent closely apposed external membrane leaflets. The substantial lipid content of these modified membrane layers insulate the underlying axon **A**, preventing ion fluxes across the axonal plasma membrane except at the nodes of Ranvier. The main bulk of the Schwann cell cytoplasm **C** encircles the myelin sheath. However a thin layer of Schwann cell cytoplasm also persists immediately surrounding the axon (arrowed).

(a)

(b)

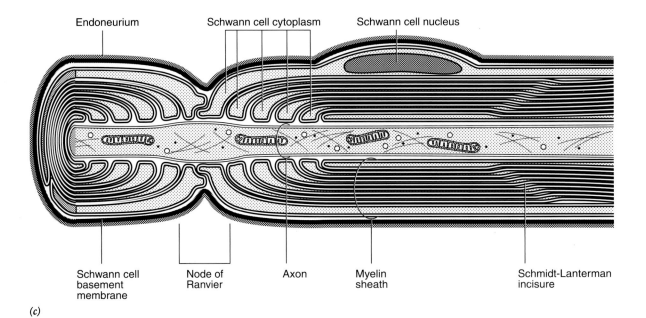

Endoneurium

Schwann cell cytoplasm

Schwann cell nucleus

Schwann cell basement membrane

Node of Ranvier

Axon

Myelin sheath

Schmidt-Lanterman incisure

(c)

(d)

(e)

Fig. 7.7 Nodes of Ranvier and Schmidt–Lanterman incisures *(illustrations (a) to (d) opposite)*

(a) Teased preparation, Sudan black × 320 (b) H & E × 320 (c) Schematic diagram (d) EM × 42 000 (e) EM × 14 000

The myelin sheath of an individual axon is provided by many Schwann cells (oligodendrocytes in the CNS), each Schwann cell covering only a segment of the axon. Between the Schwann cells there are short intervals at which the axon is not covered by a myelin sheath; these points are known as *nodes of Ranvier*.

Micrograph (a) shows a node of Ranvier **R** in a teased preparation of myelinated axons. With this method, only the lipid of the myelin has been stained, thus Schwann cell nuclei are not seen.

Micrograph (b) shows axons in longitudinal section stained with H & E. Due to a fixation artefact, myelin sheaths appear 'bubbly'; the lipid is mostly dissolved out during preparation and is therefore unstained. A node of Ranvier **R** is identifiable in the large axon in midfield. Several Schwann cell nuclei **S** can also be seen.

Diagram (c) illustrates the manner in which Schwann cells terminate at the node of Ranvier, so exposing the axon to the surrounding environment. Note the manner in which cytoplasmic processes of adjacent Schwann cells interdigitate at the node; also note the continuation of the Schwann cell basement membrane (external lamina) across the node. The myelin sheath prevents the nerve action potential from being propagated continuously along the axon and the action potential travels by jumping from node to node. This mode of conduction, known as *saltatory conduction*, greatly enhances the conduction velocity of axons. The internodal length is related to the diameter of the axon and may be up to 1.5 mm in the largest fibres.

Micrograph (e) illustrates the ultrastructure of a node of Ranvier **R**. The axon **A** is characterised by numerous neurofilaments, microtubules and elongated mitochondria. A myelin sheath **M** can be identified at each end of the field, the myelin becoming progressively thinner as it approaches the node. This is because, as it approaches the node, each compact major dense line expands to form a small membrane loop **L** containing Schwann cell cytoplasm, the loops directly abutting the axonal plasma membrane. Externally, a broader layer of Schwann cell cytoplasm **S** containing mitochondria envelops the nodal area. Note the external lamina **EL** of the Schwann cell and collagen fibrils **C** in surrounding endoneurium. Several non-myelinated axons **NMA** are seen nearby.

At certain points within the internodal myelin sheath, narrow channels of cytoplasm are retained and connect the main bulk of the Schwann cell cytoplasm peripherally to the narrow zone of Schwann cell cytoplasm adjacent to the axon. These uncompacted regions are known as *Schmidt–Lanterman incisures* or *clefts*; in longitudinal section, as in electron micrograph (d), the incisure passes obliquely across the width of the compact sheath. The axon is marked **A**, the peripheral Schwann cell cytoplasm S_1 and the periaxonal Schwann cell cytoplasm S_2. It has been suggested that the clefts are not static but rather continually moving their position providing periodic exposure of the inner faces of the myelin membranes to cytoplasm for the purpose of maintenance and molecular replacement.

Synapses and neuromuscular junctions

Synapses are highly specialised intercellular junctions which link the neurones of each nervous pathway. Similar intercellular junctions link neurones and their effector cells such as muscle fibres; where neurones synapse with skeletal muscle they are referred to as *neuromuscular junctions* or *motor end plates*. Individual neurones intercommunicate via a widely variable number of synapses depending on their location and function within the nervous system. Classically, the axon of one neurone synapses with the dendrite of another neurone (*axodendritic synapse*), but axons may synapse with the cell bodies of other neurones (*axosomatic synapses*) or other axons (*axoaxonic synapses*); dendrite-to-dendrite and cell body-to-cell body synapses have also been described. For a given synapse, the conduction of an impulse is unidirectional but the response may be either excitatory or inhibitory depending on the specific functional nature of the synapse and its location.

The mechanism of conduction of the nerve impulse involves the release from one neurone of a chemical neurotransmitter which then diffuses across a narrow intercellular space to induce excitation or inhibition in the other neurone or effector cell of that synapse. Neurotransmitters mediate their effects by interacting with specific receptors incorporated in the opposing plasma membrane.

The chemical nature of neurotransmitters and the morphology of synapses is highly variable in different parts of the nervous system, but the principles of synaptic transmission and the basic structure of synapses are similar throughout the nervous system.

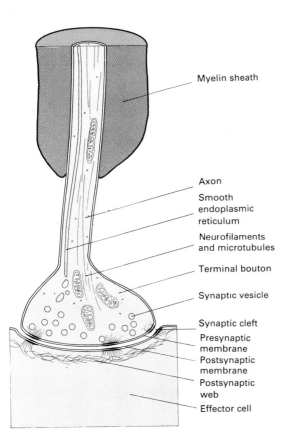

Myelin sheath

Axon

Smooth
endoplasmic
reticulum

Neurofilaments
and microtubules

Terminal bouton

Synaptic vesicle

Synaptic cleft

Presynaptic
membrane

Postsynaptic
membrane

Postsynaptic
web

Effector cell

Fig. 7.8 Synapse

This diagram illustrates the general structure of the synapse. The axon responsible for propagating the stimulus terminates at a bulbous swelling or *terminal bouton*; this is separated from the plasma membrane of the opposed neurone or effector cell by a narrow intercellular gap of uniform width (20–30 nm) called the *synaptic cleft*. The terminal boutons are not myelinated. The boutons contain mitochondria and membrane-bound vesicles of neurotransmitter substance known as *synaptic vesicles* approximately 50 nm in diameter.

Although many types of neurotransmitter substance occur in the CNS, only two types are known in the peripheral nervous system: acetyl choline and noradrenaline (norepinephrine). Acetylcholine precursors, acetate and choline, are synthesised in the perikaryon and transported to the synapse where they are conjugated. Noradrenaline synthesis takes place in both the perikaryon and the terminal bouton. Synaptic vesicles are thought to be derived by budding from the smooth endoplasmic reticulum of the axon.

Synaptic vesicles tend to aggregate towards the *presynaptic membrane* and, on arrival of an action potential, release their contents into the synaptic cleft by exocytosis. The neurotransmitter diffuses across the synaptic cleft to stimulate receptors in the *postsynaptic membrane*. Associated with synapses are a variety of biochemical mechanisms such as hydrolytic and oxidative enzymes which inactivate the released neurotransmitter between successive nerve impulses. The cytoplasm beneath the postsynaptic membrane often contains a feltwork of fine fibrils, the *postsynaptic web*, which may be associated with desmosome-like structures in maintaining the integrity of the synapse.

Fig. 7.9 Axodendritic synapse

(EM × 22 000)

This micrograph from the CNS illustrates three terminal boutons **B** (probably from different axons) forming synapses with a dendrite **D**. The dendrite can be identified as such by its content of ribosomes **R** and rough endoplasmic reticulum **rER** (which are not present in axons). Note the presence of numerous uniform-sized synaptic vesicles **V** and a few mitochondria within the terminal boutons. The *postsynaptic density* (arrowed) contributes to the structural stability of the closely apposed pre- and postsynaptic membranes.

Fig. 7.10 Autonomic synapse

(EM × 42 000)

This micrograph illustrates a synapse between an autonomic axon and a smooth muscle cell in the intestine. The terminal bouton **TB** contains mitochondria **M** and a number of synaptic vesicles **V** some of which contain a dense central core probably representing an electron-dense carrier protein; such *dense-cored vesicles* are a feature of autonomic synapses. Frequently more than one neurotransmitter substance is present in individual autonomic neurones.

The postsynaptic membrane exhibits flask-like invaginations **C** which may represent caveolae (see Fig. 6.18). Note the uniform width of the synaptic cleft between the pre- and postsynaptic membranes. The smooth muscle cell contains numerous fine actin microfilaments **A**.

Fig. 7.11 Sympathetic nerve endings

(Formalin-induced fluorescence × 80)

Noradrenaline is the main postganglionic neurotransmitter in the sympathetic nervous system. When noradrenaline combines with formalin (and some other compounds) it becomes fluorescent and can be visualised by fluorescence microscopy.

This micrograph illustrates formalin-induced fluorescence **F** in the outer layer of large and small arteries, corresponding to the presence of sympathetic noradrenergic nerve endings. Background autofluorescence outlines the general structure; note that the internal elastic lamina **L** (see Fig. 8.8) of the large artery in midfield is particularly autofluorescent.

Schwann cell nucleus

Rough endoplasmic reticulum

Synaptic vesicles

Mitochondrion

Motor nerve axon

Cytoskeleton

Myelin sheath

External lamina

Schwann cell cytoplasm

Primary synaptic cleft

Secondary synaptic cleft

Muscle cell nucleus

Myofibril

(a)

Fig. 7.12 **Motor end plates** *(illustrations (b) to (e) opposite)*

(a) Schematic diagram (b) & (c) Teased preparations: Gold impregnation method (b) × 320 (c) × 800
(d) Histochemical method for acetylcholinesterase × 320 (e) EM × 26 000

The motor end plates of skeletal muscle have the same basic structure as other synapses with the addition of several important features. Firstly, one motor neurone may innervate from a few to more than a thousand muscle fibres depending on the precision of movement of the muscle; the motor neurone and the muscle fibres which it supplies together constitute a *motor unit*.

At low magnification in micrograph (b), the terminal part of the axon of a motor neurone is seen dividing into several branches, each terminating as a motor end plate on a different skeletal muscle fibre near to its mid-point. Micrograph (c) shows the lowermost of these motor end plates at higher magnification. The axonal branch is seen to lose its myelin sheath and divides to form a cluster of small bulbous swellings (terminal boutons) on the muscle fibre surface.

As seen in the diagram, the motor end plate occupies a recess in the muscle cell surface, described as the *sole plate*, and is covered by an extension of the cytoplasm of the last Schwann cell surrounding the axon. The external lamina (basement membrane) of the Schwann cell merges with that of the muscle fibre and the delicate collagenous tissue investing the nerve (endoneurium) becomes continuous with the endomysium of the muscle fibre (not illustrated).

Each of the terminal swellings of the cluster making up the motor end plate has the same basic structure as the synapse shown in Figure 7.8 but the postsynaptic membrane of the neuromuscular junction is deeply folded to form parallel *secondary synaptic clefts*. The overlying presynaptic

membrane is also irregular and the cytoplasm immediately adjacent contains numerous synaptic vesicles. The remaining cytoplasm of the terminal bulb contains many mitochondria and a considerable amount of rough endoplasmic reticulum. The sole plate of the muscle fibre also contains a concentration of mitochondria and an aggregation of muscle cell nuclei.

The neurotransmitter of somatic neuromuscular junctions is acetyl choline, the receptors for which are concentrated at the margins of the secondary synaptic clefts. The hydrolytic enzyme acetylcholinesterase is present deeper in the clefts and is involved in deactivation of the neurotransmitter between successive nerve impulses. The histochemical technique shown in micrograph (d) defines the location of motor end plates by demonstrating acetylcholinesterase activity which appears as a brown deposit.

Micrograph (e) demonstrates the ultrastructure of a motor end plate, the terminal bouton **TB** typically lying in a depression in the skeletal muscle surface and invested externally by Schwann cell cytoplasm **S** and its external lamina **L**. Note the uniform width of the primary synaptic cleft C_1 and the branching nature of the numerous secondary synaptic clefts C_2. The underlying cytoplasm is packed with mitochondria **M**. Myofibrils **Mf** are seen in transverse section at the lower right of the field. The terminal bouton contains numerous synaptic vesicles **V** of uniform size, other membranous elements representing part of the endoplasmic reticulum and a few mitochondria.

(b)

(c)

(d)

(e)

Peripheral nervous tissues

Peripheral nerves are anatomical structures which may contain any combination of afferent or efferent nerve fibres of either the somatic or autonomic nervous systems. The cell bodies of fibres coursing in peripheral nerves are either located in the CNS or in ganglia in peripheral sites.

Each peripheral nerve is composed of one or more bundles (*fascicles*) of nerve fibres. Within the fascicles, each individual nerve fibre, with its investing Schwann cell, is surrounded by a delicate packing of loose vascular supporting tissue called *endoneurium*. Each fascicle is surrounded by a condensed layer of robust collagenous tissue called the *perineurium*. In peripheral nerves consisting of more than one fascicle, a further layer of loose collagenous tissue called the *epineurium* binds the fascicles together and is condensed peripherally to form a strong cylindrical sheath. Peripheral nerves receive a rich blood supply via numerous penetrating vessels from surrounding tissues and accompaning arteries. Larger vessels course longitudinally in the perineurium and epineurium with a rich capillary network in the endoneurium. Extensive anastomoses ensure adequate supply under normal circumstances although this can be put at risk during surgical procedures if too great a length of nerve is dissected from surrounding structures.

Fig. 7.13 Peripheral nerve (*van Gieson × 20*)

This micrograph illustrates the typical appearance of a medium sized peripheral nerve in transverse section. This specimen consists of eight fascicles **F**, each of which contains many nerve fibres. Each fascicle is invested by a condensed collagenous tissue layer, the perineurium **P**, and the nerve as a whole is encased in a loose collagenous tissue sheath, the epineurium **E**, which is condensed at its outermost aspect. Blood vessels of various sizes can be seen in the epineurium.

(a)

(b)

Fig. 7.14 Peripheral nerve (*H & E (a) ×128 (b) ×320*)

The peripheral nerve shown in longitudinal section in micrograph (a) consists of a single fascicle invested by dense perineurium **P** containing small blood vessels; a separate epineurium cannot be distinguished. Most of the nuclei seen within the fascicle are those of Schwann cells which mark the course of individual axons; axons are not readily visible in this type of preparation. Fibroblasts of the endoneurium are scattered amongst the much more numerous Schwann cells. A striking feature of peripheral nerves is that the fibres follow a zigzag longitudinal course which permits stretching during movement.

At higher magnification in micrograph (b), Schwann cell nuclei **S** are seen to be elongated in the long axis of the nerve. The relatively sparse fibroblasts **F** are distinguished by their more slender, condensed nuclei.

Fig. 7.15 Peripheral nerve *(a) H & E × 480 (b) Osmium fixation, van Gieson × 800 (c) EM × 5 000*

In routinely fixed and stained preparations, myelin is poorly preserved since it is largely composed of lipid material. Schwann cell cytoplasm is, however, well-preserved and has eosinophilic staining properties.

Micrograph (a) shows a peripheral nerve cut transversely and stained with H & E; the nerve contains axons of many different types and calibre, some of which are myelinated. Heavily myelinated fibres **M** can be identified by an unstained ring representing the myelin sheath, the centrally located axon and peripheral rim of Schwann cell cytoplasm being stained pink. Small non-myelinated fibres **N** can also be easily identified. Between these extremes are fibres of various sizes with 'bubbly', artefactually distorted myelin sheaths. Note the nuclei of Schwann cells **S** distributed among the nerve fibres. Several flattened fibroblast nuclei **F**

are also seen in the perineurium.

In osmium fixed preparations as shown in micrograph (b), the lipid constituents of myelin are well preserved and are stained black. Note the wide variation in axon diameter. The collagen of the delicate endoneurium between the individual nerve fibres and in the condensed perineurium surrounding the fascicle is stained red by the van Gieson method.

The ultrastructural features of a typical peripheral nerve are seen in micrograph (c); it contains both myelinated axons **M** and more numerous non-myelinated axons **N**, both ensheathed by Schwann cells **S**. The endoneurium mainly consists of loosely arranged collagen fibrils (difficult to identify at this magnification) lying parallel to the nerve fibres. The nuclei of two fibroblasts **F** can be identified and fibroblast processes extend through the endoneurium.

Fig. 7.16 Small peripheral nerves

(a) H & E × 480 (b) Masson's trichrome × 320 (c) Masson's trichrome × 100 (d) H & E × 150

These micrographs illustrate the appearance of a variety of small peripheral nerves in the tissues.

Micrograph (a) shows two small nerves in the dermis of the skin, each nerve consisting of a single fascicle of fibres. The nerve at the bottom of the field is cut in longitudinal section; the wavy shape of the Schwann cell nuclei reflects the course of the axons which are thereby protected from damage when the skin is stretched. The nerve in the upper part of the field is cut in oblique section. Note the dense irregular collagenous dermal tissue surrounding the nerves in this specimen.

Micrograph (b) shows a very small peripheral nerve in the loose fatty hypodermis of the skin. In contrast to the first specimen, with this technique collagen is stained blue-green.

This nerve runs a zig-zag course in the skin and the plane of section has cut it in such a way as to show it in four transverse-oblique views. Note small associated blood vessels **V** containing red-stained erythrocytes.

Micrograph (c) shows a tiny nerve bundle **N** (probably a motor nerve) in skeletal muscle. A nerve bundle of this size would be almost unrecognisable but for its numerous Schwann cell nuclei.

Finally, a neurovascular bundle from the vulva is the subject of micrograph (d). It contains a small artery **A**, arterioles **Aa**, venules **V**, a lymphatic **L**, several small peripheral nerves **N** cut in transverse section and scattered adipocytes **Ad**.

(a)   *(b)*

Fig. 7.17 Spinal ganglion *(H & E (a) × 128 (b) × 800)*

Ganglia are discrete aggregations of neurone cell bodies located outside the CNS. The spinal ganglia lie on the posterior nerve roots of the spinal cord as they pass through the intervertebral foramina; they contain the cell bodies of primary sensory neurones which are of the pseudo-unipolar form (see Fig. 7.2).

At low magnification in micrograph (a), note the fascicle **F** of nerve fibres passing to the centre of the ganglion, the ganglion cells being located peripherally. At high magnification in micrograph (b), each cell body is seen to be surrounded by a layer of flattened *satellite cells* which provide structural and metabolic support and have similar embryological origin to the Schwann cells (neural crest).

The whole ganglion is encapsulated by condensed supporting tissue which is continuous with the perineurial and epineurial sheaths of the associated peripheral nerve.

Fig. 7.18 Sympathetic ganglion

(H & E × 400)

Sympathetic ganglia have a similar structure to that of somatic sensory ganglia with a few minor differences. The ganglion cells are multipolar and thus more widely spaced, being separated by numerous axons and dendrites, many of which pass through the ganglion without being involved in synapses. As seen in this micrograph, the nuclei of the ganglion cells tend to be eccentrically located and the peripheral cytoplasm contains a variable quantity of brown-stained lipofuscin granules representing cellular debris sequestered in residual bodies. The satellite cells are smaller in number and irregularly placed due to the numerous dendritic processes of the ganglion cells.

Fig. 7.19 Parasympathetic ganglion

(H & E × 320)

The cell bodies of the terminal effector neurones of the parasympathetic nervous system are usually located within or near the effector organs. The cell bodies may form well-organised ganglia of moderate size (as in the otic ganglion) but more commonly a few cell bodies are clumped together to form tiny ganglia scattered in the supporting tissue.

This micrograph shows a minute ganglion between two smooth muscle layers in the wall of the gastrointestinal tract. Like all neurones, the ganglion cells are recognised by their large nuclei, with dispersed chromatin and prominent nucleoli, and extensive basophilic cytoplasm. As in other ganglia, the neurones are surrounded by numerous small support cells and afferent and efferent nerve fibres.

Central nervous tissues

The central nervous system consists of the brain and spinal cord, each of which can be divided macroscopically into areas of *grey matter* and *white matter*. Grey matter contains almost all the neurone cell bodies and their associated fibres (axons). White matter consists of tracts of nerve fibres in which a substantial number of the axons are myelinated, myelin appearing white in fresh tissue.

Central nervous tissue consists of a vast number of neurones and their processes embedded in a mass of support cells, collectively known as *neuroglia*, which comprise all the non-neural cells of the CNS. Central nervous tissue proper is devoid of collagenous supporting tissue which is confined to the immediate vicinity of penetrating blood vessels and to the *meninges* which invest the outer surface of the brain. The neuroglia, which form almost half the total mass of the CNS, are highly branched cells which occupy the spaces between neurones; the CNS contains little extracellular material. The neuroglia have intimate functional relationships with neurones providing both mechanical and metabolic support.

Four principal types of neuroglia are recognised: *oligodendrocytes, astrocytes, microglia* and *ependymal cells*. Oligodendrocytes are the CNS equivalent of the Schwann cells of the peripheral nervous system and are responsible for the elaboration of myelin sheaths in the CNS. Astrocytes are highly branched cells which pack the interstices between the neurones, their processes and oligodendrocytes. They provide mechanical support as well as mediating the exchange of metabolites between neurones and the vascular system. Astrocytes also play an important role in repair of CNS tissue after injury or damage by disease. Microglia are the CNS representatives of the monocyte-macrophage system and have defence and immunological functions. Ependymal cells make up a specialised epithelium which lines the ventricles and spinal canal.

Although each functional zone of the CNS has its own peculiar histological appearance, the basic organisation of grey and white matter remains consistent throughout; only the principles of organisation are discussed in this chapter. The various regions of the central nervous system are the subject of Chapter 20.

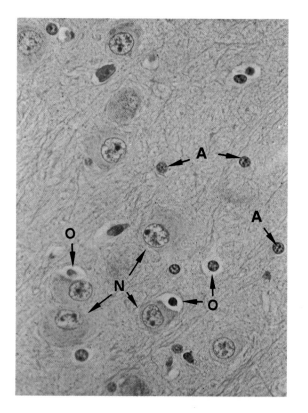

Fig. 7.20 Grey matter *(H & E × 480)*

Common staining methods usually permit neurones **N** to be readily distinguished from glial cells. Although the size and morphology of neurones varies greatly in different regions of the brain, they are usually recognisable by their large nuclei, with prominent nucleoli and dispersed chromatin, and extensive basophilic granular cytoplasm, one or more processes of which may be visible.

Neuroglia are difficult to differentiate with certainty by common staining methods. In the mature CNS, as in this specimen, oligodendroglia have small round condensed nuclei; their cytoplasm is unstained by routine methods including H & E. As described later, in grey matter oligodendrocytes are not only scattered between the nerve cell bodies along with the astrocytes but also tend to be aggregated around the neurone cell bodies. Thus the cells marked **O** can be presumed to be oligodendrocytes. Others marked **A** are probably astrocytes.

The nuclei of both neurones and neuroglia are surrounded by a feltwork of axons and dendrites arising from and converging upon the neurones. This is described as the *neuropil*. Most neuropil fibres are devoid of myelin (being so close to the neurone cell bodies) accounting for the eosinophilia of neuropil.

(a)

(b)

(c)

(d)

Fig. 7.21 Astrocytes

(a) Diagram (b) Cajal method × 400
(c) Immunoperoxidase method for glial fibrillary acidic
protein × 400 (d) EM × 12 000

Classical heavy metal impregnation methods such as that
seen in micrograph (b) identify the presence of star shaped
neuroglia, the astrocytes. These cells, which are the most
numerous glial cells in grey matter, have long branched
processes which occupy most of the interneuronal spaces. In
grey matter, many of the astrocyte processes end in terminal
expansions adjacent to the non-synaptic regions of neurones.
Other processes of the same astrocytes terminate upon the
basement membranes of capillaries, these *perivascular feet*
covering most of the surface of the capillary basement
membranes. Similar foot processes invest the basement
membrane that lies between the CNS and the innermost
layer of the meninges, the pia mater (see Fig. 7.26) forming a
relatively impermeable barrier called the *glia limitans*.

In grey matter, astrocytes thus mediate metabolic
exchange between neurones and blood and regulate the
composition of the intercellular environment of the CNS.

All astrocytes contain bundles of intracellular filaments
and microtubules. These are particularly prominent in the
astrocytes of white matter which have relatively few, straight
cytoplasmic processes and are known as *fibrous astrocytes*. By
contrast, those of grey matter have numerous short highly
branched cytoplasmic processes and are described as
protoplasmic astrocytes. The intermediate filaments consist of
a protein exclusive to astrocytes called *glial fibrillary acidic
protein (GFAP)* which is demonstrated in micrograph (c);
note the capillary **C** being embraced by astrocytic
perivascular feet.

Micrograph (d) shows an astrocyte **A** lying adjacent to a
nerve cell body **N** in the cerebral cortex. The astrocyte
cytoplasm contains many ribosomes, a little rough ER, and a
few small mitochondria and lysosomes. The origins of
several cytoplasmic extensions **C** can be identified. The
cytoplasm appears moderately electron-dense due to its
content of intermediate filaments. Typically of CNS grey
matter, the adjacent neuropil **Np** contains numerous
neuronal and glial processes in various planes of section;
some myelinated axons **M** are included in the field.

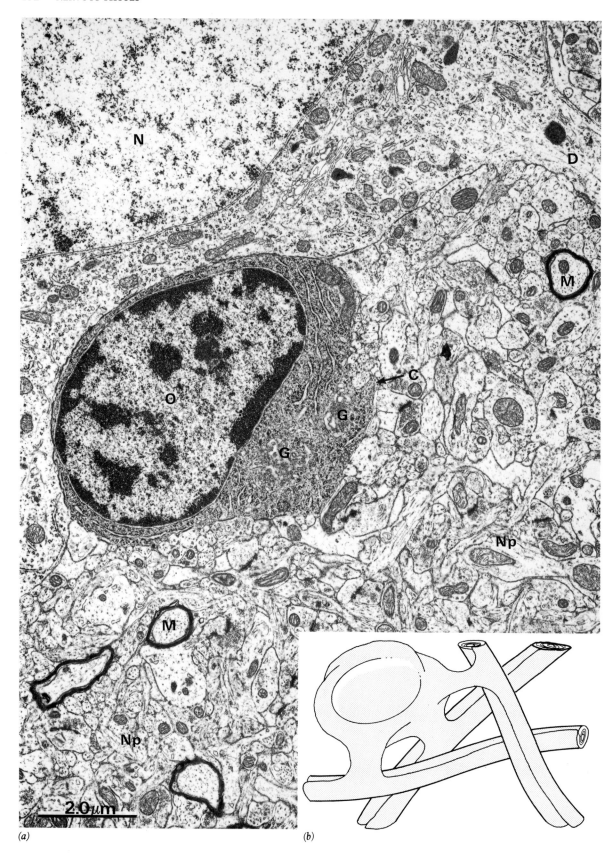

(a)   *(b)*

Fig. 7.22 Oligodendrocytes *(illustrations opposite; (a) EM × 13 000 (b) Schematic diagram)*

Oligodendrocytes were named by the early neurohistologists using classical heavy metal impregnation methods which showed that they had a small number of short, branched processes (Greek: oligos = few, dendron = tree). It is now known that oligodendrocytes are the cells responsible for myelination of axons in the CNS and the dendrites previously described are the short pedicles that connect the cell body to the myelin sheaths.

In fact, a single oligodendrocyte can contribute to the myelination of up to 50 axons which may belong to the same or different fibre tracts. Conversely, any one axon will require the services of numerous different oligodendrocytes since the myelin internodes along its length are synthesised by different cells. The mechanism of myelin sheath formation is very similar to that of Schwann cells in peripheral nerve (see Fig. 7.6). Oligodendrocytes are thus the predominant type of neuroglia in white matter as well as being abundant in grey matter. Oligodendrocytes also aggregate closely around nerve cell bodies in the grey matter where they are thought to have a support function analogous to that of the satellite cells which surround nerve cell bodies in peripheral ganglia (see Fig. 7.17).

Myelin sheath formation begins in the CNS of the human embryo at about 4 months gestational age with the formation of most sheaths at least commenced by about the age of one year. From this time, successive layers continue to be laid down with final myelin sheath thickness being achieved by the time of physical maturity.

Three types of oligodendrocytes are described, namely *light, medium* and *dark* oligodendrocytes according to their staining density with special light microscopic methods and electron microscopy. Light oligodendrocytes are capable of cell division and are highly active in myelin sheath formation and thus predominate in the fetus and neonate, whereas dark oligodendrocytes are the main form in the mature CNS. Medium oligodendrocytes represent the immature form involved in myelin sheath growth and maturation. Some light and medium forms are found in the mature CNS suggesting that there is some slow constant cell turnover and capacity for remyelination should the need arise (e.g. after demyelinating diseases such as multiple sclerosis). Reflecting their intense biosynthetic activity, light oligodendrocytes are relatively large cells with dispersed nuclear chromatin and prominent nucleoli. The cytoplasm contains numerous ribosomes, microtubules and a large Golgi apparatus. In contrast, the dark oligodendrocyte is smaller with a condensed nucleus. This micrograph shows an intermediate oligodendrocyte **O** lying adjacent to a nerve cell body **N** with a neuronal dendrite **D** at the upper right. The oligodendrocyte contains prominent rough endoplasmic reticulum, ribosomes and Golgi stacks **G**. The commencement of one cytoplasmic process **C** is seen. The remainder of the field shows the complexity of the neuropil **Np** comprising glial and neuronal processes including some myelinated axons **M**.

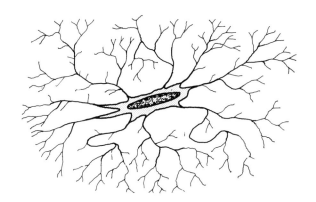

Fig. 7.23 Microglia

Microglia are small cells, relatively few in number, derived from cells of mesenchymal origin which invade the CNS at a late stage of fetal development. Microglia have small irregular nuclei and relatively little cytoplasm which forms fine, highly-branched processes. In consequence, they are difficult to identify in conventional preparations for light microscopy. In response to tissue damage, microglia transform into large amoeboid phagocytic cells and are thus considered to be the CNS representatives of the macrophage-monocyte defence system (see Fig. 3.12).

Under normal circumstances, lymphocytes and other leucocytes do not enter the brain substance proper. Considerable numbers of macrophages are however present in the space surrounding the CNS capillaries but separated from the CNS compartment proper by the perivascular feet of astrocytes.

Fig. 7.24 Ependyma *(H & E × 400)*

Ependymal cells form the simple epithelial lining of the ventricles and spinal canal. Cuboidal or low columnar in shape, the cells are tightly bound together at their luminal surfaces by the usual epithelial junctional complexes. Unlike other epithelia, however, ependymal cells do not rest on a basement membrane but, rather, the bases of the cells taper then break up into fine branches which ramify into an underlying layer of processes derived from astrocytes. At the luminal surface, there is a variable number of cilia, which may be involved in propulsion of cerebrospinal fluid within the ventricles. Microvilli are also present and probably have absorptive and secretory functions.

Fig. 7.25 Choroid plexus *(H & E × 128)*

The choroid plexus is a vascular structure arising from the wall of each of the four ventricles of the brain and responsible for the production of cerebrospinal fluid (CSF). CSF drains from the interconnected ventricular cavities via three channels connecting the fourth ventricle with the subarachnoid space which surrounds the CNS. CSF is produced at a constant rate and is reabsorbed from the subarachnoid space into the superior sagittal venous sinus via finger-like projections called *arachnoid villi*. Thus the CNS is suspended in a constantly circulating fluid medium which acts as a shock absorber.

Each choroid plexus consists of a mass of capillaries projecting into the ventricle **V** and invested by modified ependymal cells which are separated from the underlying capillaries and delicate supporting tissue by a basement membrane. Long, bulbous microvilli project from the luminal surfaces of the choroid epithelial cells and the cytoplasm contains numerous mitochondria, features which suggest that the elaboration of CSF is an active process. The capillaries of the choroid plexus are large, thin-walled and sometimes fenestrated. The mode of CSF secretion involves active secretion of sodium ions by choroid epithelial cells into the CSF, followed by passive movement of water from the choroid capillaries. Continuous tight junctions (zonula occludens) form a *blood-CSF barrier* preventing ingress of almost all other molecules. Glucose (at about 70% plasma concentration) and small amounts of protein are normal constituents of CSF but the mode of their passage into the CSF is unknown.

Fig. 7.26 Meninges *(illustrations opposite; (a) Diagram (b) H & E × 40 (c) H & E × 198 (d) H & E × 480)*

The brain and spinal cord are invested by three layers of supporting tissue collectively called the meninges. The surface of the nervous tissue is covered by a delicate layer called the *pia mater* containing collagen fibres, fine elastin fibres and occasional fibroblasts separated from the processes of underlying astrocytes by a basement membrane. The basement membrane is completely invested by astrocytic processes, the two layers forming the impermeable glia limitans (see also Fig. 7.21). Overlying the pia mater is a thicker fibrous layer, the *arachnoid mater*, which derives its name from the presence of cobweb-like strands which connect it to the underlying pia mater; since the pia and arachnoid are structurally continuous, they are often considered as a single unit, the *pia-arachnoid* or *leptomeninges*. The space between the pia and arachnoid layers is called the *subarachnoid space* and in places forms large cisterns. The subarachnoid space is connected with the ventricular system by three foramina and CSF circulates continuously from the ventricles into the subarachnoid space. The subarachnoid space (i.e. apposed surfaces of the pia and arachnoid layers, and their interconnecting fibres) is lined by flattened mesothelial cells. The outer surface of the arachnoid mater is also lined by mesothelium.

As shown in the diagram, arteries and veins passing to and from the CNS pass in the subarachnoid space loosely attached to the pia mater and invested by subarachnoid mesothelium. As the larger vessels extend into the nervous tissue, they are surrounded by a delicate sleeve of pia mater. Between the penetrating vessels and the pia there is a *perivascular space* which is continuous with the subarachnoid space.

External to the arachnoid mater is a dense fibro-elastic layer called the *dura mater* which is lined on its internal surface by mesothelium. The dura is closely applied to, but not connected with, the arachnoid layer and a potential space, the *subdural space*, containing a minute amount of fluid separates the two layers. In the cranium, the dura mater merges with the periosteum of the skull whereas around the spinal cord the dura is suspended from the periosteum of the spinal canal by the *denticulate ligaments*, the intervening *epidural space* being filled with loose, fibro-

fatty tissue and a venous plexus.

The pia and arachnoid layers of the brain meninges are illustrated in micrographs (b) and (c), the dura mater typically remaining adherent to the skull when the brain is removed from the cranial cavity. The pia mater **P** is attached to the surface of the brain and continues into the sulci **S** and around the penetrating vessels. The arachnoid mater **A** appears to be a completely separate layer and bridges the sulci. Meningeal vessels lie in the subarachnoid space. At high magnification in micrograph (c), delicate fibrous strands **F** can be discerned traversing the subarachnoid space **SS** to connect the pia and arachnoid layers. Two small vessels **V** can be seen in the subarachnoid space. A penetrating vessel is also seen surrounded by a perivascular space **PVS** which is continuous with the subarachnoid space and thus filled with CSF. The perivascular space is extremely narrow although it often appears artefactually wider as in this micrograph. The CNS contains no lymphatics and interstitial fluid is thought to drain outwards from the brain substance to join the subarachnoid CSF via the perivascular spaces and to contribute as much as 20% of its volume.

As seen in micrograph (d), the capillaries of the CNS are similar to those elsewhere in the body with flattened endothelial cells resting on a basement membrane. The endothelial cells are not fenestrated and are bound together by continuous tight intercellular junctions (zonula occludens) except in the choroid plexus where this is discontinuous. Externally, the basement membranes are completely covered by the perivascular foot processes of astrocytes (see Fig. 7.21). A thin layer of the pia mater extends down into the CNS around smaller arteries, veins, arterioles and venules but is not present around the capillaries of the CNS.

Perfusion studies show that the CNS capillaries are impermeable to certain plasma constituents especially larger molecules forming a *blood-brain barrier*. The capillary endothelium plays the central role since junctions between endothelial cells are sealed; the endothelial cells exhibit little or no pinocytosis. Luminal surface membranes contain various enzymes which destroy neurotoxic metabolites and

(a)

(b)

(c)

(d)

neuroactive humoral substances. Maintenance of barrier type endothelium appears to be under the control of astrocyte foot processes. The blood-brain barrier provides neurones with a relatively constant biochemical and metabolic environment, protection against endogenous and exogenous toxins and infective agents and insulates the neurones from circulating neurotransmitters and other humoral agents. The capillaries of the choroid plexus, the pituitary and pineal glands and the vomiting centre of the hypothalamus are, however, devoid of this barrier as befits their various functions.

Sensory receptors

Sensory receptors are nerve endings or specialised cells which convert (transduce) stimuli from the external or internal environments into afferent nerve impulses; the impulses pass into the CNS where they initiate appropriate voluntary or involuntary responses.

No classification system for sensory receptors has yet been devised which adequately incorporates either functional or morphological features. A widely used functional classification divides sensory receptors into three groups: *exteroceptors*, *proprioceptors* and *interoceptors*. Exteroceptors are those which respond to stimuli from outside the body and include receptors for touch, light pressure, deep pressure, cutaneous pain, temperature, smell, taste, sight and hearing. Proprioceptors are located within the skeletal system and provide conscious and unconscious information about orientation, skeletal position, tension and movement; such receptors include the vestibular apparatus of the ear, tendon organs and neuromuscular spindles. Interoceptors respond to stimuli from the viscera and include the chemoreceptors of blood, vascular (pressure) baroreceptors, the receptors for the state of distension of hollow viscera such as the gastrointestinal tract and urinary bladder, and receptors for such nebulous senses as visceral pain, hunger, thirst, well-being and malaise.

The structure of the receptors involved in some of these sensory modalities is poorly understood. Sensory receptors may be classified morphologically into two groups, *simple* and *compound*. Simple receptors are merely free, branched or unbranched nerve endings such as those responsible for cutaneous pain and temperature; they are rarely visible with the light microscope unless special staining methods are employed. Compound receptors involve organisation of associated non-neural tissues to complement the function of the neural receptors. The degree of organisation may range from mere encapsulation to highly sophisticated arrangements such as in the eye and ear. By tradition, the eye, ear and receptors for the senses of smell and taste are described as the *organs of special sense*; they are the subject of Chapter 21.

Fig. 7.27 Free nerve endings
(Silver/Haematoxylin × 480)

Free nerve endings are the simplest form of sensory receptor, merely consisting of numerous small terminal branches of afferent nerve fibres. Such free nerve endings are found in supporting tissues throughout the body subserving a variety of relatively unsophisticated sensory modalities such as temperature, touch and pain. The afferent fibres are of relatively small diameter with slow rates of conduction; although some of these fibres are myelinated, the nerve endings are devoid of myelin.

In the skin, free nerve endings are found along the dermo-epidermal junction. Some exhibit a terminal expansion which is intimately associated with non-neuronal cells called *Merkel cells* scattered in the basal layers of the epidermis (see Fig. 9.4). The adjacent Merkel cell cytoplasm contains vesicles with ultrastructural features similar to those found in synapses but no neurotransmitter has yet been demonstrated. Merkel nerve endings are served by large-diameter myelinated fibres and are thought to be responsible for the sensation of touch. A variety of different arrangements of free nerve endings is also incorporated in the follicles of fine and coarse hairs acting as touch receptors, the most sophisticated type being those associated with the whiskers of animals such as cats and rodents.

This thick section of skin stained by a heavy metal impregnation method shows a nerve fibre with many fine terminal branches extending as free nerve endings into the dermo-epidermal junction; Merkel cells cannot be readily identified.

(a)

(b)

Fig. 7.28 Meissner's corpuscles

(a) H & E × 320 (b) Silver method × 150

Meissner's corpuscles are small, encapsulated, sensory receptors found in the dermis of the skin, particularly of the fingertips, soles of the feet, nipples, eyelids, lips and genitalia. They are involved in the reception of light discriminatory touch, the degree of discrimination depending on the proximity of receptors to one another.

As seen in micrograph (a), Meissner's corpuscles **M** are oval in shape and are usually located in the dermal papillae immediately beneath the epidermis **E**. The receptors consist of a delicate collagenous tissue capsule surrounding a mass of plump, oval cells arranged transversely and probably representing specialised Schwann cells. Non-myelinated branches of large myelinated sensory fibres ramify throughout the cell mass in a helical manner as shown by the heavy metal impregnation technique in micrograph (b).

(a)

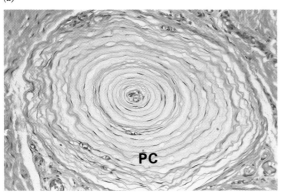

(b)

Fig. 7.29 Pacinian corpuscles

(a) Masson's trichrome × 80 (b) H & E × 100

Pacinian corpuscles **PC** are large encapsulated sensory receptors responsive to pressure or coarse touch, vibration and tension, and are found in the deeper layers of the skin, ligaments and joint capsules, in some serous membranes, mesenteries, some viscera and in some erogenous areas.

Pacinian corpuscles range from 1–4 mm in length and in section have the appearance of an onion. These organs consist of a delicate capsule enclosing many concentric lamellae of flattened cells (probably modified Schwann cells) separated by interstitial fluid spaces and delicate collagen fibres. Towards the centre of the corpuscle the lamellae become closely packed and the core contains a single large unbranched non-myelinated nerve fibre with several club-like terminals which becomes myelinated as it leaves the corpuscle. Distortion of the Pacinian corpuscle produces an amplified mechanical stimulus in the core which is transduced into an action potential in the sensory neurone.

Two other simple encapsulated mechanoreceptors are described. *Ruffini corpuscles* are robust spindle-shaped structures found particularly in the soles of the feet. *Krause end bulbs* are delicate receptors found in the lining of the oropharynx and the conjunctiva of the eye.

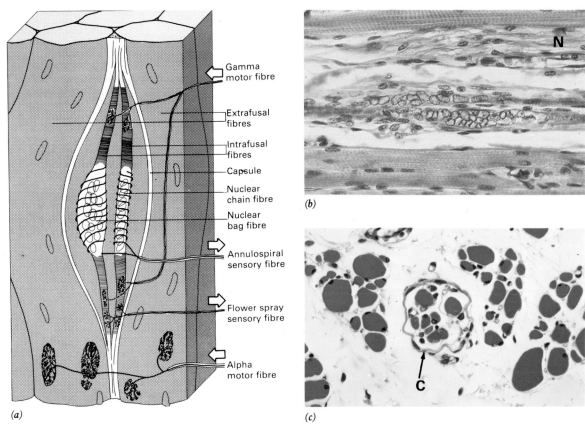

(a)

(b)

(c)

Fig 7.30 Neuromuscular spindle *(a) Schematic diagram (b) LS: H & E × 320 (c) TS: Masson's trichrome × 320*

Neuromuscular spindles are stretch receptor organs within skeletal muscles which are responsible for the regulation of muscle tone via the spinal stretch reflex. These receptors are particularly numerous in muscles involved in fine, precision movements such as the intrinsic muscles of the hand and the external muscles of the eye.

Neuromuscular spindles are encapsulated, lymph filled, fusiform structures up to 6 mm long but less than 1 mm in diameter. They lie parallel to the muscle fibres, embedded in endomysium or perimysium. Each spindle contains from 2–10 modified skeletal muscle fibres called *intrafusal fibres* which are much smaller than skeletal muscle fibres proper (*extrafusal fibres*). The intrafusal fibres have a central non-striated area in which their nuclei tend to be concentrated. Two types of intrafusal fibres are recognised. In one type, the central nuclear area is dilated, these fibres being known as *nuclear bag fibres*. In the other type, there is no dilatation and the nuclei are arranged in a single row giving rise to the name *nuclear chain fibres*.

Associated with both types of intrafusal fibres are sensory receptors of two types. Firstly, branched, non-myelinated endings of large, myelinated sensory fibres are wrapped around the central non-striated area of the intrafusal fibres forming *annulo-spiral endings*. Secondly, *flower-spray endings* of smaller, myelinated sensory fibres are located on the striated portions of the intrafusal fibres.

Together, these sensory receptors are stimulated by stretching of the intrafusal fibres which occurs when the extrafusal muscle mass is stretched. This stimulus evokes reflex contraction of the extrafusal muscle fibres via large (alpha) motor neurones of a simple two-neurone spinal reflex arc. Contraction of the extrafusal muscle mass thus removes the stretch stimulus from the intrafusal stretch receptors and equilibrium is restored.

The sensitivity of the neuromuscular spindle is modulated by higher centres via small (gamma) motor neurones arising from the extrapyramidal system. These gamma motor neurones innervate the striated portions of the intrafusal fibres thus controlling their state of contraction. Contraction of the intrafusal fibres increases the sensitivity of the intrafusal receptors to stretching of the extrafusal mass.

In any one histological section, it is impossible to demonstrate all the structural features of a neuromuscular spindle, but many of the features of the organ are shown in these micrographs. The most easily recognisable features are the discrete capsule **C** which is continuous with the endomysium of the surrounding muscle, best seen in micrograph (c), and the small size of the intrafusal muscle fibres compared with the surrounding extrafusal fibres. In micrograph (b), note the small bundle of nerve fibres **N** passing to and from the spindle.

PART THREE

Organ systems

8. Circulatory system

Introduction

The circulatory system mediates the continuous movement of all body fluids, its principal functions being the transport of oxygen and nutrients to the tissues and transport of carbon dioxide and other metabolic waste products from the tissues. The circulatory system is also involved in temperature regulation and the distribution of molecules such as hormones, and cells such as those of the immune system. The circulatory system has two functional components: the blood vascular system and the lymph vascular system.

The *blood vascular system* comprises a circuit of vessels through which flow of blood is maintained by continuous pumping of the heart. The *arterial system* provides a distribution network to the *capillaries* which are the main sites of interchange of gases and metabolites between the tissues and blood. The *venous system* returns blood from the capillaries to the heart. In contrast, the *lymph vascular system* is merely a passive drainage system for returning excess extravascular fluid, the *lymph*, to the blood vascular system. The lymph vascular system has no intrinsic pumping mechanism.

The whole circulatory system has a common basic structure:

- An inner lining comprising a single layer of extremely flattened epithelial cells called *endothelium* supported by a basement membrane and delicate collagenous tissue; this constitutes the *tunica intima*.
- An intermediate muscular layer, the *tunica media*.
- An outer supporting tissue layer called the *tunica adventitia*.

The tissues of the walls of large vessels cannot be sustained by diffusion of nutrients from their lumina and are thus supplied by small arteries called *vasa vasorum* (i.e. 'vessels of vessels') which are derived either from the main vessel itself or from adjacent arteries. The vasa vasorum give rise to a capillary network within the tunica adventitia which may extend into the tunica media.

The muscular layer exhibits the greatest variation from one part of the system to another. For example, it is totally absent in capillaries but comprises almost the whole mass of the heart. Blood flow is predominantly influenced by variation in activity of the muscular layer.

Fig. 8.1 Heart: wall of ventricle *(Monkey: Masson's trichrome × 20)*

This micrograph illustrates the three basic layers of the heart wall; monkey tissue has been chosen as that of human is too large to illustrate in this way. The tunica intima of the heart is called the *endocardium* **E**, and is difficult to see at this magnification. The tunica media of the heart is called the *myocardium* **M** and is thickest in the ventricular walls. The myocardium is made up of cardiac muscle, the structure of which meets the unique functional requirements of the heart (see Ch. 6).

The tunica adventitia of the heart, the *epicardium* **Epi** (also called *visceral pericardium*), is surrounded by a potential space, the *pericardial cavity*, enclosed by a fibrous sac, the *pericardium* (the *parietal pericardium*) which is not shown in this micrograph. The parietal pericardium is loosely fixed to the surrounding mediastinal structures. The parietal and visceral layers of the pericardium move freely against one another thus permitting relatively unimpeded movement of the heart.

Note a branch **A** of the coronary arterial system; these arteries represent the vasa vasorum of the heart. Note also *papillary muscles* **P** of the ventricle; these are extensions of the myocardium which, via the *chordae tendinae*, stabilise the cusps of the mitral and tricuspid valves.

(a)

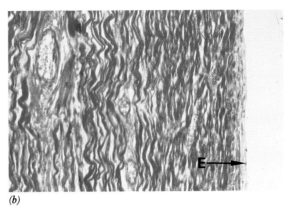

(b)

Fig. 8.2 Heart: myocardium and endocardium *(a) H & E × 128 (b) Masson's trichrome × 128*

The endocardium, the innermost layer of the heart, consists of an endothelial lining and its supporting tissue. The endothelium **E** is a single layer of flattened epithelial cells, which is continuous with the endothelium of the vessels entering and leaving the heart. The endothelium is supported by a delicate layer of collagenous tissue beneath which lies a more robust fibro-elastic layer; this accommodates movement of the myocardium without

damage to the endothelium. The deepest aspect of the endocardium may also contain a small amount of adipose tissue.

The subendothelial tissue becomes continuous with the perimysium of the cardiac muscle; this is best demonstrated in micrograph (b) in which collagen is stained blue. The endocardium contains blood vessels, nerves and branches of the conducting system of the heart.

(a)

(b)

Fig. 8.3 Heart: epicardium *(H & E (a) × 200 (b) ×480)*

The free surface of the epicardium consists of a single layer of flattened epithelial cells, the mesothelium **M**; a similar mesothelial layer lines the opposing parietal pericardial surface. The mesothelial cells secrete a small amount of serous fluid which lubricates the movement of the epicardium on the parietal pericardium.

A thin layer of fibro-elastic tissue **F** supports the mesothelium; this layer is connected to the myocardium by a broad layer of adipose tissue **A**. The coronary vessels and autonomic nerves pass in the epicardium to supply the myocardium.

(a) *(b)*

Fig. 8.4 Purkinje fibres *(H & E/Elastin (a) ×150 (b) ×400)*

The coordinated contraction of the myocardium during each pumping cycle is mediated by a specialised conducting system of modified cardiac muscle fibres. With each cardiac cycle, a wave of excitation originates in the pacemaker region of the right atrium, the *sino-atrial node*; the excitatory stimuli arise spontaneously at regular intervals, the rate being modulated by the autonomic nervous system. The wave of excitation spreads throughout the atria causing them to contract thus forcing blood into the ventricles. By this time, the wave of excitation has spread to the *atrioventricular node* from which an excitatory stimulus is passed rapidly throughout the whole ventricular myocardium via the *atrioventricular bundle* or *bundle of His*. This bundle divides within the interventricular septum to give rise to smaller branches called *Purkinje fibres* which pass in the subendocardial supporting tissue before penetrating the ventricular myocardium. This system permits coordinated contraction of the entire ventricular myocardium.

The characteristics of the specialised muscle fibres of the conducting system are demonstrated in these micrographs.

Micrograph (a) illustrates the typical subendocardial location of a bundle of Purkinje fibres **P** and the darkly staining endocardial elastin **E**. Note the broad similarity of the Purkinje bundle to the adjacent myocardium **M**.

As seen in micrograph (b), the conducting cells are larger than myocardial cells, and sometimes binucleate. The extensive pale cytoplasm contains relatively few myofibrils which are arranged in an irregular manner immediately beneath the plasma membrane of the cell. The cytoplasm is rich in glycogen and mitochondria but, in contrast to other cardiac muscle cells, there is no T tubule system. Connections between the Purkinje cells are via desmosomes and gap junctions rather than by intercalated discs as in the rest of the myocardium.

The excitatory cells of the sinoatrial and atrioventricular nodes are small specialised myocardial fibres with electrochemical stimuli being transmitted via gap junctions. The cells contain little contractile protein or glycogen and are embedded in dense vascular collagenous tissue containing numerous autonomic nerve fibres.

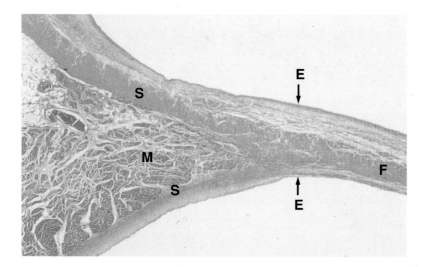

Fig. 8.5 Heart valve

(H & E × 15)

The valves of the heart consist of leaflets of collagenous tissue, the surfaces being invested with a thin endothelial layer continuous with that of the heart chambers and great vessels. This micrograph illustrates the base of a valve arising from the myocardium **M**. The tough central fibrous sheet, the *lamina fibrosa* **F**, represents a merging of the fibro-elastic supporting layers **S** beneath the endothelium **E**.

(a)

(b)

Fig. 8.6 Heart valve

(a) H & E × 60
(b) Elastic van Gieson × 60

These sections from the same specimen of heart valve are stained by different methods. The standard H & E section in micrograph (a) highlights the dense collagenous tissue of the lamina fibrosa **F** forming the main bulk of the valve. Micrograph (b) demonstrates the considerable elastin content (stained black) which is particularly concentrated in the less dense subendothelial tissue.

At the attached margins of each valve, the lamina fibrosa becomes condensed to form a fibrous ring (valve anulus) and the rings of the four valves together form a central fibrous cardiac 'skeleton' which is continuous with the collagenous tissue of the myocardium, endocardium and epicardium. The mitral and tricuspid leaflets are connected to the papillary muscles by collagenous strands, the *chordae tendinae*, which also merge with the fibrous lamina of the valve leaflet.

The arterial system

The function of the arterial system is to distribute blood from the heart to capillary beds throughout the body. The cyclical pumping action of the heart produces a pulsatile blood flow in the arterial system. With each contraction of the ventricles (systole), blood is forced into the arterial system causing expansion of the arterial walls; subsequent recoil of the arterial walls assists in maintenance of arterial blood pressure between ventricular beats (diastole). This expansion and recoil is a function of elastic tissue within the walls of the arteries. The flow of blood to various organs and tissues may be regulated by varying the diameter of the distributing vessels. This function is performed by the circumferentially disposed smooth muscle of vessel walls and is principally under the control of the sympathetic nervous system and adrenal medullary hormones.

The walls of the arterial vessels conform to the general three-layered structure of the circulatory system but are characterised by the presence of considerable elastin and the smooth muscle wall is thick relative to the diameter of the lumen. There are three main types of vessel in the arterial system:

- **Elastic arteries.** These comprise the major distribution vessels and include the aorta, the innominate, common carotid and subclavian arteries and most of the pulmonary arterial vessels.
- **Muscular arteries.** These are the main distributing branches of the arterial tree, e.g. the radial, femoral, coronary and cerebral arteries.
- **Arterioles.** These are the terminal branches of the arterial tree which supply the capillary beds.

There is a gradual transition in structure and function between the three types of arterial vessel rather than an abrupt demarcation. In general, the amount of elastic tissue decreases as the vessels become smaller and the smooth muscle component assumes relatively greater prominence.

(a)

(b)

Fig. 8.7 Elastic artery: aorta *(Elastic van Gieson (a) × 33 (b) × 320)*

The highly elastic nature of the aortic wall is demonstrated in these preparations in which the elastic fibres are stained black. In micrograph (a), the three basic layers of the wall can be seen: the tunica intima **I**, the broad tunica media **M** and the tunica adventitia **A**.

The tunica intima consists of a single layer of flattened endothelial cells (not seen at this magnification) supported by a layer of collagenous tissue rich in elastin disposed in the form of both fibres and discontinuous sheets. The subendothelial supporting tissue contains scattered fibroblasts and other cells with ultrastructural features akin to smooth muscle cells and known as *myointimal cells*. Both cell types are probably involved in elaboration of the extracellular constituents. The myointimal cells are not invested by basement membrane and are thus not epithelial (myoepithelial) in nature. With increasing age, the

myointimal cells accumulate lipid and the intima progressively thickens; in a more extreme form this represents one of the early changes of atherosclerosis.

The tunica media is particularly broad and extremely elastic. At high magnification in (b), it is seen to consist of concentric fenestrated sheets of elastin (stained black) separated by collagenous tissue (stained red) and relatively few smooth muscle fibres (stained yellow). As seen in micrograph (a), the collagenous tunica adventitia (stained red) contains small vasa vasorum **V** which also penetrate the outer half of the tunica media.

Blood flow within elastic arteries is highly pulsatile; with advancing age the arterial system becomes less elastic thereby increasing peripheral resistance and thus arterial blood pressure.

(a)

(b)

Fig. 8.8 Muscular artery

(a) H & E × 100
(b) Elastic van Gieson × 100

Muscular arteries have the same basic structure as elastic arteries but the elastic tissue is reduced to a well defined, fenestrated elastic sheet, the *internal elastic lamina* **IEL**, separating the tunica intima from the tunica media, and a less defined *external elastic lamina* **EEL** at the junction of the media and the tunica adventitia. Sometimes the internal elastic lamina is duplicated. The intima is often so thin as to be indistinguishable at low magnification. The tunica media **M** comprises a thick layer of circumferentially arranged smooth muscle, stained yellow in micrograph (b). The broad tunica adventitia **A** is mainly composed of collagen with considerable elastin, stained black in micrograph (b).

(a)   (b)

Fig. 8.9 Large arterioles *(H & E (a) TS × 128 (b) LS × 320)*

Arterioles may be defined as those vessels of the arterial system with a lumen less than 0.3 mm in diameter, although the distinction between small muscular arteries and large arterioles is somewhat artificial. Arterioles are characterised by three main features which are seen in these micrographs.

The tunic intima is very thin and comprises the endothelial lining, a little collagenous supporting tissue and a thin internal elastic lamina. The tunica media **M** is almost entirely composed of smooth muscle cells in six concentric layers or less. The tunica adventitia **A** may be almost as thick as the tunica media and merges with the surrounding

collagenous tissues. There is no external elastic lamina.

The flow of blood through capillary beds is regulated mainly by the arterioles which supply them. Contraction of the circularly arranged smooth muscle fibres of the arteriolar wall reduces the diameter of the lumen and hence blood flow. Generalised constriction of arterioles throughout the body markedly increases peripheral resistance to blood flow and the arteriolar compartment of the circulatory system thus has an important role in the regulation of systemic blood pressure.

(a)   (b)

Fig. 8.10 Small arterioles *(a) H & E × 100 (b) EM × 19 000*

Micrograph (a) illustrates two small arterioles in the dense collagenous tissue of the dermis of the skin. The tunica media **M** of each consists of two layers of smooth muscle cells. All that can be seen of the tunica intima are the nuclei of flattened endothelial cells **E**. The adventitia merges imperceptibly with the surrounding supporting tissue. Electron micrograph (b) is an example of the smallest of arterioles having only a single layer of smooth muscle **M**

which lies immediately external to the endothelium **E** and its basement membrane **BM**. Note the external lamina **EL** (equivalent to basement membrane) around the smooth muscle cell. The adjacent supporting tissue contains a tiny autonomic nerve bundle including several vesicle-containing sympathetic axons **A** and a supporting Schwann cell **S**. The adventitial layer merges imperceptibly with the surrounding loose collagenous tissue.

The microcirculation

The microcirculation is that part of the circulatory system concerned with the exchange of gases, fluids, nutrients and metabolic waste products. Exchange occurs mainly within the *capillaries*, extremely thin walled vessels forming an interconnected network. Blood flow within the capillary bed is controlled by the arterioles and muscular sphincters at the arteriolar-capillary junctions called *precapillary sphincters*. The capillaries drain into a series of vessels of increasing diameter namely *post-capillary venules*, *collecting venules* and small *muscular venules* which make up the venous component of the microcirculation.

In different tissues, the structure of the microcirculation varies to meet specific functional requirements. There are four main structural variables:

- **The diameter of the capillaries.** Diameter varies between as little as 3 to 4 μm (i.e. half the diameter of a red blood cell) and 30 to 40 μm. Large diameter capillaries are called *sinusoids*; these are found in the liver, spleen, lymph nodes and bone marrow.

- **The nature of the capillary endothelium.** Three types of capillary endothelium are found.
  Continuous capillaries: the endothelial cells form an uninterrupted lining; this is the most common type of capillary.
  Fenestrated capillaries: the endothelial cells contain numerous large pores or *fenestrations*.
  Discontinuous endothelium: the endothelial cells do not form a continuous interface between the lumen and surrounding tissues; this arrangement is found only within the sinusoids of the liver (see Fig. 15.11).

- **The presence of arterio-venous shunts.** These provide direct connections between the arterial and venous systems.

- **The abundance of the capillary network.** This depends on the functional requirements of the tissue. For example, the dense collagenous tissue of tendons has a sparse capillary network; in contrast, cardiac muscle has an extensive capillary network which pervades the interstices between the muscle fibres.

Fig. 8.11 The microcirculation

(Mesenteric spread, H & E × 120)

This micrograph demonstrates an anastomosing network of capillaries between an arteriole **A** and a venule **V**. The capillary network comprises small diameter capillaries **C**, consisting of only a single layer of endothelial cells, and larger diameter capillaries known as *metarterioles* **M**, characterised by a discontinuous outer layer of smooth muscle cells.

Note that small capillaries arise both from arterioles and metarterioles. At the origin of each capillary there is a sphincter mechanism, the precapillary sphincter, which is involved in regulation of capillary blood flow. Note also a direct wide-diameter communication between the arteriole and venule, an *arterio-venous shunt* **S**. Metarterioles also form direct communications between arterioles and venules. Contraction of the smooth muscle of the shunts and metarterioles directs blood through the network of small capillaries. Thus regulation of blood flow in the microcirculation is mediated by arterioles, metarterioles, precapillary sphincters and arterio-venous shunts. The smooth muscle activity of these vessels is modulated by the autonomic nervous system and circulating hormones, e.g. adrenal catecholamines. In addition, the concentration of oxygen and metabolites, such as lactic acid, regulate the local flow of blood within tissues; this process is called *autoregulation*.

Fig. 8.12 Capillaries *(H & E × 800)*

The vessels seen here in longitudinal section and transverse section illustrate the characteristic features of capillaries.

A single layer of flattened endothelial cells **E** lines the capillary lumen. The thin layer of cytoplasm is difficult to resolve by light microscopy. The flattened endothelial cell nuclei bulge into the capillary lumen; in longitudinal section the nuclei appear elongated whereas in transverse section they appear more rounded in shape. Muscular and adventitial layers are absent. Occasional flattened cells called *pericytes* **P** embrace the capillary endothelial cells and may have a contractile function. Note that the diameter of capillaries is similar to that of the red blood cells contained within them.

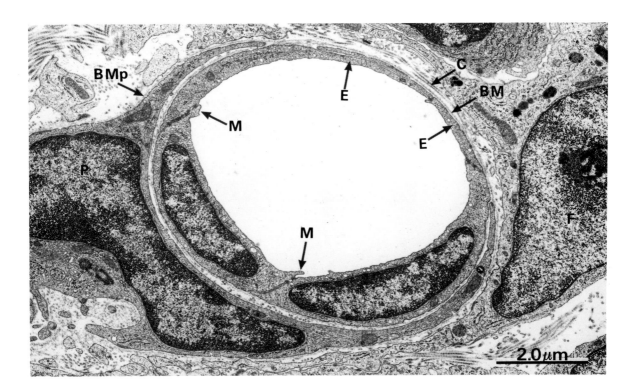

2.0 μm

Fig. 8.13 Capillary: continuous endothelium type *(EM × 12 000)*

This electron micrograph illustrates the ultrastructure of capillaries of the continuous endothelium type, the type found in most tissues.

Four endothelial cells **E** are seen to encircle the capillary lumen, their plasma membranes approximating one another very closely and bound together by scattered tight junctions of the fascia occludens type (see Fig. 5.11). Small cytoplasmic flaps called *marginal folds* **M** extend across the intercellular junctions at the luminal surface. The capillary endothelium is supported by a thin basement membrane **BM** and adjacent collagen fibrils **C**. A pericyte **P** embraces the capillary. The pericyte is supported by its own basement membrane **BMp**. In the adjacent supporting tissue, note a fibroblast **F** and larger diameter collagen fibrils cut in

transverse and longitudinal section.

Exchange between the lumen of the continuous type capillary and the surrounding tissues is believed to occur in three ways. Passive diffusion through the endothelial cell cytoplasm mediates exchange of gases, ions and low molecular weight metabolites. Proteins and some lipids are transported by pinocytotic vesicles. White blood cells pass through the intercellular space between the endothelial cells in some way negotiating the endothelial intercellular junctions. Some workers maintain that the intercellular spaces also permit molecular transport. In capillaries of the continuous endothelial type, the basement membrane is thought to present little barrier to exchange between capillaries and surrounding tissues.

(a)

(b)

0.2 µm

Fig. 8.14 Fenestrated capillary

(EM (a) × 13 000 (b) × 60 000)

Fenestrated capillaries are found in some tissues where there is extensive molecular exchange with the blood; such tissues include the small intestine, endocrine glands and the kidney.

At low magnification (a), fenestrations **F** appear as pores through attenuated areas of the endothelial cytoplasm; however, only a small proportion of these areas are fenestrated. At high magnification (b), the fenestrations appear to be traversed by a thin electron-dense line **D** which may constitute a diaphragm; the biochemical and functional nature of this is not understood. A diaphragm is not seen across the fenestrations of the glomerular capillaries of the kidney (see Fig. 16.13).

The permeability of fenestrated capillaries is much greater than that of continuous endothelium type capillaries and molecular labelling techniques have demonstrated that fenestrations permit the rapid passage of macromolecules smaller than plasma proteins from the lamina of fenestrated capillaries into surrounding tissues.

Like continuous endothelium type capillaries, all fenestrated capillaries are supported by a basement membrane **BM** which is continuous across the fenestrations. Pericytes are rarely found in association with fenestrated capillaries.

Fig. 8.15 Sinusoids *(H & E × 320)*

Sinusoids are capillaries of wide diameter found in the liver, spleen, lymph nodes, bone marrow and some endocrine glands. The endothelium of sinusoids may be continuous, fenestrated or discontinuous, the discontinuous type of endothelial lining being found only in the liver sinusoids (see Fig. 15.11). Sinusoids usually have an irregular outline which conforms to the cellular arrangement of the tissue in which they are found.

This micrograph illustrates sinusoids **S** between cords of secretory cells in the anterior pituitary. Several endothelial cell nuclei **E** can be distinguished by their flattened shape.

(a)

(b)

Fig. 8.16 Post-capillary and collecting venules

(a) H & E × 480 (b) H & E × 600 (c) EM × 6 000

The capillary beds are drained by a series of thin-walled vessels which form the first part of the venous system. Examples of each type of vessel are seen in micrograph (a).

Post-capillary venules **PCV** are the smallest of these vessels and are formed by the union of several capillaries **C** to produce a vessel similar in structure but of a wider diameter. Blood flow in post-capillary venules is sluggish and these vessels appear to be the main point at which white blood cells enter and leave the circulation. Post-capillary venules drain into *collecting venules* **CV** which are characterised by their large diameter and a greater number of enveloping pericytes. Collecting venules drain into vessels of progressively greater diameter, the walls of which contain a recognisable layer of smooth muscle and which are therefore known as *muscular venules* **MV**. This micrograph also shows a very small arteriole **A** with only a single layer of smooth muscle cells in its wall.

Micrograph (b) illustrates a post-capillary venule in the supporting tissue of a mildly inflamed organ. In early acute inflammation, leucocytes (predominantly neutrophils) are typically seen close to the endothelium at the margin of the erythrocyte stream, a phenomenon known as *margination*.

Micrograph (c) shows a lymphocyte in the process of migration from a post-capillary venule, its pseudopodium **Ps** having lifted up the marginal fold **MF** at the contact point of two endothelial cells **E**. In contrast to capillaries, intercellular junctional complexes are relatively uncommon between the endothelial cells of post-capillary venules thus facilitating leucocyte emigration.

(c)

The venous system

With the exception of the venous components of the microcirculation, the venous system merely functions as a low pressure collecting system for the return of blood from the capillary networks to the heart. Blood flow in veins occurs passively down a pressure gradient towards the heart. With each inspiratory cycle, a negative pressure is created within the chest and hence within the right atrium of the heart. Venous return from the limbs is aided by the contraction of skeletal muscles which compress the veins contained within them. During expiration, the pressure gradients are reversed and blood tends to flow in the opposite direction. This is prevented by the presence of valves in veins of medium size. The valves also overcome the problem of reverse flow due to the effects of gravity especially in the lower limbs. Valve failure is the basis for the development of varicose veins.

The structure of the venous system conforms to the general three layered arrangement elsewhere in the circulatory system, but the elastic and muscular components are much less prominent features. A major part of the total blood volume is contained within the venous system. Variations in relative blood volume, due for example to dilation of capillary beds or haemorrhage, may be compensated by changes in the capacity of the venous system. These changes are mediated by smooth muscle in the tunica media which controls the luminal diameter of muscular venules and veins.

(a)

(b)

Fig. 8.17 Muscular venules and small veins *(H & E (a) × 128 (b) × 128)*

Micrograph (a) illustrates the confluence of a small muscular venule **V₁** with a larger muscular venule **V₂** which then joins a small vein **V₃** cut in transverse section. Note the valve at the junction of the large venule and vein. Muscular venules are characterised by a clearly defined intimal layer devoid of elastic fibres and a tunica media consisting of one or two layers of smooth muscle fibres. Veins are characterised by a thicker muscular wall and a poorly developed internal elastic

lamina. Note that the tunica adventitia of these vessels is continuous with the surrounding collagenous supporting tissue.

Micrograph (b) shows a small vein cut in longitudinal section and fixed whilst still distended with blood. The wall of the vein consists of two to three layers of smooth muscle fibres. Note the wide diameter of the lumen relative to the thickness of the wall.

Fig. 8.18 Vein with valve

(Masson's trichrome × 128)

This micrograph demonstrates a valve in a small vein. The valve consists of delicate semilunar projections of the tunica intima of the vein wall; the projections are composed of fibro-elastic tissue lined on both sides by endothelium. Each valve usually consists of two leaflets, the free edges of which project in the direction of blood flow. Valves only occur in veins of more than 2 mm in diameter, particularly those draining the extremities.

Fig. 8.19 Vein *(H & E × 128)*

Small and medium size veins are characterised by the following features demonstrated in this micrograph of a medium size vein:

The tunica intima consists of little more than the endothelial lining; in veins that are not distended with blood the endothelium may be thrown up into small folds. The tunica media **M** is thin compared with that of arteries and consists of two or more layers of circularly arranged smooth muscle fibres. The tunica adventitia **A** is the broadest layer of the vessel wall and is composed of longitudinally arranged thick collagen fibres which merge with the surrounding collagenous tissue.

Note that the wall of the vein is thin relative to the diameter of the lumen. In contrast, in most arteries, the thickness of the wall approximates the diameter of the lumen.

Fig. 8.20 Large muscular vein *(Elastic van Gieson × 128)*

Large veins such as the femoral and renal veins have a relatively thick muscular wall **M** consisting of several layers of smooth muscle (stained yellow in this specimen) separated by layers of collagenous connective tissue (stained red). The tunica media and tunica intima also contain a few elastic fibres (stained black in this preparation) but there is no distinct internal elastic lamina as in arteries of comparable size.

The tunica adventitia **A** is broad and contains numerous vasa vasorum **V** reflecting the need for arterial blood by the tissues of the vein wall. Vasa vasorum as well as lymphatics also penetrate the whole thickness of the muscular wall and are much more numerous than in arterial vessels of similar size.

The largest vessels of the venous system, the *venae cavae*, have a structure similar to that just described except that the smooth muscle is disposed longitudinally rather than in a circular fashion. This arrangement may reflect the need for elongation and shortening to accommodate chest expansion and contraction during the respiratory cycle.

Fig. 8.21 Small neurovascular bundle

(H & E × 150)

The vessels supplying and draining a particular area of tissue tend to pass together, frequently accompanied by a peripheral nerve and invested by a condensation of the surrounding collagenous tissue which forms an ill-defined protective sheath. This micrograph shows such a small neurovascular bundle containing a small arteriole **A**, venules **V**, a lymphatic **L** and a nerve **N**.

The lymph vascular system

The lymph vascular system drains excess fluid, the *lymph*, from extracellular spaces and returns it to the blood vascular system. Lymph is formed in the following manner. At the arterial end of blood capillaries, the hydrostatic pressure of blood exceeds the colloidal osmotic pressure exerted by plasma proteins. Water and electrolytes therefore pass out of capillaries into the extracellular space; some plasma proteins also leak out through the endothelial wall. At the venous end of blood capillaries, the pressure relationships are reversed and fluid tends to be drawn back into the blood vascular system. In this way, about two percent of plasma passing through the capillary bed is exchanged with the extracellular tissue fluid. The rate of tissue fluid formation at the arterial end of capillaries generally exceeds the re-uptake of fluid at the venous end. The excess fluid, lymph, is drained by a system of lymph capillaries which converge to form progressively larger diameter lymphatic vessels. Lymph enters the venous system by a single vessel on each side of the body, namely the thoracic duct (on the left) and the right lymphatic duct. Movement of lymph in the lymph vascular system is similar to movement of blood in the venous system but valves are more numerous in lymphatic vessels.

Along the course of the larger lymphatic vessels are aggregations of lymphoid tissues called lymph nodes where lymph is sampled for the presence of foreign material (antigen) and where activated cells of the immune system and antibodies join the general circulation (see Ch. 11). Lymphatic vessels are found in all tissues except the central nervous system, cartilage, bone, bone marrow, thymus, placenta, cornea and teeth. The structure of lymphatic vessels conforms closely to that of vessels of similar diameter in the venous system. Lymphatic vessels may be distinguished from venous vessels by the absence of erythrocytes and the presence of small numbers of leucocytes mainly lymphocytes. Lymphatic capillaries differ from blood capillaries in several respects which reflect the greater permeability of lymphatic capillaries. In particular, the endothelial cell cytoplasm of lymphatics is extremely thin, the basement membrane is rudimentary or absent and there are no pericytes. Fine collagenous filaments known as *anchoring filaments* link the endothelium to the surrounding supporting tissue preventing collapse of the lymphatic lumen.

Fig. 8.22 Small lymphatic vessel
(H & E × 320)

This micrograph illustrates the characteristic histological differences between a small lymphatic **L** and a venule **V**. Lymphatics do not contain erythrocytes but often contain a few lymphocytes. The stained amorphous material seen in this lymphatic is the protein of lymph which becomes precipitated during tissue processing. The presence of such material is often a distinguishing feature of lymphatics in histological preparations.

Fig. 8.23 Valve of a lymphatic vessel
(H & E × 40)

A characteristic feature of the lymphatic system is the numerous delicate valves in small and medium sized vessels. The structure of these valves **V** is similar to that of valves in the venous system, but the supporting tissue core consists merely of reticulin fibres and a little ground substance. Note the presence of lymphocytes at the periphery of the lumina.

9. Skin

Introduction

The skin forms the continuous external surface or *integument* of the body. The skin is the largest organ of the body, constituting almost one sixth of the total body weight; it has four major functions:

- **Protection.** The skin provides protection against ultraviolet light and mechanical, chemical and thermal insults; its relatively impermeable surface prevents dehydration and acts as a physical barrier to invasion by micro-organisms.
- **Sensation.** The skin is the largest sensory organ in the body and contains a variety of receptors for touch, pressure, pain and temperature. These are described and illustrated in Chapter 7.
- **Thermoregulation.** In man, skin is a major organ of thermoregulation. The body is insulated against heat loss by the presence of hairs and subcutaneous adipose tissue. Heat loss is facilitated by evaporation of sweat from the skin surface and increased blood flow through the rich vascular network of the dermis.
- **Metabolic functions.** Subcutaneous adipose tissue constitutes a major store of energy, mainly in the form of triglycerides. Vitamin D is synthesised in the epidermis and supplements that derived from dietary sources.

In different regions of the body the skin varies in thickness, colour and the presence of hairs, glands and nails. Despite these variations which reflect different functional demands, all types of skin have the same basic structure.

The external surface of skin consists of a keratinised squamous epithelium called the *epidermis*, its thickness varying according to the functional forces and dehydrating influences to which it is subjected. *Thick skin* is mainly found on the palms of the hands and fingers and soles of the feet.

The epidermis is supported and nourished by a thick layer of dense, fibro-elastic tissue called the *dermis* which is highly vascular and contains many sensory receptors. The dermis is attached to underlying tissues by a layer of loose tissue called the *hypodermis* or *subcutaneous* layer which contains variable amounts of adipose tissue. The hypodermis represents the *superficial fascia* of gross anatomy. Hair follicles, sweat glands, sebaceous glands and nails are epithelial structures termed *epidermal appendages* since they originate during embryological development from downgrowths of epidermal epithelium into the dermis and hypodermis.

Fig. 9.1 Thick skin *(Masson's trichrome × 8)*

The general structure of skin is illustrated in this specimen from the fingertip. The epidermis **E** consists of a stratified squamous keratinising epithelium which has an extremely thick keratinised surface layer. A prominent feature of the skin of the fingertips, palms and soles of the feet is a pattern of surface ridges formed by the epidermis; this pattern is unique to each individual and is the basis of fingerprint identification.

The epidermis is supported by the dermis **D**, a layer of dense fibro-elastic tissue, the fibres of which are stained blue-green in this preparation. The dermis merges with the loose supporting tissue of the hypodermis **H** which consists largely of adipose tissue; in the fingertips, adipose tissue acts as a soft, shock-absorbing layer. Numerous sweat glands **S** are located in the dermis and hypodermis and discharge their secretions onto the skin surface via long excretory ducts **Dt**. Pressure receptors, Pacinian corpuscles **Pc** (see Fig. 7.28) are located deep in the dermis and are a prominent feature of fingertip skin.

The junction between the epidermis and dermis is characterised by downward folds of the epidermis called *epidermal* or *rete ridges* which interdigitate with upward projections of the dermis called *dermal papillae*. This arrangement, which is shown diagrammatically in Figure 9.9, enhances the adhesion of the epidermis to the dermis and is most prominent in skin subject to considerable frictional forces, e.g. palms of hands.

Fig. 9.2 Epidermis *(H & E × 104)*

This section of thick skin, taken from the same specimen as in Fig. 9.1, demonstrates the general features of the epidermis. Cells produced by mitosis in the germinal layer adjacent to the dermis undergo maturational changes concerned with the production of keratin. The outer keratinised layer is shed continuously and is replaced by the progressive movement and maturation of cells from the germinal layer; thus all of the cells of this lineage are often described as *keratinocytes*. The rate of mitosis in the germinal layer generally equals the rate of desquamation of keratin from the outer surface; in humans, the process of maturation of a basal cell through to desquamation takes from 25 to 50 days being more rapid in areas exposed to heavy frictional forces.

The phases of this dynamic process are represented in five morphological layers:

- The *stratum germinativum* or stratum basale **B** is the germinal layer of the epidermis. This layer is also sometimes referred to as the *stratum malpighii*.
- The *stratum spinosum* or *prickle cell layer* **S**, so named for the 'prickly' appearance of the cells at high magnification (see Fig. 9.4), contains cells which are in the process of growth and early keratin synthesis.
- The *stratum granulosum* or *granular layer* **G** is characterised by intracellular granules which contribute to the process of keratinisation.
- The *stratum lucidum* **L** is only present in extremely thick skin, and appears as a homogeneous layer between the stratum granulosum and the keratinised layer.
- The *stratum corneum* or *cornified layer* **C** consists of flattened, fused cell remnants composed mainly of the fibrous protein, keratin.

Fig. 9.3 Thin skin *(H & E × 128)*

In this preparation of thin skin from the abdomen, the individual cellular layers are more difficult to discern and a stratum lucidum is not present. In comparison with thick skin, the stratum corneum is much reduced in thickness and the combined thickness of the other layers is reduced to a lesser extent. The rete (epidermal) ridge system is much less prominent, reflecting the relatively lower shearing forces to which such thin skin is subjected.

Fig. 9.4 Epidermis *(a) Masson's trichrome × 600*

(b) Thin section, toluidine blue × 1200

The cytological details of the layers of the epidermis are illustrated in micrograph (a) whilst micrograph (b) focuses on the prickle cell layer.

Stratum basale B. The cells of this layer are cuboidal and form a single layer separated from the dermis **D** by a basement membrane too thin to be resolved by light microscopy. The basal aspect of each germinal cell is highly irregular and bound to the basement membrane by numerous hemi-desmosomes (see Fig. 5.13). Like the cells of the adjacent stratum spinosum, small cytoplasmic projections extend across the intercellular spaces to abut upon those of adjacent cells; desmosomes bind these contact points. Mitotic figures are most frequently observed in this layer but cell division also occurs to a lesser extent in the stratum spinosum.

Stratum spinosum S. The so-called 'prickle cells' of this zone are relatively large and polyhedral in shape and have numerous cytoplasmic 'prickles' bound by desmosomes to adjacent cells. Prominent nucleoli and cytoplasmic basophilia indicate active protein synthesis. A fibrillar protein *cytokeratin*, the predominant synthetic product of these cells, aggregates to form intracellular fibrils known as *tonofibrils* which converge upon the desmosomes of the cytoplasmic 'prickles'; tonofibrils are stained red in this preparation and become more prominent towards the stratum granulosum. Tonofibrils are also found in small numbers in the cells of the stratum basale.

Stratum granulosum G. The cells of this layer are characterised by numerous, dense basophilic granules which crowd the cytoplasm and tend to obscure the tonofibrils. The chemical nature of these *keratohyalin granules* is distinct from that of the fibrous protein of the tonofibrils. The process of keratinisation is thought to involve the combination of tonofibril and keratohyalin elements to form the mature keratin complex. In the outermost aspect of the stratum granulosum, cell death occurs due to rupture of lysosomal membranes; released lysosomal enzymes may play an important role in the final process of keratinisation. A **stratum lucidum** is not seen in this preparation but, when present (very thick skin only), appears as a homogeneous layer between the stratum granulosum and stratum corneum; it may merely represent a compressed transitional zone between these layers.

Stratum corneum C. The morphology and staining characteristics of this layer are strikingly different from that of the underlying layers. The dead and dying cells are flattened, devoid of nuclei and other organelles and filled with mature keratin. In the deeper aspect of this layer, the cornified cells retain their desmosomal junctions and the intracellular keratin has an ordered pattern. Towards the surface, the desmosomes and internal structure of the cells become completely disrupted, a process which precedes desquamation.

In addition to the keratinocytes, three other cell types (all poorly stained) are found in the epidermis. The most common of these are the *melanocytes* responsible for skin pigmentation (see Fig. 9.5) which are usually confined to the basal layer.

Merkel cells are associated with free nerve endings in thick skin and are presumed to serve as sensory receptors; their ultrastructural features suggest that they form part of the diffuse neuroendocrine system (see Ch. 17).

Langerhan's cells are specialised representatives of the

(a)

(b)

macrophage-monocyte system which act as antigen-presenting cells in the skin. They are found in small numbers throughout the lower epidermal layers having long dendritic processes extending between surrounding keratinocytes. Their numbers increase in atopic and other immunologically based skin disorders. When stimulated they migrate via dermal lymphatics to the paracortical zones of regional lymph nodes for presentation of antigen to T lymphocytes. In micrograph (a), a poorly stained cell can be seen in the lower prickle cell layer representing either a Merkel or Langerhan's cell.

Fig. 9.5 Skin pigmentation

(a) Caucasian abdominal skin: H & E × 320
(b) Negroid abdominal skin: H & E × 320
(c) Caucasian forearm skin: thin section, toluidine blue × 600

The colour of human skin depends on three major factors. Firstly, the skin has an inherent yellowish colour due in part to the presence of various carotene pigments in the subcutaneous fat. Secondly, the concentration and state of oxygenation of haemoglobin, and the presence of other pigments such as bile pigments in blood are reflected in skin colour. Thirdly, skin colour is determined by the amount of the pigment *melanin* present in the epidermis; this is the most important variable between parts of the body, between individuals of the same race and between members of different races.

Melanin is synthesised by *melanocytes* which are of neuro-ectodermal (neural crest) origin, migrating during development to the epidermis where they become scattered in the basal layers in contact with the basement membrane. Melanocytes have long, dendritic processes which ramify between the epithelial cells but which do not establish cell junctions with the epithelial cells. Their cell bodies are usually located between the basal epithelial cells and the basement membrane but may be seen between the epithelial cells at higher levels.

The ratio of melanocytes to basal epithelial cells varies from about one in five to one in ten in different regions of the body, being highest in the skin of the face and external genitalia. The number of melanocytes is relatively constant between different individuals irrespective of race; differences in skin colour are thus due to the amount of melanin produced rather than the number of melanocytes present.

Melanin synthesis involves conversion of the amino acid tyrosine, via intermediates including dihydroxyphenylalanine (DOPA), to melanin. Within melanocytes, melanin accumulates in immature secretory vesicles known as *premelanosomes*. These mature to form *melanosomes* which are then disseminated throughout the long, cytoplasmic processes from which they are transferred to surrounding keratinocytes cells especially in the basal layers. Hence, the pigmented cells of skin are both the melanocytes which synthesise melanin and the epithelial cells which have taken up melanin; commonly, epithelial cells contain much more melanin than the melanocytes themselves. The size, shape, and rate of production of melanosomes varies between individuals of one race and between racial groups. In blond and red-haired people there are biochemical differences in the form of melanin produced. Sunlight promotes melanin synthesis and causes darkening of previously synthesised melanin. In addition, melanin synthesis is stimulated by the pituitary hormone, *melanocyte stimulating hormone (MSH)* although the physiological importance of this in humans is not well understood (see Ch. 17).

Micrographs (a) and (b) permit comparison of Caucasian and Negroid skin. In the Caucasian, there are merely traces of melanin in the basal epithelial cells and the relatively inactive melanocytes **M** are unstained. In contrast, the basal epithelial cells of Negroid skin are packed with melanin and melanocytes themselves are difficult to identify. In thin sections, as in micrograph (c), melanocytes **M** and their major dendritic processes are readily distinguishable from the surrounding epithelial cells.

(a)

(b)

(c)

(a)

(b)

(c)

Fig. 9.6 Dermis

(a) H & E × 60 (b) H & E × 100 (c) Elastic van Gieson × 150

The dermal layer of the skin provides a robust supporting base for the epidermis as well as incorporating a generous vascular system necessary for the metabolic support of the avascular epidermis and for thermoregulation.

As seen in micrograph (a), the dermis is divided into two zones. Superficially, the dermal papillae and immediately subjacent tissue comprise the *papillary dermis* **P** which is relatively loose and highly vascular with fine interlacing collagen fibres. It accommodates the subpapillary arterial, venous and lymphatic plexuses and papillary vascular loops; these are described in Fig. 9.18. It also contains the fine axonal connections of free sensory nerve endings in the epidermis (see Fig. 7.27) and, in highly sensitive areas, the small encapsulated Meissner's corpuscles (see Fig. 7.28).

The main bulk of the dermis comprises the *reticular layer* **R**, so named for the interlacing (reticular) arrangement of its collagen fibres. As seen in micrograph (b), the collagen fibres are coarse and disposed in thick irregular bundles cut in many different planes. As seen in micrograph (a), the reticular dermis contains blood vessels **V** connecting the subpapillary plexuses with the cutaneous plexuses, the latter located at the junction of the dermis and hypodermis. Two arterioles **A** in various planes of section, can be identified in micrograph (b), snaking their way towards the surface. A small peripheral nerve **N** can be also identified.

Elastin is an important constituent of both layers of the dermis and is highlighted in micrograph (c) in which it stains black amongst the red-stained collagen. The elastin forms a fine interlacing network of fibres in the papillary dermis **P** whereas in the reticular layer **R** the elastin forms long thick fibres which follow the path of the coarse interlacing collagen bundles.

The cells of the dermis are mainly fibroblasts responsible for elaboration of the collagen, elastin and ground substance. Various white blood cells, mast cells and tissue macrophages involved in non-specific defence and immune surveillance functions are also present.

(a)

(b)

(c)

Fig. 9.7 Epidermis *(illustration (a) opposite)*

EM (a) × 8 000 (b) × 8 000 (c) × 17 000

These micrographs illustrate the ultrastructure of thin skin from an albino rat.

The full thickness of the epidermis is shown at low magnification in micrograph (a); this demonstrates the transition of keratinocytes from a cuboidal form in the basal layer **B** through the prickle shape of the stratum spinosum **S** to the flattened form in the granular layer **G**. Towards the surface, cellular outline and nuclei are lost with the formation of the homogeneous keratinised stratum corneum **C**; at the surface is a flake of keratin **K** in the process of desquamation. Basement membrane **BM** separates the stratum basale from the underlying papillary dermis **D** which contains a fibroblast **F**, a capillary **Cap** and extensive fine collagen fibrils **Co**.

Micrograph (b) shows another part of the basal layer at higher magnification and includes parts of the cell bodies of two melanocytes **M** typically located adjacent to the basement membrane **BM**. As this is a specimen of non-pigmented skin, the melanocytes are devoid of melanosomes. Numerous fine cytoplasmic processes ramify between the keratinocytes providing the means of transfer of melanin from the melanocytes to the keratinising cells. The intimate relationship of these melanocytic processes **Mp** is shown at greater magnification in micrograph (c). Note the hemidesmosomes **H** (see Fig. 5.13) which bind the basal cells to the basement membrane **BM** and thence to the fibres of the extracellular matrix of the underlying dermis **D**. A cytoplasmic process of a fibroblast **F** can be seen in the dermis.

(a)

(b)

Fig. 9.8 Epidermis *(illustration (a) opposite; (a) EM × 15 000 (b) EM × 58 000)*

Micrograph (a) illustrates the transition of cells from the stratum spinosum **S** to the stratum granulosum **G**. The polygonal-shaped cells of the stratum spinosum exhibit numerous cytoplasmic spines (prickles) which are tightly bound to those of adjacent cells by desmosomes **D**, shown at high magnification in micrograph (b). The desmosomes are the anchorage points for numerous bundles of intermediate filaments called *tonofibrils* **T** composed of the protein cytokeratin, the arrangement conferring great resistance to potentially disruptive abrasive forces at the epidermal surface. Between the cytoplasmic spines are numerous fine interdigitating cytoplasmic processes **P** separated by narrow extracellular spaces and probably involved in exchange and diffusion of metabolites (bearing in mind the absence of blood vessels in the epidermis). Apart from tonofibrils, the most obvious feature of the prickle cell cytoplasm is the numerous ribosomes involved in cytokeratin synthesis.

Referring back to micrograph (a), the cells of the stratum granulosum are flattened and devoid of 'prickles' and interdigitating cytoplasmic processes, the intercellular space having by now been almost obliterated. The cytoplasm is characterised by numerous non-membrane bound electron-dense granules of the protein keratohyalin **K**. As seen here, in the upper part of the stratum granulosum, the cell outlines are barely distinguishable and the cytoplasm contains an increasingly amorphous mass of keratohyalin and tonofibrillar material. Beyond this point the keratinocytes die, the release of lysosomal enzymes catalysing some form of polymerisation of the keratohyalin granules and cytokeratin filaments to form the amorphous mass of surface keratin. The cells of the granular layer also produce a hydrophobic glycophospholipid which acts as an intercellular cement preventing disaggregation of the surface squames and rendering the skin surface impermeable to water.

Epidermis

Dermal papillae

Dermis

Arrector pili

Merocrine sweat gland

Hypodermis

Sebaceous gland

Hair follicle

Hair bulb

Fig. 9.9 Skin appendages

Skin has a variety of appendages, principally hairs, sebaceous glands and sweat glands, which are derived embryonically from the surface epithelium (epidermis). The distribution, arrangement and detailed structure of the appendages varies from one part of the skin to another but nevertheless the general structure conforms to a basic pattern. The three-dimensional arrangement shown in this diagram has been deduced from studies of serial sections of skin; individual sections of skin rarely demonstrate all these features.

Hairs. Hairs are highly modified keratinised structures produced by *hair follicles* which are essentially cylindrical downgrowth of the surface epithelium ensheathed by collagenous tissue. Hair growth takes place within a terminal expansion of the follicle, the *hair bulb*, which consists of actively dividing epithelial cells surrounding a papilla of vascular tissue, the *dermal papilla*.

A bundle of smooth muscle cells, the *arrector pili* muscle, is attached to the follicular sheath and is inserted into the dermal papillary zone. Contraction of the arrector pili causes the hair to become erect and pulls down its point of insertion, producing the effect known as 'goose-flesh'.

The arrector pili muscles are innervated by the sympathetic nervous system and pilo-erection is activated by cold or fear. In furry animals, hair erection traps a thicker layer of air over the skin surface thus increasing insulation against heat loss; hair erection also makes the animal appear larger and is thus a protective mechanism in dangerous circumstances. These functions are probably of little physiological significance in humans. However, contraction of the arrector pili may play some part in expulsion of sebum from sebaceous glands.

Sebaceous glands. One or more sebaceous glands are associated with each hair follicle; these glands secrete an oily substance called *sebum* onto the hair surface in the upper part of the follicle. Sebum acts as a waterproofing and moisturising agent for the hair and skin surface. In regions of transition from the skin to the body tracts such as the lips, eyelids, glans penis, labia minora and nipples, sebaceous glands are found independent of hair follicles and secrete directly on to the skin surface.

Sweat glands. In most areas of the skin, sweat glands are simple, coiled tubular glands which secrete a watery fluid onto the skin surface by the process of merocrine secretion (see Ch. 5). The coiled, secretory portions of these glands are an important component of the thermoregulatory mechanism in humans. When the body requires to lose heat, skin blood flow and sweat production are increased; evaporation of sweat causes cooling of the skin surface and loss of heat from the underlying vascular bed. Merocrine sweat glands are innervated by cholinergic fibres of the sympathetic nervous system; sweating is stimulated not only by excessive body heat but also by fear-provoking stimuli.

A different type of sweat gland is found in the skin of the axilla and genital regions of humans. In contrast to the merocrine sweat glands, these glands are believed to secrete by the apocrine process (see Ch. 5) and are thus called *apocrine sweat glands*. They also differ in that they produce a viscid secretion which is discharged into hair follicles rather than directly on to the surface. Apocrine sweat glands are innervated by adrenergic fibres of the sympathetic nervous system.

(a)

(b)

(c)

Fig. 9.10 Regional variations of skin structure

(a) Scalp skin: Masson's (green) trichrome × 12 (b) Abdominal skin: Masson's (blue) trichrome × 12 (c) Pubic skin: H & E × 12

The structure of the skin differs considerably from one part of the body to another, the principal differences being in epidermal thickness, the size, density and state of activity of the hair follicles, and the nature and density of sweat glands and sensory receptors. These micrographs illustrate three extremes of structure in hairy skin.

As seen in micrograph (a), the skin of the scalp is robust due to a thick, densely collagenous dermis (stained blue-green in this preparation), and the hair follicles **F** are numerous and closely packed. In fair-haired people, the follicles are fewer in number and somewhat smaller in size, producing finer hair. The follicles of the scalp are particularly long and have more numerous sebaceous glands **S** than those of other areas. Note the arrector pili muscles **A** extending from the base of the follicles towards the upper dermis. Merocrine sweat glands **G** are numerous though less prominent than in the skin of the trunk and limbs due to the profusion of other appendages.

Micrograph (b) illustrates the typical histological appearance of the skin which covers most of the body. The hair follicles **F** and associated sebaceous glands **S** are sparse and merocrine sweat glands **G** are relatively shorter; the hairs produced are finer.

The skin of the axillae and pubic region, shown in micrograph (c), exhibits a moderate density of hair follicles **F** which, unlike those of the scalp, tend to be oriented obliquely to the skin surface and are often curved rather than straight causing the hairs to be curled. Apocrine sweat glands **A** are a common feature of this type of skin and are seen typically associated with hair follicles into which they discharge their secretions.

GM
Cu
M
Cx
IRS
ERS
CT

DP

(a)   *(b)*

Fig. 9.11 Hair follicle *(a) H & E × 120 (b) Explanatory diagram*

The hair follicle is a tubular structure consisting of five concentric layers of epithelial cells. At the base, there is a bulbous expansion, the hair bulb, enclosing the dermal papilla **DP**. As they are pushed towards the skin surface from the hair bulb, the inner three epithelial layers undergo keratinisation to form the hair shaft whilst the outer two layers form an epithelial sheath. At the hair bulb, all the layers merge to become indistinguishable from one another; the mass of cells destined to form the hair is known as the *hair matrix*.

During active hair growth, the epithelial cells surrounding the dermal papilla proliferate to form the four inner layers of the follicle whilst the outermost layer merely represents a downward continuation of the stratum germinativum of the surface epithelium. The whole epithelial mass surrounding the dermal papilla constitutes the *hair root*.

The cells of the innermost layer of the follicle undergo moderate keratinisation to form the *medulla* **M** or core of the hair shaft; the medullary layer is often not distinguishable in fine hairs. The medulla is surrounded by a broad, highly keratinised layer, the *cortex* **Cx**, which forms the bulk of the hair. The third cell layer of the follicle undergoes keratinisation to form a hard, thin *cuticle* **Cu** on the surface of the hair. The cuticle consists of overlapping keratin plates, an arrangement which is said to prevent matting of the hair.

The fourth layer of the follicle constitutes the *internal root sheath* **IRS**; the cells of this layer become only lightly keratinised and disintegrate at the level of the sebaceous gland ducts leaving a space into which sebum is secreted around the maturing hair. The outermost layer, the *external root sheath* **ERS**, does not take part in hair formation; this layer is separated from the sheath of connective tissue **CT** surrounding the follicle by a thick, specialised basement membrane known as the *glassy membrane* **GM**.

In the growing follicle, large active melanocytes (see Fig. 9.5) are scattered amongst the proliferating cells with melanin being incorporated in the cortex of the hair shaft. Black, brown and yellow forms of melanin are produced in various combinations to determine final hair colour. In infancy, childhood and females, body hair is fine and soft and known as *vellus* in contrast to the coarser hair of the scalp which is known as *terminal hair*. Male sex hormone production at puberty is responsible for the development of further terminal pubic and axillary hair in both sexes and for the replacement of vellus hair with terminal hair on the mature male body.

The cross-sectional shape of hairs also varies between races. The straight hair of the Mongol races is round in cross-section, the wavy hair characteristic of Europeans is oval and the curly hair of black skinned peoples is more kidney-shaped.

In addition, the structure of hair follicles depends on the type of hair being produced. For example, the follicles of the scalp and other terminal hairs tend to be long and straight, whereas those of the body, which produce fine, downy hair (vellus), are relatively short and plump; curly hair may be produced by curved follicles or follicles in which the hair bulb lies at an angle to the hair shaft.

Fig. 9.12 Hair follicle

(H & E × 198)

This is a slightly oblique, transverse section through the lower part of a hair follicle. The broad external root sheath **E** is separated from the collagenous root sheath **S** by the glassy membrane **G**. Passing inwards, the internal root sheath **I** is recognised by its content of eosinophilic (keratohyalin) granules; the outermost cells of the internal root sheath have a more homogeneous appearance. Deep to the internal root sheath is the thin, pale-stained cuticle layer **Cu** which surrounds the strongly stained cortex **Cx**. A medulla is not present in this specimen.

Fig. 9.13 Hair bulb *(Masson's trichrome × 198)*

This staining method permits clear delineation of the epithelial and collagenous elements of the hair follicle. The dermal papilla **DP** is highly vascular and is separated from the epithelial cells by a basement membrane which is continuous with the glassy membrane **G** surrounding the follicle externally. The sheath of the follicle is also rich in blood vessels and contains a delicate plexus of sensory nerve endings which are receptive to minute movements of the hair follicle and thus act as highly sensitive touch receptors.

Note the five cell layers of the hair follicle merging with the proliferating cells of the hair root. Note also the large amount of pigment in the basal layer extending up into the cortical layer and produced by melanocytes scattered along the basement membrane of the hair root.

Individual hair follicles undergo cycles of growth and quiescence and this is reflected in changes in their structure. In the *growing phase*, follicles penetrate deeply into the hypodermis and the hair bulb is prominent, whereas during the *resting phase*, follicles are shorter and the hair bulb is smaller and lacking in a dermal papilla; quiescent follicles are known as *club hairs*.

This cyclical growth pattern is the factor which determines the limits of length reached by hairs in different parts of the body. For example, the growth phase of head hairs is of the order of two years or more, each hair being shed during a follicular resting phase lasting a matter of months. Only a small proportion of follicles are normally in the resting phase at any one time thus maintaining a continuous crop of hair. In contrast, body hairs, eyebrows, eyelashes, etc. have a relatively short growth phase and longer resting phase preventing inappropriate overgrowth. This explains why pubic hair does not reach the knees!

(a)

(b)

(c)

Fig. 9.14 Sebaceous glands

(H & E (a) × 33 (b) × 150 (c) × 198)

Micrograph (a) illustrates the relationship of a sebaceous gland **G** and an arrector pili muscle **M** to a hair follicle **F**. At a point about one-third of its length from the surface, each hair follicle is surrounded by one or more sebaceous glands which discharge their secretions on to the hair shaft and thence on to the skin surface. As seen in micrograph (b), sebaceous glands lie within the sheath surrounding the hair follicle and the glandular epithelium represents an outgrowth of the external root sheath.

The arrector pili muscle of each follicle consists of a bundle of smooth muscle fibres. The muscle inserts at one end into the sheath of the follicle at a point below the sebaceous glands, and at the other end into the dermal papillary area beneath the epidermis. Each hair follicle and its associated arrector pili muscle and sebaceous glands is known as a *pilosebaceous unit*. Note that the bulk of the sebaceous glands and the arrector pili muscle lie on that aspect of the hair to which the hair follicle inclines.

More detail of sebaceous gland structure can be seen in micrograph (c). Each sebaceous gland has a branched acinar form, the acini converging upon a short duct which empties into the hair follicle beside the maturing hair. Each acinus consists of a mass of rounded cells which are packed with lipid-filled vacuoles; during tissue preparation the lipid is largely removed leaving the cytoplasm of these cells poorly stained. Towards the duct, the lipid content of the acinar cells increases greatly and the distended cells degenerate, so releasing their contents, sebum, into the duct by the process known as holocrine secretion (see Ch. 5). Cells lost by holocrine secretion are replaced by mitosis in the basal layer of the acinus.

(a)

(b)

Fig. 9.15 Merocrine (eccrine) sweat glands *(H & E (a) × 198 (b) × 480)*

Merocrine sweat glands are distributed in the skin of most parts of the body with the exception of areas such as the margins of the lip and the glans penis. Merocrine sweat glands secrete a watery fluid, hypotonic with respect to plasma, the evaporation of which plays an important role in thermoregulation. Sweat contains significant quantities of sodium and chloride ions, some other ions, urea and small molecular weight metabolites; thus sweating may be considered as a minor mode of excretion.

Merocrine sweat glands are unbranched tubular glands, the secretory portion forming a compact coil in the more superficial part of the fatty hypodermis. In histological section, the glands appear as a mass of tubules cut in various planes; secretory portions are interspersed with sections of the first part of the excretory duct. The secretory portion **S** consists of a single layer of large cuboidal or columnar cells, whereas the excretory duct **D** is lined by two layers of smaller cuboidal cells. The surrounding dermis contains a rich capillary plexus.

At higher magnification, the secretory portions **S** of merocrine sweat glands are seen to be mainly composed of pale-stained, pyramidal cells which rest on a prominent basement membrane. These cells are believed to pump sodium ions into the gland lumen; this is followed by passive diffusion of water. A second less numerous, darkly-stained cell type, which is difficult to identify with light microscopy, has ultrastructural features typical of protein secreting cells. The dark cells are believed to secrete a glycoprotein, nevertheless the content of such in sweat is very low. Myoepithelial cells **M** form a discontinuous layer between the secretory cells and the basement membrane; contraction of these cells expels sweat into the excretory ducts.

Sections of the excretory duct **D** are readily distinguishable from sections of the secretory portion. The excretory duct has a narrower lumen, a double layer of small cuboidal cells, no underlying myoepithelial cells and a characteristically eosinophilic luminal aspect which may result from adsorption of the glycoprotein product of the dark secretory cells. The duct epithelium is thought to reabsorb sodium ions from the basic secretion, thus making it hypotonic with respect to plasma. When seen at low magnification, the ducts pursue a helical course through the dermis to discharge at the skin surface via a *sweat pore* located on an epidermal ridge.

Fig. 9.16 Apocrine sweat glands
(H & E × 128)

Apocrine sweat glands are mainly confined to the areolae of the breasts, axillae and genital regions where they produce a viscid, milky secretion which becomes malodorous after the action of skin commensal bacteria.

Apocrine sweat glands are large glands which always secrete into an adjacent hair follicle via a duct which is histologically similar to that of merocrine sweat glands. The secretory portion of the gland is of the coiled, tubular type with a widely dilated lumen. The secretory cells are usually low cuboidal and have an eosinophilic cytoplasm. The budding appearance of the apical cytoplasm of some cells gave rise to the belief that the mode of secretion was of the apocrine type but recent evidence suggests that this appearance may be due to a fixation artefact and that the original interpretations were erroneous. Like merocrine sweat glands, apocrine glands have a discontinuous layer of myoepithelial cells between the base of the secretory cells and the prominent basement membrane.

Apocrine sweat glands do not become functional until puberty and in women undergo cyclical changes under the influence of the hormones of the menstrual cycle.

Apocrine glands are analogous to the odiferous glands of many mammals but their biological significance in humans is unknown.

(a)

(b)

Fig. 9.17 Fingernail *(Monkey: H & E (a) × 5 (b) × 20)*

The dorsal skin surface of the tip of each finger and toe forms a highly specialised appendage, the nail **N**, consisting of a dense keratinised plate, the *nail plate*, which rests on a stratified squamous epithelium called the *nail bed*. The proximal end of the nail, the *nail root* **R**, and the underlying nail bed, extend deeply into the dermis to lie in close apposition to the distal interphalangeal joint, and the dermis beneath the nail plate is firmly attached to the periosteum of the distal phalanx **DP**.

Nail growth occurs by proliferation and differentiation of the epithelium underlying the nail root (known as the *nail matrix*), and the nail plate slides distally over the rest of the nail bed which does not actively contribute to nail growth. Reflecting its proliferative activity, the nail matrix is thicker than that of the rest of the nail bed and exhibits pronounced epidermal ridges as seen in micrograph (b); on the surface, the distal part of the nail matrix is marked by the white crescent shaped *lunular* at the base of the nail.

The skin overlying the root of the nail is known as the *nail fold* **F** and its highly keratinised free edge is known as the *eponychium* **E**. The skin beneath the free end of the nail is known as the *hyponychium* **H**.

Papillary loops

Arteriovenous anastomosis

Sweat gland

Arterial supply

Subpapillary plexus

Sebaceous gland

Cutaneous plexus

Venous drainage

Fig. 9.18 The skin circulation

The circulation of the skin has an unusual arrangement which accommodates several different, sometimes conflicting, functional requirements: nutrition of the skin and appendages, increased blood flow to facilitate heat loss in hot conditions, and decreased blood flow to minimise heat loss in cold conditions whilst nevertheless maintaining adequate nutritional flow.

The arteries supplying the skin are located deep in the hypodermis from which they give rise to branches passing upwards to form two plexuses of anastomosing vessels. The deeper plexus lies at the junction of the hypodermis and dermis and is known as the *cutaneous plexus*; the more superficial plexus lies just beneath the dermal papillae and is known as the *subpapillary plexus*. Branches of the cutaneous plexus supply the fatty tissue of the hypodermis, the deeper

aspect of the dermis and capillary networks which envelop the hair follicles and deep sebaceous glands and sweat glands. The subpapillary plexus supplies the upper aspect of the dermis and the capillary networks around the superficial appendages. The subpapillary plexus also gives rise to a capillary loop in each dermal papilla. The venous drainage of the skin is arranged into plexuses broadly corresponding to the arterial supply.

Numerous shunts provide direct arterio-venous communications which play an important role in thermoregulation by controlling blood flow to the appropriate part of the dermis.

The skin has a rich lymphatic drainage which forms plexuses corresponding to those of the blood vascular system.

Fig. 9.19 Glomus body *(H & E × 128)*

In the dermis of the finger tips, and other odd peripheral sites prone to excessive cold such as the external ear, the flow in arterio-venous shunts is controlled by structures called *glomus bodies*. The glomus consists of a highly convoluted segment of an arterio-venous shunt enveloped by condensed collagenous tissue. In histological section, one or more convolutions of the arterial **A** and venous **V** elements of the shunt are usually seen. Just before the arterio-venous junction, the wall of the artery becomes greatly thickened and its smooth muscle cells assume an epithelioid appearance.

10. Skeletal tissues

Introduction

The skeletal system is composed of a variety of specialised forms of supporting/connective tissue. Bone provides a rigid protective and supporting framework for most of the soft tissues of the body, whereas cartilage provides semi-rigid support in limited sites such as the respiratory tree and external ear. Cartilage formation is also a precursor in the processes of bone formation by either the membranous or endochondral ossification processes. Joints are composite structures which join the bones of the skeleton and, depending on the function and structure of individual joints, permit varying degrees of movement. Ligaments are robust but flexible bands of collagenous tissue which contribute to the stability of joints. Tendons provide strong, pliable connections between muscles and their points of insertion into bones.

The functional differences between the various tissues of the skeletal system relate principally to the different nature and proportion of the ground substance and fibrous elements of the extracellular matrix. The cells of all the skeletal tissues, like the cells of the less specialised supporting/connective tissues, have close structural and functional relationships and a common origin from primitive mesenchymal cells (see Ch. 4).

Cartilage

Cartilage is a semi-rigid form of supporting tissue, the characteristics of which mainly stem from the nature and predominance of ground substance in the extracellular matrix. Proteoglycans (see Ch. 4), disposed in *proteoglycan aggregates* of one hundred or more molecules, make up the ground substance and account for the solid, yet flexible, consistency of cartilage. Sulphated glycosaminoglycans (chondroitin sulphate and keratan sulphate) predominate in the proteoglycan aggregates with molecules of the non-sulphated GAG, hyaluronic acid, forming the central backbone of the complex.

Within the ground substance are embedded varying proportions of collagen and elastic fibres giving rise to three main types of cartilage: *hyaline cartilage*, *fibrocartilage* and *elastic cartilage*.

Cartilage formation commences with the differentiation of stellate-shaped, primitive mesenchymal cells (see Fig. 4.2) to form rounded cartilage precursor cells called *chondroblasts*. Subsequent mitotic divisions give rise to aggregations of closely packed chondroblasts which grow and begin synthesis of ground substance and fibrous extracellular material. Secretion of extracellular material traps each chondroblast within the cartilaginous matrix thereby separating the chondroblasts from one another. Each chondroblast then undergoes one or two further mitotic divisions to form a small cluster of mature cells separated by a small amount of extracellular material. Mature cartilage cells, known as *chondrocytes*, maintain the integrity of the cartilage matrix. This differentiation and maturation sequence is most advanced in the centre of a mass of growing cartilage. Towards the periphery of the cartilage, chondroblasts at progressively earlier stages of differentiation merge with the surrounding loose supporting tissue. On completion of growth, the cartilage mass consists of chondrocytes embedded in a large amount of extracellular matrix. At the periphery of mature cartilage is a zone of condensed supporting tissue called *perichondrium* containing chondroblasts with cartilage-forming potential. Growth of cartilage occurs by *interstitial growth* from within and *appositional growth* at the periphery.

Most cartilage is devoid of blood vessels and consequently the exchange of metabolites between chondrocytes and surrounding tissues depends on diffusion through the water of solvation of the ground substance. This limits the thickness to which cartilage may develop whilst maintaining viability of the innermost cells; in sites where cartilage is particularly thick (e.g. costal cartilage), *cartilage canals* convey small vessels into the centre of the cartilage mass.

In mature mammals, cartilage has a limited distribution, whereas in immature mammals cartilage forms a template for most of the developing bony skeleton.

(a)

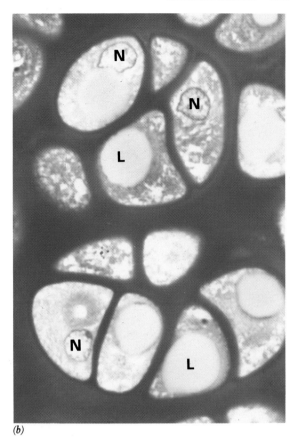

(b)

Fig. 10.1 Hyaline cartilage *(a) H & E × 150 (b) Thin section, toluidine blue × 1200*

Hyaline cartilage is the most common type of cartilage and is found in the nasal septum, larynx, tracheal rings, most articular surfaces and the sternal ends of the ribs. It also forms the precursor of bone in the developing skeleton. Mature hyaline cartilage is characterised by small aggregations of chondrocytes embedded in an amorphous matrix of ground substance reinforced by collagen fibres.

In the preparation of mature hyaline cartilage shown in micrograph (a), two zones are evident: an inner, strongly basophilic zone and a narrow, pale-stained peripheral zone which merges with adjacent supporting tissue containing adipocytes **A**, capillaries **C** and small nerves **N**. The chondrocytes of the inner zone are arranged in characteristic clusters usually consisting of two or four fully differentiated cells. The clusters are separated by a large mass of amorphous cartilage matrix whilst the cells of each cluster are separated by only a thin layer of matrix. In standard histological preparations, considerable shrinkage distorts the cellular detail of the chondrocytes so that they may appear not to fully occupy their spaces within the matrix.

Extending from the inner zone towards the outer surface of the cartilage, the chondrocytes are progressively less differentiated so that the cells of the *perichondrium* **P** at the surface resemble mature fibroblasts. Note that the cells of the peripheral cartilage have not divided to form clusters. The morphological gradation of cartilage cells from the perichondrium to the most mature chondrocytes of the inner zone represents the progressive changes that occur during the development of cartilage. In adult cartilage, cell differentiation in the perichondrium and cartilage periphery is suspended unless growth is stimulated. When growth is stimulated, isolated chondrocytes divide to form clusters thereby promoting interstitial growth whilst, at the same time, chondroblasts of the perichondrium differentiate into chondrocytes resulting in appositional growth.

The matrix of hyaline cartilage appears fairly amorphous since the ground substance and collagen have similar refractive properties. With the exception of articular cartilage, the collagen of hyaline cartilage, designated as collagen Type II (see Ch. 4), is not cross-banded and is arranged in an interlacing network of fine fibrils; this collagen cannot be demonstrated by light microscopy. The variable staining intensity of the cartilage matrix reflects the concentration of acidic, sulphated proteoglycans which is greatest around the clusters of fully differentiated cells and least in the perichondrium.

With the technique employed in micrograph (b), the cellular detail of chondrocytes is preserved. Note that the chondrocytes fully occupy the spaces in the matrix, each space containing a single chondrocyte. Mature chondrocytes are characterised by small nuclei with dispersed chromatin and basophilic, granular cytoplasm reflecting a well developed rough endoplasmic reticulum. Lipid droplets **L**, often larger than the nuclei **N**, are a prominent feature of larger chondrocytes; the cytoplasm is also rich in glycogen. These characteristics reflect the active role of chondrocytes in synthesis of both the ground substance and fibrous elements of the cartilage matrix. In fully formed cartilage, the constituents of the extracellular matrix are continuously turned over, the integrity of the matrix being thus absolutely dependent on the viability of the chondrocytes.

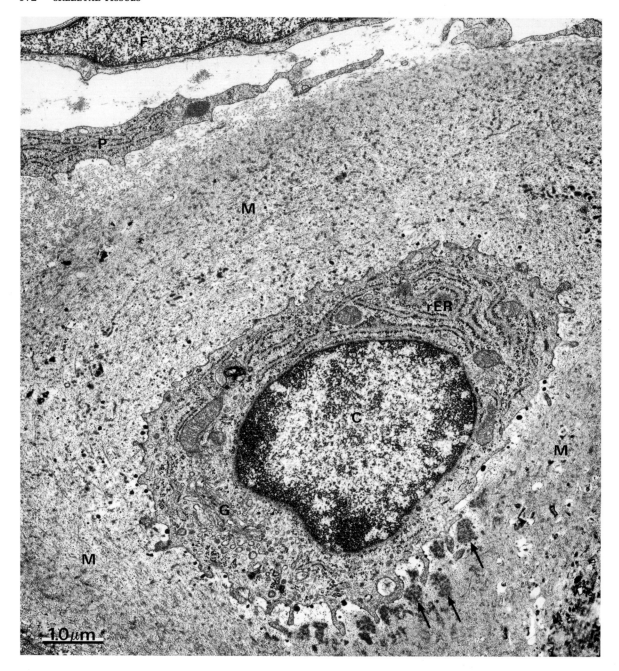

Fig. 10.2 Chondrocytes *(EM × 16 000)*

This micrograph illustrates a chondrocyte **C** lying within its lacuna and surrounded by cartilage matrix **M**. At the surface, part of the cytoplasm of a flattened perichondrial chondrocyte **P** can also be seen. Beyond this lies the nucleus and surrounding cytoplasm of a fibroblast **F** in the adjacent supporting tissue. Typical of cells active in protein synthesis (in this case matrix turnover), chondrocytes have prominent rough endoplasmic reticulum **rER** which is distended with secretory material. By contrast, note the absence of rER in

the fibroblast in this micrograph. A well developed Golgi apparatus **G** is present. Glycogen granules are scattered in the cytoplasm. Note that the chondrocyte completely fills its lacuna within the matrix. Small cytoplasmic extensions mediate the constant interaction between chondrocytes and matrix. At this magnification, the fibrous elements of the matrix can just be discerned. The electron-dense material adjacent to the deep aspect of the cell (arrowed) represents recently secreted matrix material.

Fig. 10.3 Fibrocartilage *(H & E/Alcian blue × 320)*

Fibrocartilage, which has features intermediate between cartilage and dense fibrous supporting tissue, is found in the intervertebral discs, some articular cartilages, the pubic symphysis, and in association with dense collagenous tissue in joint capsules, ligaments and the connections of some tendons to bone. Fibrocartilage consists of alternating layers of hyaline cartilage matrix and thick layers of dense collagen fibres oriented in the direction of the functional stresses.

This micrograph is taken from the same specimen of intervertebral disc illustrated in Fig. 10.29. Pink-stained collagen characteristically permeates the blue-stained cartilage ground substance. Chondrocytes **C** are typically arranged in rows between the dense collagen layers within lacunae in the glycoprotein matrix.

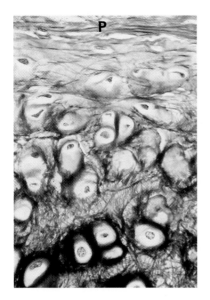

Fig. 10.4 Elastic cartilage *(Elastic van Gieson × 128)*

Elastic cartilage occurs in the external ear and external auditory canal, the epiglottis, parts of the laryngeal cartilages and the walls of the Eustachian tubes.

The histological structure of elastic cartilage is similar to that of hyaline cartilage, its elasticity, however, being derived from the presence of numerous bundles of branching elastic fibres in the cartilage matrix; this network of elastic fibres (stained black in this preparation) is particularly dense in the immediate vicinity of the chondrocytes. Collagen (stained red) is also a major constituent of the cartilage matrix and makes up the bulk of the perichondrium **P** intermingled with a few elastic fibres.

Development and growth of elastic cartilage occurs by both interstitial and appositional growth in the same manner as for hyaline cartilage.

Bone

Bone is a specialised form of supporting tissue in which the extracellular components are mineralised, thus conferring the property of marked rigidity and strength whilst retaining some degree of elasticity. Bone also constitutes a store of calcium and other inorganic ions, and actively participates in the maintenance of calcium homeostasis in the body as a whole. The structure of individual bones provides for the maximum resistance to mechanical stresses whilst maintaining the least bony mass. To accommodate changing mechanical stresses and the demands of calcium homeostasis, all bones in the body are in a dynamic state of growth and resorption throughout life.

Like other supporting/connective tissues, bone is composed of cells and an organic extracellular matrix containing proteoglycan ground substance and collagen fibres. Inorganic salts, predominantly *calcium hydroxyapatite* crystals, form the mineral component of bone matrix. Ground substance constitutes only a small proportion of the organic extracellular matrix of bone and contains proteoglycans similar to those found in cartilage except that the proportion of sulphated glycoproteins is much less than in cartilage. The fibrous component of the extracellular material is mainly Type I collagen which exhibits a similar banding pattern to that of common collagenous supporting tissues (see Ch. 4).

The cells found in bone are of three types: *osteoblasts*, *osteocytes* and *osteoclasts*, the first two cells types being derived from mesenchymal-type cells called *osteoprogenitor cells*. Osteoblasts are responsible for the synthesis and secretion of the organic component of the extracellular matrix of new bone, a substance known as *osteoid*; osteoid rapidly undergoes mineralisation to form bone. Osteoblasts become trapped within bone as osteocytes and are then responsible for maintenance of the bone matrix. Osteoclasts are multinucleate cells probably derived from the macrophage-monocyte system (see Fig. 3.9); they are actively involved in resorptive processes associated with continuous remodelling of bone.

Bone exists in two main forms: *woven bone* and *lamellar bone*. Woven bone is an immature form and is characterised by a random (woven) organisation of its collagen, the fibres of which are much coarser than those of lamellar bone. During bone development, woven bone is the first form of bone to be produced; it is then remodelled to form lamellar bone, the form which constitutes most of the mature skeleton. Lamellar bone is composed of successive layers each of which has a highly organised infrastructure. Lamellar bone may be formed as a solid mass, when it is described as *compact bone*, or may be disposed in an open sponge-like manner, described as *cancellous bone*.

The mineralised component of bone makes it too brittle to be cut into ordinary histological sections. Consequently, for routine histological purposes, bone is first decalcified in acid solutions prior to sectioning and staining. With this method, cellular detail and the organic component of the matrix is preserved though the stains are taken up less readily than normal. More recently, acrylics have become available for embedding bone without prior decalcification; using diamond-edged knives, sections can be cut and then stained, preserving detail in both the cells and the calcified matrix. Such methods are used in the study of the mineralisation process and its disorders.

Finally, for the study of the morphology of the mineralised matrix, *ground sections* are made. This involves sawing undecalcified bone into relatively thick sections which are then ground thin and smooth with grinding stones. All cellular detail is lost in such preparations.

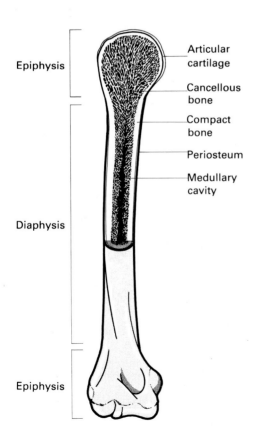

Epiphysis

Articular cartilage

Cancellous bone

Compact bone

Periosteum

Medullary cavity

Diaphysis

Epiphysis

Fig. 10.5 Long bone

This diagram illustrates the general structure of long bones in the mature skeleton and the gross morphological appearance of the two types of lamellar bone found in the mature skeleton, i.e. compact bone and cancellous (spongy) bone.

Compact bone forms the dense walls of the shaft or *diaphysis* while cancellous bone occupies part of the large central *medullary cavity*. Cancellous bone consists of a network of fine, irregular plates called *trabeculae* separated by intercommunicating spaces. In immature animals, the medullary cavities of most bones contain active (red) marrow which is responsible for the production of the cellular elements of blood. In the adult, active marrow is restricted to a few sites (see Ch. 3); the medullary cavities of other bones are filled with inactive (yellow) marrow which is largely composed of adipose tissue.

The articular (joint) surfaces of the expanded ends, or *epiphyses*, of long bones are protected by a layer of specialised hyaline cartilage called *articular cartilage*. The external surface of the bone is invested in a dense fibrous layer called the *periosteum* into which are inserted muscles, tendons and ligaments. The inner surfaces of the bone, including the trabeculae of cancellous bone, are invested by a delicate layer called the *endosteum*. The endosteum and periosteum contain cells of the osteogenic series which are responsible for growth, continuous remodelling and repair of bone fractures.

Prior to the attainment of skeletal maturity, the long bones grow in length by the process of endochondral ossification which occurs at a *growth* or *epiphysial plate* situated at each end of the bone at the junction of the diaphysis (shaft) and epiphysis. The *metaphysis* (not illustrated) is defined as the junction of the shaft with the growth plate.

Lacuna
Cortical bone
Haversian canal
Interstitial system
Lamellae

Volkmann's canal

Periosteum

Lacuna

Haversian canal

Fig. 10.6 Compact bone

Compact bone is made up of parallel bony columns which, in long bones, are disposed parallel to the long axis, i.e. in the line of stress exerted on the bone. Each column is made up of concentric bony layers or *lamellae* disposed around a central channel containing blood vessels, lymphatics and nerves. These neurovascular channels are known as *canals of Havers* or *Haversian canals*, and with their concentric lamellae form *Haversian systems*. The neurovascular bundles interconnect with one another, and with the endosteum and periosteum, via *Volkmann's canals* which pierce the columns at right angles (or obliquely) to the Haversian canals.

Each Haversian system begins as a broad channel, at the periphery of which osteoblasts lay down lamellae of bone. With the deposition of successive lamellae, the diameter of the Haversian canal decreases and osteoblasts are trapped as osteocytes in spaces called *lacunae* in the matrix. The

osteocytes are thus arranged in concentric rings within the lamellae. Between adjacent lacunae and the central canal are numerous minute interconnecting canals called *canaliculi* which contain fine cytoplasmic extensions of the osteocytes.

As a result of the continuous resorption and redeposition of bone, complete, newly formed Haversian systems are disposed between partly resorbed systems formed earlier. The remnants of lamellae no longer surrounding Haversian canals form irregular *interstitial systems* between intact Haversian systems.

At the outermost aspect of compact bone, Haversian systems give way to concentric lamellae of dense *cortical bone* laid down at the bone surface by osteoblasts of the periosteum. At the inner medullary aspect, similar but irregular circumferential lamellae merge with trabeculae of cancellous bone (not illustrated).

(a)

Fig. 10.7 Compact bone *(Ground sections, unstained)*

(a) TS × 80 (b) TS × 600 (c) LS × 150

These ground sections illustrate many of the features
described in the preceding figure. In micrograph (a), the
bone has been cut transversely thereby demonstrating newly
formed Haversian systems H_1 and older, partly resorbed
Haversian systems H_2; irregular interstitial systems I,
representing the remnants of former Haversian systems, fill
the spaces between the Haversian systems. Concentric rings
of flattened lacunae can be seen to surround the central
Haversian canals which appear as very dark areas in this
preparation.

Micrograph (b) focuses on a single Haversian system, the
central canal being surrounded by concentric lamellae of
bone matrix containing empty lacunae L. Fine canaliculi C
radiate from each lacuna to anastomose with those of
adjacent lacunae. In life, the osteocytes do not completely
fill the lacunae, the remaining narrow space being filled with
extracellular bone fluid. Fine cytoplasmic processes of the
osteocytes pass in the canaliculi to communicate via gap
junctions with the processes of osteocytes in adjacent
lamellae. The canaliculi provide passages for circulation of
extracellular fluid and diffusion of metabolites between the
lacunae and vessels of the Haversian canals.

Osteocytes maintain the structural integrity of the
mineralised matrix and mediate short-term release or
deposition of calcium for the purpose of calcium
homeostasis in the body as a whole. The activity of
osteocytes in calcium regulation is controlled directly by
plasma calcium concentration and indirectly by the
hormones parathormone and calcitonin secreted by the
parathyroid and thyroid glands respectively (see Ch. 17).
Osteoblasts and osteocytes also appear to respond to minute
piezo-electric currents induced by bone deformation
increasing or decreasing local bone formation as appropriate
and inducing complementary activity in local osteoclasts via
the secretion of local humoral factors. In this fashion bone is
remodelled to adapt to mechanical stresses imposed on it.

Micrograph (c) shows compact bone cut in longitudinal
section, the plane of section including some Haversian
canals HC. These appear dark in colour as in micrograph (a)
due to an optical artefact related to air trapped in the section.
For the same reason, the tiny osteocyte lacunae appear as
brown specks elongated in shape and arranged in concentric
layers around the Haversian canals.

(b)

(c)

Fig. 10.8 Compact bone *(TS: H & E × 198)*

The morphology of the cells and organic components of bone may be studied in standard decalcified preparations, as in this micrograph. Several Haversian systems **H** are seen in transverse section separated by irregular interstitial systems **I**. The matrix of decalcified mature bone is strongly eosinophilic because of its high content of collagen. The collagen of the lamellae is disposed in a helical manner around the long axes of the Haversian systems.

At its outer aspect, the Haversian bone gives way to lamellae of cortical bone **C** which provides a more dense, protective outer surface to most bones. Where the Haversian systems and cortical lamellae abut one another, fine basophilic cement lines **L** are seen, rich in proteoglycan ground substance. Note the fibrous periosteum **P** investing the surface of the cortical bone.

Osteocytes **O** have densely stained, irregular nuclei and pale, basophilic cytoplasm which undergoes considerable shrinkage in routine preparations such as this. Unlike the chondrocytes of cartilage, osteocytes do not usually completely occupy their lacunae in the bone matrix but rather they and their cytoplasmic processes are surrounded by a narrow space filled with extracellular fluid. Recent evidence suggests that this *bone fluid* may be of different composition to that of extracellular fluid of other tissues, the surface osteocytes and osteoblasts forming some form of 'bone membrane' separating the bone fluid from other extracellular fluid. Canaliculi, containing the fine cytoplasmic processes of osteocytes, are not usually visible in this type of preparation. Within the Haversian canals, note the presence of small blood vessels and nuclei representing endosteal osteoblasts.

(a)

(b)

Fig. 10.9 Mature periosteum *(a) H & E × 128 (b) Masson's trichrome × 200*

The outer surface of most bone is invested by a layer of condensed fibrous tissue, the periosteum **P**, which contains numerous osteoprogenitor cells which are practically indistinguishable from fibroblasts. During bone growth or repair, the osteoprogenitor cells differentiate into osteoblasts which are responsible for the deposition of concentric lamellae of cortical bone by appositional growth. The periosteum is bound to the underlying bone by bundles of collagen fibres called *Sharpey's fibres* which may penetrate the whole thickness of the cortical bone; collagen is stained blue-green in micrograph (b). The periosteum is richly supplied with blood vessels from adjacent tissues.

Periosteum is not present on the articular surfaces of bone, the sites of insertion of tendons and ligaments, and at several other discrete sites such as the subcapsular area of the neck of the femur. The periosteum plays an important role in the repair of bone fractures and its absence may lead to delay or failure of healing particularly of subcapsular fractures of the femoral neck.

Fig. 10.10 Muscular insertion into bone

(Phosphotungstic acid/ Haematoxylin × 480)

Muscle may be attached directly to bone, in which case the area of attachment is relatively extensive, or alternatively, the muscle may be inserted into a tendon which is attached to bone over a more localised area.

This micrograph shows the direct attachment of skeletal muscle **M** to bone **B**. The ends of the muscle fibres abut onto the periosteum **P**, the collagenous fibres of which extend between the muscle fibres to mingle with the collagen of the endomysium **E**; collagen stains red with this staining method. In areas of muscle attachment, the surface of the cortical bone tends to be roughened and the periosteal Sharpey's fibres **S** are robust and extend deeply into the bony cortex.

(a)

(b)

Fig. 10.11 Active periosteum *(H & E (a) ×200 (b) ×480)*

These micrographs illustrate highly active periosteum from a developing fetal long bone. The periosteum consists of plump, basophilic osteoblasts **O**, two to three cells deep on the surface of the developing bone, and a thin layer of immature, loose collagenous tissue **C**. The cytoplasmic basophilia of active osteoblasts reflects their large content of rough endoplasmic reticulum involved in synthesising the collagen, ground substance and other organic constituents of bone matrix. When appositional bone growth at the periosteal surface is complete, osteoblasts revert to quiescent, osteoprogenitor cells which closely resemble fibroblasts. Note that the bone of the developing shaft is of the woven type; the process of remodelling, to form lamellar bone, occurs at a later stage (see Fig. 10.21).

(a)

(b)

Fig. 10.12 Osteoblasts and osteoid *(a) H & E × 320 (b) Undecalcified section, Goldner's trichrome × 320*

These micrographs illustrate active osteoblasts in the process of laying down the organic components of bone matrix; before mineralisation occurs, the organic matrix is known as *osteoid*. In comparison with mature osteocytes, osteoblasts are large cells with abundant basophilic cytoplasm, a large Golgi apparatus and a pale stained nucleus with a prominent nucleolus. These features reflect a high rate of protein and proteoglycan synthesis.

In normally developing bone, as seen in micrograph (a), osteoid becomes calcified soon after deposition. Under conditions in which adequate calcium and phosphate ions are not available (e.g. rickets, chronic renal failure), there is a lag in mineralisation of osteoid; under such circumstances osteoid tissue accumulates. Osteoid is readily demonstrated in undecalcified sections as shown in micrograph (b), a biopsy specimen from a man with chronic renal failure. With this staining method, osteoid appears as a red-stained zone between a layer of active osteoblasts and the mineralised bone (stained blue). In normal subjects the amount of unmineralised matrix is minimal.

(a)

(b)

Fig. 10.13 Osteoclasts

(a) H & E × 400
(b) Undecalcified section, Goldner's trichrome × 320

Resorption of bone is performed by large multinucleate cells called osteoclasts **O** which are often seen lying in depressions resorbed from the bone surface called *Howship's lacunae* **H**. The aspect of the osteoclast in apposition to bone is characterised by fine microvilli which form a *ruffled border* which is readily visible with the electron microscope. The ruffled border secretes several organic acids which dissolve the mineral component whilst lysosomal proteolytic enzymes are employed to destroy the organic matrix.

In decalcified preparations as in micrograph (a), osteoclasts tend to shrink and become detached from the bone surface; the intimate relationship of osteoclasts with bone is seen better in micrograph (b).

Osteoclastic resorption contributes to bone remodelling in response to growth or changing mechanical stresses upon the skeleton. Osteoclasts also participate in the long-term maintenance of blood calcium homeostasis by their response to parathyroid hormone and calcitonin (see Ch. 17). Parathyroid hormone stimulates osteoclastic resorption and the release of calcium ions from bone, whereas calcitonin inhibits osteoclastic activity.

The specimen shown in micrograph (b) is from a woman with a low serum calcium level. This condition stimulates release of parathyroid hormone which promotes excessive osteoclastic resorption in an attempt to restore serum calcium levels. In addition, under these circumstances there is a lag in mineralisation of newly deposited bone matrix which is manifest by the presence of osteoid **Os**.

Fig. 10.14 Cancellous bone

(H & E × 50)

Cancellous (spongy) bone is composed of a network of bony trabeculae separated by a labyrinth of interconnecting spaces containing bone marrow. The trabeculae are thin and composed of irregular lamellae of bone with lacunae containing osteocytes (not seen at this magnification). Spongy bone does not usually contain Haversian systems and the osteocytes exchange metabolites via canaliculi with blood sinusoids in the marrow. The trabeculae are lined by a delicate layer of tissue called endosteum which contains osteoprogenitor cells, osteoblasts and osteoclasts.

Bone matrix and mineralisation

Mature compact bone is made up of about 70% inorganic salts and 30% organic matrix by weight. Collagen makes up over 90% of the organic component, the remainder being ground substance proteoglycans and a group of non-collagen molecules which appear to be involved in regulation of bone mineralisation.

The collagen of bone represents about half of the total body collagen and is almost exclusively in the form of type 1 fibres, a polymer of numerous elongated overlapping tropocollagen subunits (see Ch. 4). Spaces within this three-dimensional structure often referred to as *hole zones* are the initial site of mineral deposition.

Ground substance proteoglycans contribute a much smaller proportion of the matrix than in cartilage and mainly consist of chondroitin sulphate and hyaluronic acid in the form of proteoglycan aggregates. As well as controlling the water content of bones, ground substance is probably involved in regulating formation of collagen fibres in a form appropriate for subsequent matrix mineralisation. The remaining non-collagen organic material includes *osteocalcin* (*Gla protein*), involved in binding calcium during the mineralisation process, *osteonectin* which may serve some bridging function between collagen and the mineral component, *sialoproteins* (rich in sialic acid) and certain proteins which appear to be concentrated from plasma.

The mineral component of bone mainly consists of calcium and phosphate in the form of hydroxyapatite crystals. These are conjugated to a small proportion of magnesium carbonate, sodium and potassium ions but also have affinity for heavy metal and radioactive environmental pollutants.

Collagen and the other organic matrix constituents are synthesised by the rough endoplasmic reticulum of osteoblasts, packaged by the Golgi and secreted from the cell surface resulting in the production of osteoid. After a maturation phase lasting several days, amorphous (non-crystalline) calcium phosphate salts begin to precipitate in the 'hole zones' of the collagen. These mineralisation foci expand and coalesce into hydroxyapatite crystals by further remodelling. Nevertheless, 20% or more of the mineral component remains in the amorphous form providing a readily available buffer in whole body calcium homeostasis.

The concentration of calcium and phosphate ions in bony extracellular fluid is greater than required for spontaneous deposition of calcium salts and a variety of inhibitors including *pyrophosphate* play a crucial role in controlling bone mineralisation. The deposition of calcium appears to be associated with membrane bound vesicles derived from osteoblast plasma membrane called *matrix vesicles*; these contain *alkaline phosphatase* and other phosphatases which may play a role in neutralising the inhibitory effect of pyrophosphate.

(a) *(b)*

Fig. 10.15 Bone marrow *(H & E (a) × 128 (b) × 480)*

The intertrabecular spaces of all bones are filled with bone marrow containing the primitive stem cells from which all the cellular elements of blood are derived (see Ch. 3). Active bone marrow is crammed with precursors of mature blood cells and the predominance of maturing erythrocytes confers a deep red colour on active marrow and hence the name *red marrow*. In the newborn, all bone marrow is involved in haemopoiesis; however with increasing age, the marrow of peripheral long bones becomes less active and is progressively dominated by adipocytes. In mature mammals, therefore, much of the marrow is inactive and yellow in colour; *yellow marrow* may, however, be reactivated if the need arises for increased haemopoiesis.

These preparations from a 7-year-old child contain much active haemopoietic tissue and scattered adipocytes **A**. Note two thin trabeculae **T** of cancellous bone in micrograph (a). Micrograph (b) shows a moderate sized artery and one of its branches passing through the marrow.

The marrow has two sources of blood supply, the *nutrient artery* and *periosteal capillaries*. The nutrient artery is a relatively large vessel which reaches the marrow cavity via the *nutrient canal* which pierces the cortical bone. On entering the marrow, the nutrient artery divides into proximal and distally directed branches which in turn give rise to radial branches which run towards the inner aspect of the cortex; here they pass through the endosteum ramifying into a system of capillaries which permeate the cortical bone. Periosteal capillaries, which are derived from arteries in surrounding muscles, penetrate the outer cortex and anastomose with the nutrient artery-derived vessels before re-entering the marrow cavity to form a sinusoidal plexus extending throughout the marrow cavity. The marrow sinusoids drain into a large *central sinus* which drains from the bone as the *emissary vein* via the nutrient canal.

Bone development and growth

The fetal development of bone occurs in two ways, both of which involve replacement of primitive collagenous supporting tissue by bone. The resulting woven bone is then extensively remodelled by resorption and appositional growth to form the mature adult skeleton which is made up of lamellar bone. Thereafter, resorption and deposition of bone occur at a much reduced rate to accommodate changing functional stresses and to effect calcium homeostasis. The long bones, vertebrae, pelvis and bones of the base of the skull are preceded by the formation of a continuously growing cartilage model which is progressively replaced by bone; this process is called *endochondral ossification* and the bones so formed are called *cartilage bones*. In contrast, the bones of the vault of the skull, the maxilla and most of the mandible are formed by the deposition of bone within primitive mesenchymal tissue; this process of direct replacement of mesenchyme by bone is known as *intramembranous ossification* and the bones so formed are called *membrane bones*. Bone development is controlled by growth hormone, thyroid hormone and the sex hormones.

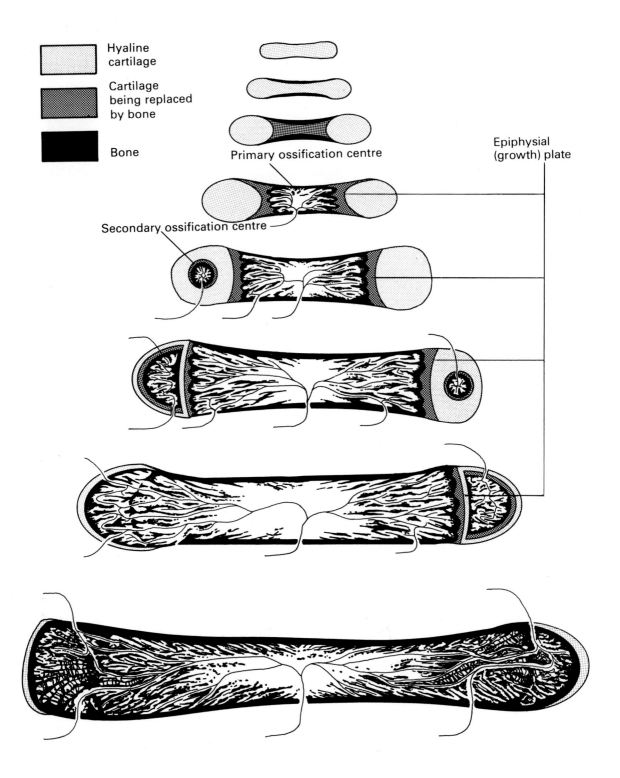

Hyaline cartilage

Cartilage being replaced by bone

Bone

Primary ossification centre

Epiphysial (growth) plate

Secondary ossification centre

Fig. 10.16 Endochondral ossification *(illustration opposite)*

Endochondral ossification is a method of bone formation which permits functional stresses to be sustained during skeletal growth. It is well demonstrated in the development of the long bones.

A small model of the long bone is first formed in solid hyaline cartilage. This undergoes mainly appositional growth to form an elongated, dumb-bell shaped mass of cartilage consisting of a shaft (diaphysis) and future articular portions (epiphyses) surrounded by perichondrium.

Within the shaft of the cartilage model the chondrocytes enlarge greatly, resorbing the surrounding cartilage so as to leave only slender perforated trabeculae of cartilage matrix. This cartilage matrix then becomes calcified and the chondrocytes degenerate leaving large, interconnecting spaces. During this period, the perichondrium of the shaft develops osteogenic potential and assumes the role of periosteum. The periosteum then lays down a thin layer of bone around the surface of the shaft. At the same time, primitive mesenchymal cells and blood vessels invade the spaces left within the shaft after degeneration of the chondrocytes. The primitive mesenchymal cells differentiate into osteoblasts and blood-forming cells of the bone marrow. The osteoblasts form a layer of cells on the surface of the calcified remnants of the cartilage matrix and commence the formation of irregular, woven bone.

The ends of the original cartilage model have by now become separated by a large site of *primary ossification* in the shaft. The cartilaginous ends of the model, however, continue to grow in diameter. Meanwhile, the cartilage at the ends of the shaft continues to undergo regressive changes followed by ossification so that the developing bone now consists of an elongated, bony diaphysial shaft with a semilunar cartilage epiphysis at each end. The interface between the shaft and each epiphysis constitutes a *growth or epiphysial plate*. Within the growth plate, the cartilage proliferates continuously, resulting in progressive elongation of the bone. At the diaphysial aspect of each growth plate, the chondrocytes mature and then die, the degenerating zone of cartilage being replaced by bone. Thus the bony diaphysis lengthens and the growth plates are pushed further and further apart. On reaching maturity, hormonal changes inhibit further cartilage proliferation and the growth plates are replaced by bone causing fusion of the diaphysis and epiphyses.

In the meantime, in the centre of the mass of cartilage of each developing epiphysis, regressive changes and bone formation similar to that in the diaphysial cartilage occur along with appositional growth of cartilage over the whole external surface of the epiphysis. This conversion of central epiphysial cartilage to bone is known as *secondary ossification*. A thin zone of hyaline cartilage always remains at the surface as the articular cartilage.

Under the influence of functional stresses, the calcified cartilage remnants and the surrounding irregular woven bone are completely remodelled so that the bone ultimately consists of a compact outer layer with a medulla of cancellous bone. By maturity, the medullary bone is almost completely resorbed to leave a large medullary space filled with bone marrow.

Fig. 10.17 Epiphysis

(H & E/Alcian blue × 12)

This micrograph illustrates the head of a kitten femur at an advanced stage of development.

The cartilaginous epiphysis **E** is separated from the diaphysis **D** by the epiphysial growth plate **GP**. Note the thickening compact bone **C** at the outer aspect of the diaphysis and the trabeculae of bone in the medulla. Note also the centre of secondary ossification **SC** in the epiphysial cartilage.

Epiphysial growth plates provide for growth in length of long bones whilst accommodating functional stresses in the growing skeleton. The next three micrographs focus, at higher magnification, on particular areas of the epiphysial plate.

Fig. 10.18 Epiphysial growth plate *(H & E/Alcian blue × 40)*

At higher magnification, the epiphysial growth plate **GP** shows a progression of morphological changes between the epiphysial cartilage **E** and the newly forming bone **B** of the diaphysis. Similar, but less stratified, morphological changes are seen between the epiphysial cartilage and the centre of secondary ossification **SC** within the epiphysis although this does not represent a growth plate. The Alcian blue counter stain has been employed as it has particular affinity for the ground substance of cartilage. Note blood vessels **V**, cut in transverse section, passing into the secondary ossification centre via cartilage canals.

Fig. 10.19 Epiphysial growth plate

(H & E/Alcian blue × 120)

The dynamic process of endochondral ossification is summarised in this micrograph of the epiphysial growth plate at high magnification. The transition between epiphysial cartilage and new bone occurs in six functional and morphological stages:

- *Zone of reserve cartilage* **R**: this consists of typical hyaline cartilage (see Fig. 10.1) with the chondrocytes arranged in small clusters surrounded by a large amount of moderately stained matrix.
- *Zone of proliferation* **P**: the clusters of cartilage cells undergo successive mitotic divisions to form columns of chondrocytes separated by strongly stained matrix rich in proteoglycans.
- *Zone of maturation* **M**: cell division has ceased and the chondrocytes increase in size.
- *Zone of hypertrophy and calcification* **H**: the chondrocytes become greatly enlarged and vacuolated and the matrix becomes calcified.
- *Zone of cartilage degeneration* **D**: the chondrocytes degenerate and the lacunae of the calcified matrix are invaded by osteogenic cells and capillaries from the marrow cavity of the diaphysis.
- *Osteogenic zone* **O**: the osteogenic cells differentiate into osteoblasts which congregate on the surface of the spicules of calcified cartilage matrix where they commence bone formation. This transitional zone is known as the *metaphysis*.

Fig. 10.20 Endochondral ossification: metaphysis *(H & E/Alcian blue × 198)*

In the metaphysis seen in this preparation, the blue-stained spicules of calcified cartilage matrix are surrounded by osteoblasts and newly formed woven bone which is stained pink. Further growth of metaphysial woven bone is followed by extensive remodelling to produce mature compact and spongy bone.

At physical maturity the process of endochondral ossification ceases. This stage is recognised by the fusion of the diaphysis with the epiphysis, resulting in the obliteration of the growth plates. From this point onwards no further endochondral ossification is possible. Although endochondral ossification is the means of growth in length of a long bone, growth in diameter of the shaft occurs by appositional growth at the periosteal surface and complementary osteoclastic resorption at the endosteal (medullary) aspect.

Fig. 10.21 Bone remodelling and repair
(H & E × 480)

This micrograph illustrates an irregular spicule of woven bone from a fetus. Some of the surfaces of the spicule exhibit osteoblastic deposition **Ob** whereas other surfaces are in the process of being resorbed by osteoclasts **Oc**.

Woven bone is not only the first type of bone to be formed during skeletal development but is also the first bone to be laid down during the repair of a fracture. At the fracture site, a blood clot initially forms, later being replaced by highly vascular collagenous tissue (*granulation tissue*) which becomes progressively more fibrous. Mesenchymal cells then differentiate into chondroblasts and progressively replace this *fibrous granulation tissue* with hyaline cartilage. This firm but still flexible bridge is known as the *provisional callus*. The provisional callus is then strengthened by deposition of calcium salts within the cartilage matrix. Meanwhile, osteoprogenitor cells in the endosteum and periosteum are activated and lay down a meshwork of woven bone within and around the provisional callus; the provisional callus thus becomes transformed into the *bony callus*. *Bony union* is achieved when the fracture site is completely bridged by woven bone. Under the influence of functional stresses, the bony callus is then slowly remodelled to form mature lamellar bone.

Fig. 10.22 Intramembranous ossification
(H & E × 75)

Intramembranous bone formation occurs within 'membranes' of condensed, primitive mesenchymal tissue. Mesenchymal cells differentiate into osteoblasts which begin synthesis and secretion of osteoid at multiple *centres of ossification*; mineralisation of osteoid follows closely. As osteoid is laid down, osteoblasts are trapped in lacunae to become osteocytes and their fine cytoplasmic extensions shrink to form the fine processes contained within the canaliculi. Osteoprogenitor cells at the surface of the centres of ossification undergo mitotic division to produce further osteoblasts which lay down more bone. Progressive bone formation results in the fusion of adjacent ossification centres to form bone which is spongy in gross appearance.

The collagen fibres of developing bone are randomly arranged in interlacing bundles, giving rise to the term woven bone. The woven bone then undergoes progressive remodelling by osteoclastic resorption and osteoblastic deposition to form mature compact or spongy bone. The primitive mesenchyme remaining in the network of developing bone differentiates into bone marrow.

This preparation from the developing skull vault of a cat fetus illustrates spicules of woven bone **B**, separated by primitive mesenchymal tissue. Note the condensed primitive mesenchyme **M** which delineates the outer margin of the developing bone.

Fig. 10.23 Skull *(Cat: H & E × 30)*

This micrograph shows a full thickness view of the skull vault of a mature cat which, as in humans, is formed by the process of intramembranous ossification. The skull vault consists of cancellous bone which is condensed at its internal and external aspects to form continuous, relatively smooth surfaces. The external surface of the skull is invested by periosteum **Px** which merges with the deep layers of the overlying scalp. The internal surface of the skull is also lined by periosteum **Pi**; this layer also constitutes the outermost membranous covering of the brain, the dura mater.

During skeletal growth, the skull vault expands in response to the pressure of the growing brain within. The developing skull bones, which are bound together by *sutures* of periosteum, are pushed outwards and new membrane bone is laid down at the sutural margins. At the same time, periosteal deposition of new bone on the outer surfaces, and corresponding osteoclastic resorption at the inner surfaces, provides for the necessary recontouring of the skull bones which become progressively flatter. At skeletal maturity the sutures between the skull bones become almost closed and filled with dense fibrous tissue which represents the periosteal layers of opposing bones. With advancing age the sutures tend to ossify.

Joints

Joints may be classified into two main functional groups, *synovial* and *non-synovial*, both of which may show wide morphological variations.

Synovial joints. In this type of joint there is extensive movement of the bones upon one another at the articular surfaces. The articular surfaces are maintained in apposition by a fibrous capsule and ligaments, and the surfaces are lubricated by *synovial fluid*. Synovial joints are known as *diarthroses*. In some diarthroses such as the temporomandibular and knee joints, plates of fibrocartilage may be completely or partially interposed between the articular surfaces but remain unattached to the articular surfaces.

Non-synovial joints. These joints have limited movement, the articulating bones having no free articular surfaces rather being joined by dense collagenous tissue. This may be of three types:

- *Dense fibrous tissue:* this forms the sutures between the bones of the skull and permits moulding of the fetal skull during its passage through the birth canal. The sutures are progressively replaced by bone with advancing age. Such fibrous tissue joints are called *syndesmoses*, and when replaced by bone are called *synostoses*.

- *Hyaline cartilage:* this type of joint, called a *synchondrosis* or *primary cartilaginous joint*, unites the first rib with the sternum and is the only synchondrosis found in the human adult.

- *Fibrocartilage:* the opposing surfaces of some bones are covered by hyaline cartilage but instead of a synovial space, are directly connected to each other by a plate of fibrocartilage. Such fibrocartilaginous joints are called *symphyses* or *secondary cartilaginous joints* and occur in the pubic symphysis and at the intervertebral discs. The fibrocartilage disc of the pubic symphysis develops a central cavity and the intervertebral discs have a fluid-filled central cavity.

Fig. 10.24 Synovial joint *(Monkey: H & E × 12)*

This micrograph illustrates a typical synovial joint, in this case, the distal interphalangeal joint of the finger. The articular surfaces of the terminal phalanx **T** and the middle phalanx **M** are covered by hyaline cartilage **C**. The joint space is artefactually widened. In vivo, the articular surfaces are maintained in close contact by a fibrous capsule **Cp** which is inserted into the articulating bones at some distance beyond the articular cartilages. The *synovium* **S** is a specialised layer of collagenous tissue which lines the inner aspect of the capsule. Note the extensor tendon **E** which inserts into the base of terminal phalanx.

Fig. 10.25 Articular cartilage *(H & E × 20)*

This micrograph focuses on the opposing articular cartilages **AC** of the synovial joint shown in the previous micrograph.

Each articular cartilage is bonded to its long bone at a region called the *bony end plate* **BP**; this region is composed of an unusual type of bone which lacks Haversian systems and canaliculi and in which osteocytes occupy particularly large lacunae. The articular cartilage is sharply demarcated from the underlying bony end plate by a thick layer of glycoprotein-rich substance **G** which resembles the cement lines of Haversian bone.

Fig. 10.26 Articular cartilage *(H & E × 128)*

This micrograph shows the lower rim of the articular cartilage **AC** of the middle phalanx of the joint shown in Fig. 10.24. Articular cartilage differs from other hyaline cartilage in two respects. Firstly, the articular surface is not covered by perichondrium. Secondly, the collagen fibres of the articular cartilage matrix are of type I, exhibiting the characteristic cross-banding of the collagen fibres typical of supporting tissue and bone. In contrast, the collagen fibres of hyaline cartilage elsewhere (type III collagen) are not cross-banded (see Ch. 4).

Articular cartilage, like other hyaline cartilage, is avascular; it is nourished by diffusion from the synovial fluid of the joint cavity. Note part of the synovial layer **S** of the joint capsule.

(a)

(b)

Fig. 10.27 Synovium *(H & E (a) × 100 (b) × 400)*

The inner surface of the capsule of synovial joints and tendon sheaths is lined by a specialised collagenous tissue, the synovium, which is responsible for the elaboration of the synovial fluid which lubricates the movement of articular surfaces. Depending on the location, the bulk of the synovial tissue may be of loose collagenous type (*areolar synovium*), of more dense collagenous type (*fibrous synovium*) or predominantly composed of fat (*adipose synovium*) as in the case of intra-articular fat pads.

As seen in micrograph (a), the surface of the synovium **S** is thrown up into folds and smaller villi which may extend for some distance into the joint cavity **JC**. The synovial tissue contains numerous blood vessels **V**, lymphatics and nerves.

As seen in micrograph (b), the free surface of the synovium is characterised by a discontinuous layer of cells up to four cells deep. These *synovial cells* are not connected by junctional complexes and do not rest on a basement membrane and the synovial surface, therefore, does not constitute an epithelium. The synovial cells are of mesenchymal origin. The majority are plump with an

extensive Golgi complex and numerous lysosomes, features suggestive of macrophages (*type A synovocytes*). The remainder have profuse rough endoplasmic reticulum and represent fibroblasts (*type B synovocytes*). Also in this micrograph, note the rich network of capillaries and the thick strands of collagen which would define this as fibrous synovium.

In the normal joint, the synovial fluid is little more than a thin film covering the articular surfaces. In that the articular space is not demarcated from the synovium by an epithelium, the synovial fluid represents a highly specialised fluid form of synovial extracellular matrix, rather than a secretion in the usual sense. Its major constituents are hyaluronic acid and associated glycoproteins secreted by the type B synovocytes and its fluid component is a transudate from synovial capillaries. This arrangement facilitates the continuous exchange of oxygen, carbon dioxide and metabolites between blood and synovial fluid which is the major source of metabolic support for articular cartilage. Normal synovial fluid also contains a small number of leucocytes (less than 100/mm³), predominantly monocytes.

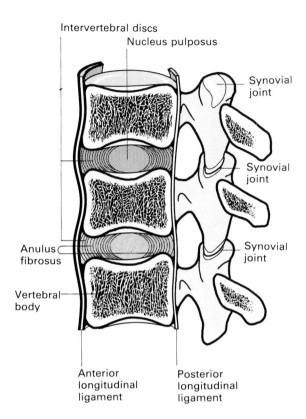

Intervertebral discs
Nucleus pulposus
Synovial joint
Synovial joint
Synovial joint
Anulus fibrosus
Vertebral body
Anterior longitudinal ligament
Posterior longitudinal ligament

Fig. 10.28 The intervertebral joints

The vertebrae articulate by means of two different types of joints:

- The vertebral bodies are united by symphysial joints, the *intervertebral discs*, which permit movement between the vertebral bodies whilst maintaining a union of great strength. The fibrocartilage of each intervertebral disc is arranged in concentric rings forming the *anulus fibrosus*. Within the disc, there is a central cavity containing a viscous fluid, the *nucleus pulposus*, which acts as a shock absorber. The anulus fibrosus is reinforced peripherally by circumferential ligaments. A thick ligament extending down the anterior aspect of the spinal column merges with and further reinforces the anulus fibrosus and a similar, but thinner, ligament reinforces the posterior aspect.
- The vertebral arches articulate with each other by pairs of synovial joints known as facet or zygoapophyseal joints. Strong elastic ligaments connecting the bony processes of the vertebral arches contribute to the stability of the spinal column.

(a)

(b)

Fig. 10.29 Intervertebral disc

(Rat: H & E/Alcian blue (a) × 20 (b) × 128)

An intervertebral disc is shown in these micrographs of the tail of an immature rat; this has been chosen since the much larger intervertebral discs of mature mammals and humans would not be amenable to sectioning and photomicroscopy in this manner.

The intervertebral disc lies between the articular surfaces **A** of adjacent vertebral bodies. The disc consists of concentric layers of fibrocartilage, constituting the anulus fibrosus **AF**, which surrounds the central nucleus pulposus **NP**. This staining method distinguishes the collagen component of the fibrocartilage, which is stained pink, from the ground substance component, which is stained blue.

At high magnification, the nucleus pulposus is seen to consist of an unusual fluid form of supporting tissue; this is the only remnant of the embryonic notochord persisting in adult mammals. The cells of the nucleus pulposus, called *physaliphorous cells* **P**, are scattered in irregular clumps throughout an extracellular matrix **M** which consists of ground substance only.

The intervertebral disc functions in the manner of a hydraulic shock absorber, the nucleus pulposus acting as hydraulic fluid. With advancing age, the fibrocartilage of the anulus fibrosus becomes thinned and weakened and the nucleus pulposus tends to be extruded, particularly at the postero-lateral aspect where the disc is least reinforced by surrounding ligaments. This gives rise to the inappropriately named condition, 'slipped disc'.

(a)

(b)

Fig. 10.30 Tendon *(H & E (a) × 128 (b) × 128)*

Tendons are tough inextensible but flexible straps which connect certain muscles to various skeletal structures allowing the muscular forces to be exerted at some distance from the body of the muscle itself and, in some cases, in a different direction.

Tendon is the densest form of collagenous supporting tissue, consisting of bundles of coarse collagen fibres among which are scattered rows of fibroblasts with elongated nuclei. Each tendon is composed of small bundles of this dense tissue bound together by a small amount of looser collagenous supporting tissue which contains the scanty blood supply and tiny nerve fibres from the tendon stretch receptors. The tendon surface is smooth and condensed with minimal connections with the surrounding tissue so as to allow relatively unimpeded movement of the tendon.

In some sites, as shown in micrograph (a), tendons are invested in a fibrous sheath lined by synovium **S**, movement of the tendon within the sheath being lubricated by synovial fluid.

Micrograph (b) shows the insertion of two masses of skeletal muscle **M** into a common tendon **T**; in this case, the tendon will exert the muscular force in a direction different from the direction of pull of the individual skeletal muscles attached to it.

Ligaments are dense bands of fibrous tissue which reinforce joint capsules and maintain bones in the correct anatomical arrangement. Ligaments are histologically similar to tendons but have a less ordered arrangement of the collagen fibres and a variable content of elastic fibres.

11. Immune system

Introduction
All living tissues are subject to the constant threat of invasion by disease-producing foreign agents and micro-organisms (*pathogens*), i.e. bacteria, viruses, fungi, protozoa and multicellular parasites, which may enter via breaches in the skin or linings of the gut, respiratory and genitourinary tracts. Three main lines of defence have consequently evolved:

- *protective surface mechanisms*
- *non-specific tissue defences*
- *specific immune responses.*

Protective surface mechanisms
In humans, these provide the first line of defence. The skin constitutes a relatively impenetrable barrier to most micro-organisms unless breached by injury such as abrasion or burning. The sero-mucous surfaces of the body, such as the conjunctivae and oral cavity, are protected by a variety of antibacterial substances including the enzyme *lysozyme*, secreted in tears and saliva. The respiratory tract is protected by a layer of surface mucus which is continuously removed by ciliary action and replaced by goblet cell activity. The maintenance of an acidic environment in the stomach, vagina and to a lesser extent the skin, inhibits the growth of pathogens in these sites. When such defences fail, the two other main types of defence mechanisms are activated.

Non-specific tissue defences
Damage to tissues usually excites a non-specific response called *inflammation* (which may be *acute* or *chronic*) aimed at removal of any dead tissue and foreign matter, replacement of lost tissue by scar and in some cases regeneration of normal tissue. Acute inflammation is characterised by vascular changes including capillary dilatation, enhanced permeability and increased blood flow resulting in the production of a fibrin-rich inflammatory exudate. Neutrophils, and later macrophages, migrate into the damaged tissues, their phagocytic activity removing tissue debris, deleterious foreign material and pathogens; phagocytosis is often greatly enhanced by involvement of immunological mechanisms as described later. Destroyed tissue is initially replaced by proliferation of capillary-rich *granulation tissue* which is then slowly replaced by fibroblast proliferation and collagen deposition with the eventual formation of a relatively avascular and acellular *fibrous scar*. Some tissues such as liver, skin and epithelial linings are able to regenerate to a greater or lesser degree. In the case where actual tissue damage is minimal, phagocytic activity may occur with little if any overt vascular, exudative and reparative response.

Complement is a series of plasma proteins constituting an enzyme cascade analogous to the clotting system. The cascade can be activated via either the *classical pathway* (usually involving antigen-antibody complexes, see below) or the *alternative pathway* (direct activation by certain organisms). The various peptides and proteins so generated mediate a diverse range of processes including vascular changes (dilatation and increased permeability), cell lysis, *opsonisation* (coating of organisms with complement which enhances phagocytosis by leucocytes), leucocyte attraction (*chemotaxis*) and activation. The alternative pathway probably evolved first as a non-specific defence system with the classical pathway evolving later as an effector mechanism linked to the immune response.

The immune system
This highly specific system depends upon the recognition of exogenous materials as being foreign to the body, any particular foreign substance so recognised being known as an *antigen*; some normal body components may also act as antigens in autoimmune reactions. This results in the activation of the immune system with the purpose of neutralising or destroying the antigen. Lymphocytes play the central role in the immune response. The process is highly antigen-specific but usually depends on phagocytic cells of the monocyte-macrophage system in *presentation of antigen* to lymphocytes. Components of the non-specific defence system (i.e. complement, neutrophils, macrophages) are frequently employed in final destruction of antigen. As any one

micro-organism is usually made up of many different antigens (i.e. peptides, proteins, polysaccharides), the immunological response may involve a combination of responses.

The cells of the immune system, particularly lymphocytes, are scattered throughout the body either as isolated cells, as non-encapsulated aggregations in the gastrointestinal, respiratory and other tracts (*mucosa associated lymphoid tissue* or *MALT*) or within the lymphoid organs namely the *thymus, lymph nodes* and *spleen*. This chapter begins with an overview of the function of the immune system which is an essential prerequisite for understanding the structure and function of the different lymphoid tissues.

The immune system is traditionally divided into two branches namely *cell-mediated immunity* and *humoral immunity* corresponding to two types of lymphocytes identified by early immunological research. *B lymphocytes* are responsible for antibody production and mediate the humoral response. In cell mediated immunity, *T lymphocytes* function as cytotoxic cells directly killing abnormal body cells. More recent research has revealed a more sophisticated system making this classification a gross oversimplification. Lymphocyte subtypes such as T helper and T suppressor cells control B and T cell responses. *Antigen presenting cells* (APCs) of various types including macrophages and B lymphocytes control the activation of T cells. The entire system forms an exquisitely balanced mechanism which can be switched on and off in response to antigen challenge and which can respond with a varied armamentarium to different pathogens.

The specificity of the immune system is entirely attributable to the remarkable chemical structure of antigen receptors on lymphocytes, namely *surface immunoglobulin* (*sIg*) on B cells and the *T cell receptor* (*TCR*) on T cells. The ability of this system to respond to the huge variety of antigens confronting it depends on rearrangement of the genes for these receptors by DNA splicing to generate an enormous diversity of receptor structures in a random manner.

Lymphocytes

Lymphocytes comprise some 20–50% of leucocytes in the circulation, their numbers increasing in response to viral infections. Most circulating lymphocytes measure 6–9 μm (i.e. about the same size as erythrocytes) and are called *small lymphocytes*. About 3% are *large lymphocytes* measuring 9–15 μm.

The light and electron microscopic appearance of circulating lymphocytes has been illustrated in Chapter 3 (Fig. 3.8). Lymphocyte nuclei are ovoid or kidney-shaped with dense chromatin typical of cells with relatively little biosynthetic activity. Nucleoli are not visible with the usual Romanowsky stains of light microscopy but can be demonstrated using the methyl green/pyronin method.

In small lymphocytes, the nucleus occupies about 90% of cell volume, the cytoplasm forming only a narrow rim. The cytoplasm exhibits pale basophilia (i.e. stains light blue) due to a considerable number of free ribosomes; rough endoplasmic reticulum is minimal. With the electron microscope, the Golgi apparatus appears rudimentary and a few lysosomes can be seen. The glycogen content is variable. The plasma membrane exhibits small cytoplasmic projections which, with the scanning electron microscope, appear as short microvilli; these are much more numerous on B lymphocytes. With phase contrast microscopy, lymphocytes exhibit slow amoeboid movement without the cytoplasmic spreading seen in monocytes.

In the case of large lymphocytes, the increase in size is due to a greater amount of cytoplasm. The majority of large lymphocytes seen in blood represent activated B lymphocytes en route to the tissues where they will become antibody-secreting *plasma cells* (see Fig. 11.2).

Investigation of blood cells for spontaneous cytotoxic responses towards various target cells has revealed that this *natural killer activity* appears to be confined to some members of the population of large circulating lymphocytes; cells with this property have been designated as *natural killer (NK) cells*. The cytoplasm of natural killer cells exhibits numerous azurophilic granules containing acid hydrolases and these cells are thus described by some authors as *large granular lymphocytes (LGL)*. NK cells have some but not all features of T lymphocytes and may constitute a separate lymphocyte subset in addition to T and B lymphocytes.

The role of T lymphocytes

As outlined above, lymphocytes play the central role in the immune system differentiating into two main functional types described as *T lymphocytes (T cells)* and *B lymphocytes (B cells)*.

Immunologically immature T lymphocytes migrate from the bone marrow to the thymus where they develop into mature T (thymus-dependent) lymphocytes. Immature T cells proliferate in the thymus acquiring a variety of surface markers (see Fig. 11.3) to become mature albeit *naive lymphocytes*, having as yet had no contact with antigen. It is at this stage of development that T lymphocytes with the ability to react to the body's own normal constituents ('self antigens') are either destroyed or suppressed resulting in *self tolerance*. Clones of mature T cells then populate the peripheral lymphoid tissues (lymph nodes, mucosa-associated lymphoid tissues and spleen) and from here continuously circulate via the bloodstream in a constant quest for antigen. On encountering antigen, T lymphocytes effect antigen destruction either by direct cytotoxic activity or indirectly via activation of B lymphocytes or macrophages.

T lymphocytes, are divided into several functional subsets known as *T helper cells, cytotoxic T cells* and *suppressor T cells*. These subsets can be identified by the presence of different surface markers.

- **T helper cells** (T_H cells). These T lymphocytes 'help' other lymphocytes to perform their effector functions by secreting a variety of peptide or protein chemical messengers called *interleukins*. Such functions include activation of B cells to produce antibody, regulation of cytotoxic T cell function and activation of macrophages to mount a chronic granulomatous inflammatory (delayed-type hypersensitivity) response. It seems likely that subsets of T_H cells, designated T_{H1} and T_{H2}, secrete different interleukins and preferentially activate macrophages or 'help' B cells respectively. T_H cells are characterised by the presence of the surface marker CD4 as well as the *pan-T cell markers* (CD2, CD3 and the T cell receptor) which are present on all mature T cells (see Fig. 11.3).

- **Cytotoxic T cells** (T_C cells). These lymphocytes function in the killing of virus-infected and malignant cells. Most carry the surface marker CD8 as well as the pan-T cell markers. They require interaction with T_H cells to become activated and to undergo proliferation for cytotoxic functions.

- **Suppressor T cells** (T_S cells). The existence of this functional subset is still controversial although suppressor function can be demonstrated by CD8-bearing lymphocytes in experimental animals. These cells are thought to be responsible for switching off the immune response when the initiating stimulus is removed and for suppressing immune responsiveness to self antigens. However other mechanisms are known which can carry out at least some of these functions and the exact role of suppressor cells in vivo is thus unknown. Because they carry the CD8 marker, cytotoxic and suppressor cells are often lumped together in one subgroup designated suppressor/cytotoxic cells.

The role of B lymphocytes

B lymphocytes are derived from precursors in the bone marrow but also undergo maturation in the bone marrow. B cell maturation was first studied in birds in which it occurs in a gut-associated organ called the *Bursa of Fabricius*; this bursal involvement is the origin of the designation 'B' lymphocyte. Exposure to antigen results in clonal proliferation in the peripheral lymphoid tissues with the production of antibody-secreting plasma cells and *B memory cells*.

B lymphocytes are characterised by their ability to synthesise antibodies, glycoproteins which bind to specific antigens. These glycoproteins, also known as *immunoglobulins*, fall into five different structural classes, namely IgG, IgA, IgD, IgM and IgE. In some cases, immunoglobulins are secreted and circulate in the blood. In others, they remain bound to the surface of the B lymphocyte where they behave as antigen receptors, activating the B cell when the appropriate antigen is encountered and binds with the antibody. As a general rule, activation of B cells requires the 'help' of a T helper cell (see above) responding to the same antigen.

Once activated, the B cell undergoes mitotic division to produce a clone of cells, able to synthesise immunoglobulin of the same antigen specificity (though of more than one immunoglobulin class). Most of the B cells of such a clone mature into plasma cells which are capable of synthesis and secretion of large quantities of immunoglobulin. When an antigen is encountered for the first time, this is described as the *primary immune response*. A few cells from the same clone mature to become memory cells, small long-lived circulating lymphocytes which are able to respond quickly to any subsequent challenge with the same antigen. Antibody production during this *secondary immune response* occurs much more rapidly, is of much greater magnitude and produces IgG rather than IgM. This phenomenon explains the lifetime immunity which follows many common infections; it is also the general principle on which vaccination is based.

Antibodies neutralise or destroy invading organisms by a number of methods, all of which involve binding of antibody to one or more antigens associated with the organism; further details are given in Fig. 11.4.

Fig. 11.1 Lymphocytes and antigen presenting cell *(illustration opposite: EM × 18 000)*

This micrograph illustrates several lymphocytes and an antigen presenting cell (APC) in a lymph node. Lymphocytes and antigen presenting cells exhibit similar features in other lymphoid tissues.

The lymphocytes **L** are relatively small with a round nucleus and moderately condensed chromatin which tends to be clumped around the periphery. Cell outlines are fairly regular with occasional surface projections. The cytoplasm is homogeneous and electron-dense due to extensive free ribosomes. There are modest numbers of mitochondria but little rough or smooth endoplasmic reticulum and few lysosomes or secretory granules.

The centre of the field is occupied by the large cell body of an antigen presenting cell **APC** in this case an *interdigitating cell*. These have numerous long branched cytoplasmic extensions **CE** reaching out between the surrounding lymphocytes and almost completely filling the spaces between them. Its nucleus is deeply indented with dispersed chromatin; in this example, the plane of section has resulted in a small nuclear extension appearing to be separate from the main part of the nucleus. Typically, the APC cytoplasm is very heterogeneous containing numerous small lysosomal granules **G**, larger phagosomes **P** and scattered profiles of rough endoplasmic reticulum and cytoskeletal microtubules.

Many of the antigen presenting cell types found in lymphoid tissue are probably derived from circulating monocytes and form part of the macrophage-monocyte system described with Fig. 3.9. Antigen-presenting cells take up foreign material and *process* the antigen by breaking it down into molecular fragments of a form capable of recognition by T lymphocytes.

Processed antigen is then passed to the plasma membrane for *presentation* to appropriate lymphocytes. This process is enhanced by the intimate relationship of the lymphocyte plasma membranes to those of the APC cytoplasmic extensions. The shapes of APCs vary according to the arrangement of cells in the different lymphoid tissues, and a variety of names are therefore applied, e.g. interdigitating cells and follicular dendritic cells of lymph node, interdigitating cells of thymus; regrettably a standard terminology has yet to be developed. Some APCs are mobile, such as the Langerhans cells of the skin which migrate from their site of antigen uptake in the skin to regional lymph nodes where they become paracortical interdigitating dendritic cells.

Antigen presentation is not exclusively the function of cells derived from the macrophage-monocytic system. B lymphocytes, and, in certain circumstances, a variety of other cells including vascular endothelial cells, dermal fibroblasts, thyroid epithelial cells and brain astrocytes may present antigen to T lymphocytes.

2.0 μm

Fig. 11.2 Plasma cell *(EM × 10 000)*

When B lymphocytes are stimulated by antigen, they differentiate to form plasma cells which produce large quantities of antibody. Plasma cells are not usually found in the circulation but function in the tissues, in particular the medullary cords of lymph nodes, the white pulp of the spleen, supporting tissues of mucosal surfaces (e.g. lamina propria of intestine) and the bone marrow (comprising 1% of cells in marrow aspirates). Some plasma cells may appear in lymphatics and the bloodstream following strong antigen stimulation, in certain viral infections (e.g. glandular fever, mumps) and in certain other disease states.

Antibody production involves the synthesis of the immunoglobulin polypeptide chains on rough endoplasmic reticulum. The basic antibody unit is made up of two identical light chains and two identical heavy chains. These are then transferred to the Golgi apparatus where synthesis is completed and the immunoglobulin is packaged into small vesicles before secretion into the extracellular space by exocytosis.

Differentiation of a B lymphocyte into an antibody-secreting plasma cell involves three essential steps: activation, proliferation and maturation.

Two types of antigen can activate B cell responses, T cell-dependent and T cell-independent. The former require T cell help mediated by T_H cell-secreted interleukins. The latter are usually large molecular weight polymers with simple repeating structures which induce cross linking of cell surface receptors. T cell-dependent antigens are by far the most important in physiological terms.

Several cell divisions are involved in the process of transformation from resting lymphocyte to *plasmablast* and thence to mature plasma cell. Immature plasma cells can undergo successive waves of mitosis in the medullary cords of lymph nodes to enlarge the clone of cells still further.

Each stage of this process requires several signals including recognition of appropriate antigen by the surface immunoglobulins (sIg) of naive **B** cells (see Fig. 11.3) and secretion by activated T_H cells of soluble factors including interleukins 4, 5 and 6. Interleukin release by T_H cells is dependent on simultaneous activation and clonal expansion of T_H cells.

Morphology

Plasma cells are large with an eccentric round or oval nucleus **N** with the chromatin coarsely clumped in a characteristic 'cart-wheel' or 'clock face' pattern; this dispersed chromatin pattern and the presence of nucleoli (not seen in this plane of section) are typical of cells active in protein synthesis.

In light microscopy, the cytoplasm is deeply basophilic due to its large content of ribosomal RNA (see Fig. 1.20). With electron microscopy, the ribosomes are seen to be associated with an extensive rough endoplasmic reticulum **rER**. For the same reason, the cytoplasm stains red with *methyl green-pyronin* (see Fig. 11.17) whilst the nucleus stains a pale blue green with a prominent nucleolus. A well developed Golgi **G** displaces the nucleus to one side of the cell and by light microscopy is represented by a perinuclear halo (see Fig. 1.20). The light and heavy chains of immunoglobulin are synthesised in the rER with the carbohydrate element being added by the Golgi. Secretory vesicles **V** then convey the antibody to the surface where it is promptly secreted rather than being stored. In the centre of the cell and surrounded by the Golgi complex is the centrosome **C** from which radiate the microtubules of the cytoskeleton. Note the fine cytoplasmic extensions of fibroblasts **F** in the surrounding tissues.

Lymphocyte Stage	T Lymphocytes		B Lymphocytes	
	Marker	Function	Marker	Function
Immature	CD2 CD25 CD1,CD5 CD3 TCR CD4 CD8	Receptor for LFA-2 and sheep erythrocytes Receptor for interleukin 2 ? Transmembrane signalling element of TCR T cell antigen receptor Marks T_H subset. Also HIV receptor Marks T_C/T_S subset	surface IgM sIgA/sIgG,IgD MHC Class II MHC Class I CD19 CD20 CD21	B cell antigen receptor Antigen receptor B cell committed to IgA or IgG production Presents antigenic peptides to T_H cells Presents antigenic peptides to T_C cells B cell marker ? function May be part of regulated Ca++ channel Complement receptor
Mature	CD2,CD3,CD4/8 MHC Class I	As above As above	CD19,20,21 MHC Class I & II sIgM,sIgD,sIgA/G	As above As above
Activated	CD2,3,4/8,25 MHC Class I & II CD54,58	As above As above Accessory adhesion molecules	CD25 CD30	As above ?
Memory	CD2,11a,54,58	Accessory adhesion molecules	sIgG/sIgA,CD19	As above

Fig. 11.3 Lymphocyte surface antigens

A wide variety of membrane antigens are found on lymphocyte plasma membranes, the antigens changing according to their state of maturation and functional activity. These molecules are customarily referred to as antigens because they were originally detected using monoclonal antibodies. These antigens are used in research for the identification of particular lymphocytes and are thus also referred to as *surface markers*. The function of many of these surface proteins and glycoproteins is still unknown. They can be divided into 4 groups as outlined below and detailed in the table above.

Immunoglobulins. B lymphocytes are constantly being produced in the bone marrow, each cell subsequently acquiring the ability to recognise a single particular chemical configuration, i.e. a particular antigen to which it might be exposed at some time in the future. This occurs by the random rearrangement of segments of the genes which code for the variable region of the immunoglobulin molecule. By the time the B lymphocyte is mature, it exhibits on its surface IgM, IgD and either IgA or IgG. Nevertheless, the B lymphocyte has yet to encounter the antigen for which it is programmed and is thus described as a naive mature B lymphocyte. Most circulating B cells are in this category.

Binding of antigen to the surface immunoglobulin sIg signals the B lymphocyte to divide, differentiate into a clone of plasma cells and secrete immunoglobulin of the same antigen specificity as the surface immunoglobulin.

T cell receptor (TCR). This molecule, found on the surface of T cells, bears some structural similarity to immunoglobulin and is also produced with a wide range of binding affinities by random DNA rearrangements.

MHC (major histocompatibility) antigens. These are the major antigens that differentiate tissues of one individual from another and were first discovered in the context of organ transplant rejection; in humans, the system is called *HLA (human leuçocyte antigen)*.

The MHC antigens are of three different classes designated Class I, Class II and Class III. *Class I MHC antigens* are present on the surfaces of virtually all cells in the body with the important exception of erythrocytes. *Class II MHC antigens* are normally present only on B lymphocytes, immunologically-activated T lymphocytes and antigen presenting cells. Certain MHC antigens are associated with certain diseases (e.g. HLA B27 in ankylosing spondylitis). The function of MHC molecules is to present antigen to Tlymphocytes. Small peptide fragments of non-self (and

self) proteins bind to the MHC molecule within the cell and the complex then appears on the cell surface where the combination is available for recognition by a T lymphocyte bearing an appropriate receptor; T lymphocytes can only recognise antigen if bound to MHC protein whereas B lymphocytes can recognise soluble antigen.

Class I MHC molecules present non-self proteins synthesised intracellularly (e.g. viral proteins and abnormal proteins produced by neoplastic cells) thus activating cytotoxic T lymphocytes to destroy the infected or neoplastic cell. Class II MHC molecules bind peptide products of phagocytosis and lysosomal breakdown of exogenous protein (e.g. bacterial products) which are recognised by the helper T cells necessary for the activation of B lymphocytes and production of antibody.

Surface antigens defined by the CD system. These antigens have been characterised by monoclonal antibodies and represent a diverse group of surface proteins with a wide variety of functions. Historically, monoclonal antibodies were developed by a number of different commercial and research groups who used their own naming systems, e.g. OKT4, OKT8; many of these antibodies were found to react with the same antigen, although not necessarily the same epitope (chemical formation of the antigen), leading to great terminological confusion. Subsequent international collaboration resulted in the development of the **CD** (cluster of differentiation) system of standard nomenclature which is updated every few years.

The characterisation of surface antigens using monoclonal antibodies and the technique of *flow cytometry* have shown that B and T lymphocytes express different CD antigens at different stages of maturation and activation.

The CD naming system has been used to name many surface molecules on lymphocytes (and on other leucocytes). CD surface antigens have the following functions:

- receptors for complement components, the Fc portions of immunoglobulin molecules, transferrin, interleukins
- intercellular adhesion molecules such as ICAM-1
- transmembrane signalling protein complexes such as CD3 which transmits the message to the interior of the T cell that antigen has bound to the TCR
- many other surface molecules whose function has not been elucidated but which are characteristic of a particular lymphocyte subclass or stage of maturation, e.g., CD4, CD8, CD1.

CYTOTOXIC T CELL ACTIVATION

B CELL ACTIVATION

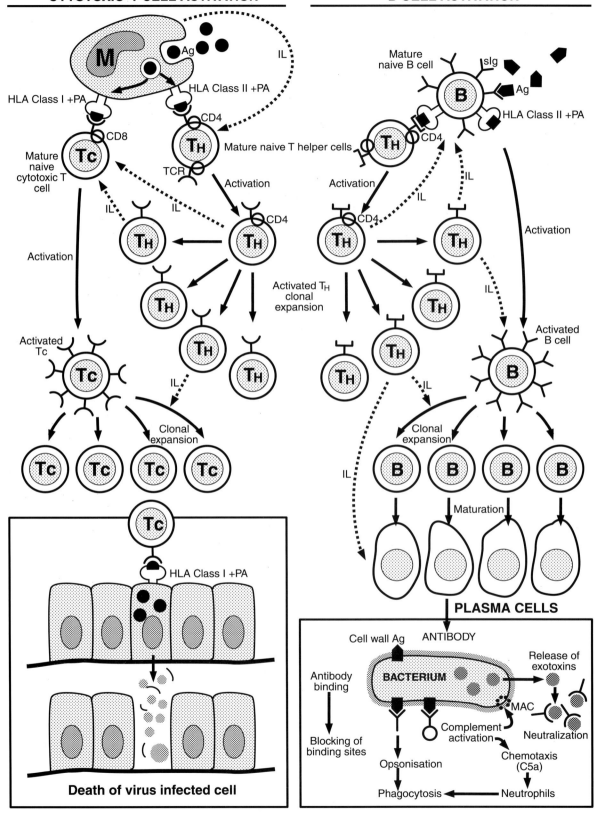

Death of virus infected cell

PLASMA CELLS

Fig. 11.4 Essential immunological processes *(illustration opposite)*

The essential processes in development of immunological responses are summarised below and the better understood pathways are illustrated in simplified form in the diagram.

Activation of the immune system

Initiation of an immune response first requires contact between antigen **Ag** and mature lymphocytes; in the case of T cells, this requires an antigen presenting cell. There are several mechanisms of immunological activation:

1. Interaction of a B cell with a protein or polysaccharide antigen which has a repeating chemical structure (e.g. polysaccharide coat of bacteria such as pneumococcus). Few antigens are of this type (not illustrated).
2. Antigen is taken up by an antigen presenting cell (e.g. macrophage **M**, B lymphocyte **B** via binding to surface immunoglobulin **sIg**, Langerhans cells of skin) and processed (e.g. in the case of a protein, chemically and enzymatically broken down into peptides). Processed antigen **PA** is then bound to an HLA protein to be expressed on the cell surface. Here the HLA protein is incorporated in the cell membrane such that part of the molecule including the bound antigenic peptide is exposed to the outside milieu. If the antigen in that form comes in contact with a mature T lymphocyte which bears a T cell receptor **TCR** with appropriate specificity, it will activate an immune response. The nature of the response depends on whether the peptide is presented bound to HLA of class I or II (see Fig. 11.3) as these only interact with CD8- or CD4-bearing T lymphocytes respectively. Antigenic peptides bound to Class II HLA molecules thus induce a T helper cell T_H response, which is then available to 'help' B cells to respond to the same antigen with the production of immunoglobulins. T cell 'help' involves production of a range of interleukins **IL** which mediate activation, clonal expansion and maturation of the B cell response. The architecture of lymph nodes and other lymphoid tissues and the routes of circulation of T lymphocytes are designed to bring as many lymphocytes as possible into contact with each antigen.
3. Antigen synthesised within a body cell (e.g. tumour cell, virus-infected cell) is incorporated in the cell membrane (bound to a class I HLA protein) where it is available for recognition by CD8-bearing cytotoxic T lymphocytes T_c. T_H activation is also required for a T_c response to be mounted. Activation of both T_c and T_H probably requires processing and presentation of antigen by a macrophage **M**.
4. Cells that bear different HLA proteins on their cell surfaces (i.e. transplanted tissues) are able to excite an immune response which involves at least T helper cells and either cytotoxic T cells or macrophages (not illustrated).

During activation of the immune response, the surface antigens on the lymphocytes alter; for simplicity only essential markers are included in this diagram (see Fig. 11.3).

Generation of the means of antigen destruction

1. *Production of antibodies* by clonal expansion of B cells and maturation into plasma cells. Mechanisms of antibody-mediated antigen elimination are as follows:

- Antibody binding to surface molecules on an organism may prevent binding of that organism to the specific receptor on the host tissue which would otherwise permit invasion of the host.
- Antibody bound to its antigen is able to bind complement and activate the complement cascade. This causes lysis of the membrane of the invading organism by the membrane attack complex **MAC** and augments the acute inflammatory response by producing peptides chemotactic for neutrophils.
- Bound antibody (especially if complement is also bound) 'opsonises' the surface of an organism, i.e. makes it easier for neutrophils to bind to and phagocytose the organism.
- Bound antibody can also mediate *'antibody dependent cell cytotoxicity'* (*ADCC*); in this case, a cytotoxic cell is only able to kill the organism if it has antibody bound to its surface, facilitating binding of the cytotoxic cell to its target (not illustrated).
- Antibody is also able to inactivate toxins released by some organisms and, by binding them into immune complexes, both inhibits the action of the toxin and facilitates their clearance from the body by the cells of the monocyte-macrophage system.

2. *Cell-mediated cytotoxicity* is the destruction of altered or abnormal cells by cytotoxic cells which may be either classical cytotoxic T cells T_c, natural killer cells or cytotoxic cells which require specific antibody to carry out their cytotoxic function (ADCC).
3. Certain types of antigens (e.g. of mycobacteria) interact with T lymphocytes promoting the secretion of certain lymphokines; such lymphokines activate macrophages to kill organisms which they have previously ingested but which they are otherwise unable to destroy; this is the mechanism of chronic granulomatous inflammation (not illustrated).

Termination of the immune response

There are a number of mechanisms for switching off the immune response when the need for it has been removed; these include the idiotype-antiidiotype antibody networks, cross-linking of surface immunoglobulins to Fc receptors by antigens, down-regulation by immune complexes, suppressor T cells and factors they may produce, and neuroendocrine interactions.

Immunological memory

When activated lymphocytes undergo clonal expansion during an immune response, some of the cells generated mature to become memory T and B cells. These lymphocytes have a similar appearance to naive lymphocytes but are able to produce a faster and more effective response to a smaller quantity of antigen encountered at a later date. B memory cells are known to have higher affinity receptors for antigen (surface immunoglobulin) than naive B cells and to produce IgG earlier in the response.

Thymus

The thymus is a large flattened lymphoid organ located in the upper anterior mediastinum and lower part of the neck. The thymus is most active during childhood after which it undergoes slow involution.

In the embryo, the thymus originates from epithelial outgrowths of the ventral wing of the third pharyngeal pouch on each side. These merge in the midline forming a single organ comprising two lobes subdivided into numerous fine lobules. The epithelium develops into a sponge-like structure containing a labyrinth of interconnecting spaces which become colonised by lymphocytes derived from haemopoietic tissue elsewhere in the developing embryo. Towards the centre of the organ, the epithelial framework has a coarser structure with smaller interstices and a much smaller lymphocyte population so that, on microscopic examination, the gland has a highly cellular outer *cortex* and a less cellular central *medulla* which is continuous throughout the gland.

The epithelial cells of the thymus not only provide a mechanical supporting framework for the lymphocyte population but in the cortex tend to envelop the lymphocytes performing some kind of 'nurse' function promoting T cell differentiation, proliferation and subset maturation. Furthermore, the epithelial cells secrete at least three different hormones and a variety of other humoral factors which regulate T cell maturation and proliferation within the thymus and in other lymphoid organs and tissues.

Functions of the thymus

The prime functions of the thymus include:

- Development of immunocompetent T lymphocytes from lymphocytes derived from bone marrow. This involves differentiation of the two T cell subsets, T helper cells and T cytotoxic/suppressor cells.
- Proliferation of clones of mature naive T cells to supply the circulating lymphocyte pool and peripheral tissues.
- Development of immunological self tolerance.
- Secretion of hormones and other soluble factors which regulate T cell maturation, proliferation and function within the thymus and peripheral tissues. Thymic hormones also regulate the development of peripheral lymphoid organs and tissues. There are at least three polypeptides with hormonal characteristics namely *thymulin*, *thymopoietin* and *thymosin alpha 1*.
- Haemopoiesis is an important function of the thymus during fetal development.

Involution of the thymus

The thymus continues to grow from birth until puberty but after this it slowly involutes so that in later life, the thymus is often difficult to differentiate macroscopically from surrounding fibrofatty tissue.

Involution involves two distinct processes, fatty infiltration and lymphocyte depletion; these appear to occur independently and on a different time scale. Adipocytes first begin to appear at birth, their numbers slowly rising until puberty when the rate of fatty infiltration increases markedly. The process involves the supporting tissue component of the organ which is mainly located around the blood vessels. Consequently, fatty infiltration of the interlobular septa occurs first, spreading out into the cortex and later the medulla.

Lymphocyte numbers begin to fall from about one year of age, the process continuing thereafter at a constant rate. Despite this, the thymus continues to provide a supply of mature T lymphocytes to the circulating pool and peripheral tissues. Lymphocyte depletion results in collapse of the epithelial framework. However cords of epithelial cells persist and continue to secrete thymic hormones throughout life.

The normal process of slow thymic involution associated with ageing should be distinguished from *acute thymic involution* which may occur in response to severe disease and metabolic stress associated with pregnancy, lactation, infection, surgery, malnutrition, malignancy and other systemic insults. Stress involution is characterised by greatly increased lymphocyte death and is probably mediated by high levels of corticosteroids; thus the size and activity of the adult thymus is often underestimated if examined after prolonged illness.

(a)   *(b)*

Fig. 11.5 Thymus *(H & E (a) ×15 (b) ×40)*

As seen in micrograph (a), the thymus is a highly lobulated organ invested by a loose collagenous capsule **C** from which short interlobular septa **S** containing blood vessels radiate into the substance of the organ. The thymic tissue is divided into two distinct zones, a deeply basophilic outer cortex **Cx** and an inner eosinophilic medulla **M**; distinction between the two is most marked in early childhood as in this specimen.

Micrograph (b) shows part of a pubertal thymus at higher magnification. The cortex **Cx** is packed with lymphocytes accounting for its basophilia whereas the medulla **M** contains fewer lymphocytes. Note the collagenous capsule **C** which is continuous with an interlobular septum **S** terminating at the cortico-medullary junction.

The epithelial framework of the medulla is relatively coarse and bulky, the interstices being much smaller than those of the cortex and therefore accommodating fewer lymphocytes. The eosinophilia of the epithelial framework, and the relative paucity of lymphocytes, explains the pale pink staining characteristics of the medulla.

The epithelial framework of the cortex is more delicate and finely branched than that of the medulla, and is sometimes described by the term 'reticular'; there is however no evidence that the cells are phagocytic or represent part of the so-called reticuloendothelial system (see Ch. 4). At an ultrastructural level, the epithelial cells are found to have typical desmosomes at their points of contact and the cytoplasm contains bundles of intermediate filaments of the protein keratin.

In the centre of the medulla are eosinophilic lamellated structures known as *Hassal's corpuscles* **H** representing degenerate epithelial cells (see Fig. 11.7).

Numerous small branches of the internal thoracic and inferior thyroid arteries enter the thymus via the interlobular septa branching at the cortico-medullary junction to supply the cortex and medulla. The cortical capillaries are of the continuous endothelium type whereas those of the medulla and septa may be fenestrated. Post capillary venules in the cortico-medullary region have a specialised cuboidal endothelium similar to that of the high endothelial venules of the lymph node (see Fig. 11.15) which allows passage of lymphocytes into and out of the thymus. The venous and lymphatic drainage follows the course of the arterial supply; there are no afferent lymphatics.

The inner surface of the thymic capsule and septa is invested by a continuous layer of thymic epithelial cells resting on a basement membrane. The epithelium also forms sheaths around the blood vessels forming a barrier to the entry of antigenic material into the system of spaces within the epithelial framework. This is known as the *blood-thymus barrier*.

Sympathetic and parasympathetic fibres derived respectively from the sympathetic chain and phrenic nerves accompany the blood vessels into the thymus. Some serve vasomotor functions but many terminate in the medulla in association with a variety of cells of possible neuroendocrine function; their secretory products include vasoactive intestinal peptide (VIP), oxytocin, vasopressin, neurophysin and acetyl-cholinesterase but their function in the thymus is not understood.

Fig 11.6 Thymic cortex *(H & E × 480)*

The thymic cortex is predominantly populated by lymphocytes of the T cell lineage, those of the outer cortex being larger than those deeper in the cortex. The large lymphocytes are *lymphoblasts* which divide by mitosis to produce clones of smaller T cells which undergo further maturation as they are pushed deeper into the cortex towards the medulla. Several mitotic figures **Mt** can be seen in the outer cortex in this micrograph. At the cortico-medullary junction they enter the blood vessels and lymphatics to join the pool of circulating T lymphocytes and populate the T lymphocyte domains of other lymphoid organs where they attain immunological maturity. Of the vast number of lymphocytes produced, the majority die before ever leaving the thymus. This extraordinary wastage may be the means by which lymphocytes programmed to recognise the body's own indigenous constituents (i.e. self antigens) are eliminated, retaining only those programmed to recognise foreign antigens.

The thymic cortex also contains pale stained vacuolated macrophages **M** which engulf dead lymphocytes. Macrophages containing little phagocytosed material are common in the cortico-medullary region and medulla, some having the form of *dendritic interdigitating cells* which may act as antigen presenting cells.

Note also in this micrograph, a small capillary lined by flattened endothelial cells **E** entering the cortex from the capsule **C**. Around the capillary can be discerned the basement membrane **BM** of epithelial cells at the interface between the thymic framework and supporting tissue elements; these cells constitute the blood-thymus barrier. The cells of the cortical epithelial framework stain poorly and cannot be distinguished, being obscured by the mass of lymphocytes.

Fig. 11.7 Thymic medulla *(H & E × 480)*

The dominant feature of the thymic medulla is the robust epithelial component **E**, the cells having large pale stained nuclei, eosinophilic cytoplasm and prominent basement membranes.

A particular feature are the concentrically lamellated *Hassal's corpuscles* **H** which first appear in fetal life and increase in number thereafter. Initially, the corpuscles begin as a single medullary epithelial cell which enlarges and then degenerates to form a vacuolated eosinophilic (pink-stained) mass. The process is repeated in surrounding epithelial cells with the formation of a lamellated mass surrounded by flattened degenerating epithelial cells. In this micrograph, a smaller mass of large atypical epithelial cells **D** may represent an early Hassal's corpuscle. Some authorities maintain that macrophages, laden with debris from degenerate cortical lymphocytes, become incorporated in the Hassal's corpuscles and the number and size of the corpuscles increase at times of intense lymphocytic destruction.

Although the thymus is usually considered a specifically T cell organ, occasional mature B lymphocytes, B cell germinal centres and rarely plasma cells can be found in the thymus particularly in children. Ultrastructural studies have shown that these lie outside the epithelial enclosure and within the perivascular spaces of the medulla, cortico-medullary junction and septa and this has led to a concept of two functional compartments of the thymus, namely an intraepithelial compartment and an extraepithelial (perivascular) compartment.

Lymph nodes

Mature lymphocytes are distributed throughout the body where they are arranged in aggregations which exhibit various degrees of structural organisation. Isolated lymphocytes are found in most loose supporting tissues and amongst epithelial cells, particularly the epithelium of the gastrointestinal and respiratory tracts; in addition, large non-encapsulated aggregations of lymphocytes are found in the walls of these tracts. Most lymphocytes are, however, located in encapsulated, highly organised structures called *lymph nodes*, which are interposed along the larger regional vessels of the lymph vascular system. Lymph nodes tend to occur in groups, particularly in areas where the lymphatics converge to form larger trunks as in the neck, axillae, groins, lung hila and para-aortic areas.

Four interrelated functions occur within lymph nodes:

- Non-specific filtration of particulate matter and microorganisms from lymph by the phagocytic activity of macrophages, thus preventing exogenous material from reaching the general circulation.
- Interaction of circulating lymphocytes with antigen-containing lymph as it is filtered through the narrow confines of the node; initiation of an immune response may require the involvement of antigen presenting cells.
- Aggregation, activation and proliferation of B lymphocytes; in response to appropriate antigenic stimulation, this leads to plasma cell formation and antibody production.
- Aggregation, activation and proliferation of T lymphocytes with induction of cytotoxic immune responses after appropriate antigenic stimulation.

Cell types in the lymph node

The cells of the lymph node can be divided into three functional types:

- **Lymphoid cells.** These are lymphocytes of all types and their derivatives. All originate from bone marrow with some cell populations being expanded in the thymus and other peripheral lymphoid tissues (e.g. MALT); the majority of lymphocytes enter the node via the bloodstream with a small proportion entering via lymph draining from the tissues .
- **Immunological accessory cells.** These are a variety of macrophages and other phagocytic antigen processing and presenting cells and cells with non-specific effector functions. These cells originate in the bone marrow and pass to the peripheral tissues before reaching the lymph node in lymph; they probably constitute part of the mononuclear phagocyte (monocyte-macrophage) system.
- **Stromal cells.** These include lymphatic and vascular endothelial cells and fibroblasts responsible for elaboration of the lymph node supporting framework. The lymphendothelium is highly active in phagocytosis of particulate material from afferent lymph and this was responsible for the now outdated reticulo-endothelial concept (see Ch. 4). This phagocytic activity appears to be an entirely non immunologically-specific process which is quite distinct from the activity of bone marrow-derived accessory cells.

With conventional microscopy and staining techniques, identification of different cell types in the lymph node is not possible with any degree of accuracy partly due to the changing morphology of cells according to functional activity. Furthermore, the terminology is fraught with inconsistencies due to the rapidity of new discoveries which have mainly employed enzyme histochemical and immunohistochemical methods and in particular the use of monoclonal antibodies.

Fig. 11.8 Lymph node *(illustrations opposite) (a) Structure and vascular organisation (b) H & E × 8*

Lymph nodes are small bean-shaped organs situated in the course of the regional lymphatic vessels such that lymph draining back to the bloodstream passes through one or more lymph nodes. Relatively inactive nodes are only a few millimetres long, increasing greatly in size when mounting an active immunological response. The outer part of the lymph node is highly cellular and is known as the *cortex* whilst the central area is less cellular and is known as the *medulla*.

The lymph node is encapsulated by dense collagenous tissue from which *trabeculae* extend for a variable distance into the substance of the node. *Afferent lymphatic vessels* divide into several branches outside the node, then pierce the capsule to drain into a narrow space called the *subcapsular sinus* extending around beneath the convex surface of the node. From here, a labyrinth of channels called *cortical sinuses* passes towards the medulla through the cortical cell mass; sinuses adjacent to the trabeculae pursue a more direct course towards the medulla but nevertheless form part of the cortical sinus system. The dominant feature of the medulla is the network of broad interconnected lymphatic channels called *medullary sinuses* which converge upon the hilum in the concavity of the node. Lymph drains from the hilum into one or more *efferent lymphatic vessels* which in turn drain into more proximal nodes before eventually joining the bloodstream via the *thoracic duct* or *right lymphatic duct*.

The parenchyma of the lymph node consists of an open meshwork of reticulin fibres which provides support for an ever changing population of lymphocytes. The *cortex* consists of densely-packed lymphocytes and forms extensions called *medullary cords* which project into the medulla between the medullary sinuses.

In the outer cortex, lymphocytes form a variable number of densely packed *lymphoid follicles* many of which show less dense *germinal centres*. The deep cortex (*paracortical zone*) is devoid of lymphoid follicles.

The blood supply of the lymph node is derived from one or more small arteries which enter at the hilum and branch in the medulla, giving rise to extensive capillary networks corresponding to the cortical follicles, paracortical zone and medullary cords. Lymphocytes enter lymph nodes mainly via the arterial system, gaining access by migrating across the walls of specialised post-capillary venules as described later. The post-capillary venules drain into small veins which leave the node via the hilum.

The micrograph illustrates the main histological features of a lymph node. The node is seen to comprise an outer, densely staining cell-rich cortex **Cx** and a pale stained inner medulla **M** which is continuous with the hilum **H**. The superficial cortex contains a number of dense cellular aggregations, the follicles **F**, many of which have a pale stained germinal centre. The deeper cortex or paracortical zone **P** is also densely cellular but has a more homogeneous staining appearance. At the left of the field, some lymphoid follicles appear to be located deep in the paracortex; this is not the case but is a product of the plane of section which passes at that point through the superficial cortex. Extensions of the cortical cell mass extend into the medulla as medullary cords **MC**. The superficial cortex, the paracortex and medulla represent the three different centres of immunological activity in the lymph node being dominated by B lymphocytes, T lymphocytes and plasma cells respectively.

Several trabeculae **T** extend from the capsule **C** into the substance of the node. Beneath the capsule can be seen the subcapsular sinus **S** which is continuous with the trabecular sinuses; these are all that can be seen of the cortical sinuses which are generally difficult to visualise because of their highly convoluted shape and numerous fine extensions which penetrate the cellular mass of the cortex. Some particulate matter is probably taken up and disposed of by lymphendothelial cells without evoking any immune response. Antigens are phagocytosed by various types of antigen presenting cells exposed to the lymph (described in more detail later), processed and then passed via their cytoplasmic extensions to be presented to lymphocytes. Lymphocytes entering the node in afferent lymph constitute less than 10% of all lymphocytes entering the node except in mesenteric nodes where they may constitute up to 30%.

The vascular system provides the main route of entry of lymphocytes into the node as well as supplying its metabolic requirements. Within the paracortex, the post-capillary venules have a cuboidal endothelium specialised for the exit of lymphocytes; these are often described as *high endothelial venules (see Fig. 11.15)*. The recognition by lymphocytes of these exit sites appears to involve the presence of specific complementary *adhesion molecules* on the surface of the endothelial cells and lymphocytes. High endothelial cells have a prominent Golgi apparatus and have been shown to secrete glycolipids and glycoproteins in amounts correlating with, but lagging by days or weeks, periods of high lymphocyte migration into the lymph nodes; the functional significance of this is obscure. The vessels of the superficial cortex and medullary cords are not thought to be specialised and do not appear to allow exit of lymphocytes.

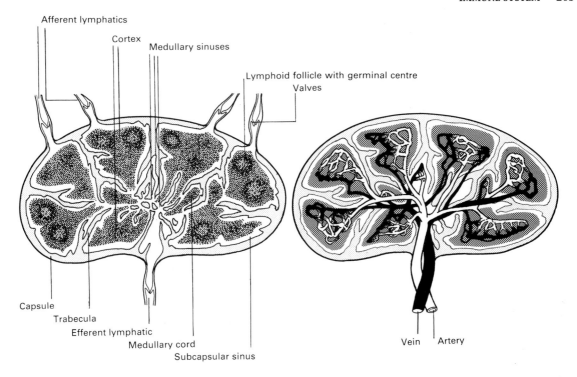

Afferent lymphatics

Cortex

Medullary sinuses

Lymphoid follicle with germinal centre
Valves

Capsule

Trabecula

Efferent lymphatic

Medullary cord

Subcapsular sinus

Vein   Artery

(a)

(b)

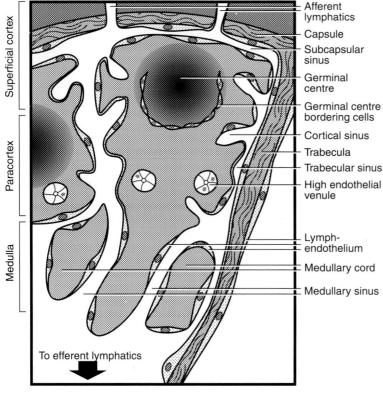

Afferent lymphatics

Capsule

Subcapsular sinus

Germinal centre

Germinal centre bordering cells

Cortical sinus

Trabecula

Trabecular sinus

High endothelial venule

Lymph-endothelium

Medullary cord

Medullary sinus

Superficial cortex

Paracortex

Medulla

To efferent lymphatics

Fig. 11.9 Functional compartments of the lymph node

This diagram illustrates the three functional compartments within the lymph node.

- **A network of lymphatic sinuses** lined with lymphatic endothelium and continuous with the lumen of the afferent and efferent lymphatic vessels.
- **The blood vascular compartment** represented by the microvascular network of the node; its specialised *high endothelial venules* are the site of entry of circulating lymphocytes into the node.
- **The interstitial compartment**, into which pass circulating lymphocytes in the quest for antigen; lymphocytes which do not recognise antigen leave the node within a few hours via the lymphatic compartment and efferent lymph to rejoin the general circulation.

The lymphatic and vascular endothelia thus define the boundaries of the three compartments and control passage of cells and molecules between the different compartments.

The germinal centre is partly encapsulated by flattened stromal cells called *germinal centre bordering cells*, the 'capsule' being open towards the subcapsular sinus; the role of this 'capsule' is discussed in Fig. 11.13.

Fig. 11.10 Lymphocyte domains in the lymph node *(H & E × 30)*

The interstitial compartment of the lymph node has three functional domains, each populated by different types of lymphocytes.

The lymphocytes of the superficial cortex are mainly arranged in spheroidal lymphoid follicles **F** and these are the major sites in which B lymphocytes localise and proliferate. Traditionally, lymphoid follicles have been classified as 'primary follicles' if a central pale area is absent and 'secondary follicles' if such an area is present. The pale central areas are the site of B lymphocyte proliferation and are thus termed germinal centres; the 'primary' follicles probably represent quiescent 'secondary' follicles.

The deep cortical zone or paracortex **P**, consists mainly of T lymphocytes which are never arranged as follicles.

The medullary cords **MC** mainly contain B lymphocytes and plasma cells involved in immunoglobulin synthesis.

The number of cortical lymphoid follicles and the depth of the paracortex vary greatly according to the immunological state of the particular lymph node and the individual as a whole. A predominantly cytotoxic immunological response is associated with paracortical thickening whereas a predominantly humoral response is shown by the appearance of many cortical follicles with pale germinal centres.

(a)

(b)

Fig. 11.11 Supporting tissue of the lymph node *(Reticulin method × 30)*

This technique shows the fine reticular architecture of the lymph node; reticulin fibres are stained black and lymphocyte nuclei appear brown.

The main structural support for the lymph node is derived from the collagenous capsule **Cap** and trabeculae **T** which extend into the body of the node. From these, a fine meshwork of reticulin fibres extends throughout the node providing an open supporting framework for the mass of lymphocytes and accessory cells within the cortex and medullary cords. The reticular network is particularly dense in the cortex except for the follicular areas where it is relatively sparse. The subcapsular sinus **SS**, trabecular sinuses **TS**, other cortical sinuses **CS** and medullary sinuses **MS** are kept patent by a fine skeleton of reticulin fibres which traverse the sinuses and are completely invested by lymphendothelial cells.

The reticulin framework and collagen of the capsule and trabeculae are laid down by fibroblasts as in other supporting tissues and a few fibroblast-like cells are found on the reticulin network. Numerous macrophages are draped over the whole reticular meshwork, their long dendritic cytoplasmic processes providing a large surface area for the clearance of particles, organisms and soluble antigens from the afferent lymph.

Fig. 11.12 Capsule and subcapsular sinus *(H & E (a) × 128 (b) × 320)*

As seen in micrograph (a), the fibrous capsule **Cap** of the lymph node is pierced by branches of afferent lymphatic vessels **A** with valves **V** ensuring one-way flow. Beneath the capsule is the subcapsular sinus **S** which drains via the cortical sinuses towards the medulla.

Micrograph (b) focuses on the subcapsular sinus **S** at high magnification. A fine eosinophilic line **E** can been seen representing the lymphendothelial lining of the sinus and demarcating the lymph compartment from the interstitial compartment. The lymph node sinuses are traversed by fine reticulin strands which are invested by attenuated pale staining endothelial cells which are very difficult to identify with ordinary light microscopical methods. The reticulin strands provide support for large eosinophilic *sinus macrophages* **M**. These macrophages engulf particles, soluble antigens and other debris from afferent lymph. Some do this in a non-specific manner whilst others process antigen for presentation to T lymphocytes of the cortex. Antigens may also be sampled in peripheral tissues by macrophages which then migrate to regional lymph nodes via afferent lymph for presentation to lymphocytes located in the node. Cortical lymphocytes may also sample antigen directly as it percolates through the node.

Scanning electron microscopy has demonstrated the presence of phagocytic cells with a highly irregular 'veiled' cell surface within afferent lymph and the subcapsular sinus. Known as *veiled cells* they appear to be the precursors of the interdigitating cells of the paracortex (see Fig. 11.15).

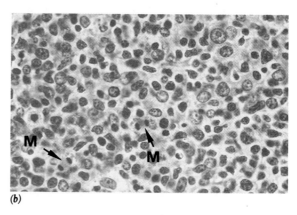

Fig. 11.13 Lymphoid follicle and germinal centre *(H & E (a) ×64 (b) ×480)*

Micrograph (a) shows a lymphoid follicle with a less intensely stained germinal centre **GC**; the more intensely stained periphery is described as the *lymphocyte corona* **LC**. B lymphocytes are the predominant cell type in the lymph node follicles along with a small number of helper T lymphocytes (mainly located in the corona) and various types of immunological accessory cells. The B lymphocytes in the superficial cortex are mainly naive B cells and B memory cells. B lymphocytes enter the lymph node via high endothelial venules of the paracortex passing outwards towards the superficial cortex. Their duration of stay is variable, some passing out of the node within a matter of hours with others remaining for a prolonged period. B cell activation within the follicles results in *blast transformation*, the cells enlarging and increasing in cytoplasmic RNA content prior to cell division. The resulting lymphoblasts of the germinal centres are also known as *follicle centre cells* and are illustrated in micrograph (b). The centre of the follicle is less intensely stained than the corona because the cells are not only much larger but also less closely packed together. Note two mitotic figures **M**. The product of follicular B lymphocyte activation and proliferation is an expanded population of B memory cells and not the formation of plasma cells as previously believed. It was formerly thought that the germinal centres were the site of proliferation and differentiation of antibody-secreting plasma cells but this is now believed to occur as a result of T cell/B cell interaction in the paracortex with the antibody-secreting cells migrating directly to the medullary cords where they are conveniently situated for secretion of antibody into the efferent lymph.

At the periphery of the germinal centres is a capsule-like structure of flattened stromal cells called *germinal centre bordering cells* open at its superficial aspect (see Fig. 11.9). This appears to prevent the entry of circulating T cells to the germinal centre. On the other hand, activated lymphocytes entering the node via afferent lymph pass readily into the germinal centres which may explain why the structure is open at its superficial aspect.

Immunological accessory cells of various types are found in the superficial cortex, all appearing to be involved in antigen processing. These cells cannot be readily distinguished by light microscopy but require sophisticated ultrastructural and other research techniques. In consequence, their functions are not well understood and the nomenclature is not yet standardised.

The main accessory cell types described in the cortical follicles are summarised as follows:

- *Tingible body macrophages:* these cells contain numerous lysosomes and are named for their content of ingested cellular remnants; they are mainly found within the germinal centres.
- *Follicular dendritic cells:* these cells have numerous hair-like branching surface projections covered by electron-dense material and are found in the superficial or *cap region* of the follicles. Although not apparently phagocytic, in the presence of specific antibody and complement, these cells will retain antigen on their surface for many months; their origin and immunological role is not understood but they appear to be continuous with the germinal centre bordering cells.
- *Marginal zone macrophages:* these are one type of morphologically diverse phagocytic cells situated within the follicular interstitium immediately beneath the subcapsular sinus.
- *Natural killer cells:* these cells which have the ability to kill target cells without previous sensitisation are found in small numbers in the follicles and in appearance resemble large lymphocytes; they appear to play a role in surveillance for tumour and virus-infected cells.

(a)

(b)

Fig. 11.14 Cortical distribution of T and B lymphocytes

(Immunoperoxidase methods (a) B cells × 40 (b) T cells × 40)

Micrograph (a) employs an immunoperoxidase method for a B lymphocyte surface marker which stains the plasma membrane brown. Nuclei are counterstained blue with haematoxylin. Note that the B lymphocytes are concentrated in the germinal centres of the lymphoid follicles.
Micrograph (b) employs the same method, in this case utilising a T cell marker. Note that the brown deposit is mainly concentrated in the area between the follicles. There is also some concentration of marker in the corona of each follicle representing helper T cells involved in B cell activation.

(a)

(b)

Fig. 11.15 Paracortical zone *(a) H & E × 320 (b) Thin section, toluidine blue × 800*

T lymphocytes are the main cell type in the paracortical zone.

Circulating T lymphocytes of both helper and cytotoxic/suppressor subsets enter the lymph node in arterial blood then migrate through the walls of high endothelial venules **V** into the paracortical zone; they rejoin the circulation some 6 to 16 hours later, passing out of the lymph node in efferent lymph.

When activated, T lymphocytes enlarge to form lymphoblasts, histologically similar to their B cell counterparts in the follicular germinal centres, before mitotic proliferation to produce expanded clones of activated T lymphocytes. Indeed in a T cell-dominated immunological response, the paracortical zone may be vastly expanded into the medulla, producing the so-called *paracortical reaction.* Activated T cells are then disseminated via the circulation to peripheral sites where much of their activity occurs. Within the paracortex, they may modulate the role of B cells en route from the high endothelial venules to the superficial cortex or medullary cords.

The cell population of the paracortex is predominantly on the move, the more permanent cells being mainly T lymphoblasts and an accessory cell type known as *interdigitating cells.* These are named for their numerous cytoplasmic processes which interdigitate with those of other similar cells as well as making numerous contacts with other cell types in the vicinity; because of their similar surface markers, it is believed that the veiled cells of the subcapsular sinuses may represent the precursors of the interdigitating cells. Another type of accessory cell found in the paracortex are macrophages with their cytoplasm packed with lipid (possibly engulfed cellular membrane) and nuclear debris.

Post-capillary venules of the paracortex have an unusual structure which facilitates the passage of T lymphocytes from the blood circulation into the lymph node. Micrograph (b) illustrates a high endothelial venule which is lined by tall cuboidal rather than the usual squamous endothelial cells. Several lymphocytes **L** can be seen in various stages of progress through the wall between the high endothelial cells.

(a)   *(b)*

Fig. 11.16 Medullary cords and sinuses *(a) H & E × 20 (b) Reticulin method/neutral red × 20*

Micrograph (a) illustrates the structure of the lymph node medulla with branching medullary cords **MC** separated by irregular medullary sinuses **MS**. Throughout the medulla are trabeculae **T** extending from the collagenous supporting tissue of the capsule and hilum and conveying afferent and efferent blood vessels.

The medullary cords largely contain plasma cells and their precursors although a few macrophages and T lymphocytes may also be present. As in the cortex, the cells of the medullary cords are supported on a reticulin framework as seen in micrograph (b), the black-staining reticulin being condensed around trabecular blood vessels **V**. As in the subcapsular and trabecular sinuses, fine reticular strands traverse the medullary sinuses providing support for highly active sinus macrophages.

The dominant cell population of the medullary cords is plasma cells and their smaller precursors, the *plasmablasts* (see Fig. 11.2). B lymphocyte activation, proliferation and maturation of antibody-secreting cells appears to occur in the paracortex rather than in the superficial cortical follicles as once thought. Plasma cells synthesise antibody which is carried from the node to the general circulation via efferent lymph; some mature plasma cells probably also migrate from the node likewise.

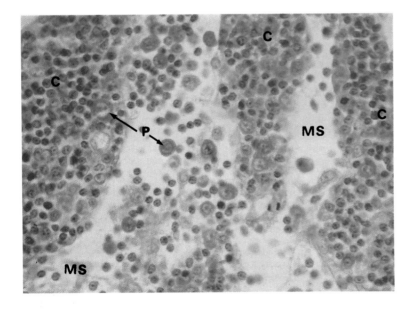

Fig. 11.17 Medullary cords and sinuses

(Methyl green/Pyronin × 480)

This preparation, taken from a lymph node undergoing an intense antibody-mediated response, has been stained by a technique to demonstrate plasma cells. The plasma cells **P** are large with an extensive, red stained cytoplasm and a pale stained nucleus with a prominent nucleolus. The red dye pyronin has a marked affinity for ribosomal RNA and hence stains the plasma cell cytoplasm strongly since it is packed with ribosomes involved in antibody synthesis. Note the presence of numerous plasma cells in both the medullary cords **C** and sinuses **MS**.

Classical macrophages are the main accessory cell type found in the medulla, being located in the sinuses and deriving support from the traversing reticulin fibres.

Fig. 11.18 Efferent lymph *(H & E × 320)*

This micrograph shows efferent lymph in a medullary sinus. Efferent lymph differs from afferent lymph in several important respects. Afferent lymph contains particulate matter (often including microorganisms), soluble antigens, relatively few lymphocytes and some antigen presenting cells migrating from peripheral tissues. In contrast, efferent lymph contains little particulate matter or soluble antigens but contains large numbers of recirculating T lymphocytes and a variable number of B lymphocytes and plasma cells. Antibody is also carried in efferent lymph to the general circulation and thence to the site of antigenic stimulation.

Mucosa-associated lymphoid tissue (MALT)

Lymphoid tissue is distributed throughout the gastrointestinal tract either as a diffuse lymphocytic infiltrate or as large discrete non-encapsulated aggregations such as in the tonsils and intestinal Peyer's patches. In the large aggregations, follicles may form with germinal centres similar to those of lymph nodes. Smaller follicular aggregations and diffuse lymphocytic infiltrates are also seen in the tracheo-bronchial tree (see Fig. 12.9) and genitourinary tract.

The total mass of lymphoid tissue in the gastrointestinal and respiratory tracts is enormous but until recently its function was unknown and largely discounted. This mass of lymphoid tissue is now considered to be a lymphoid organ in its own right and is collectively known as *mucosa-associated lymphoid tissue (MALT)*. The larger aggregations function in a manner analogous to lymph nodes, sampling antigenic material entering the tracts and mounting both antibody-mediated and cytotoxic immune responses where appropriate; they contain discrete B and T cell zones as well as antigen-processing accessory cells.

The diffusely scattered lymphocytes seen in the lamina propria of the gut and respiratory tree are mainly B lymphocytes some of which mature into antibody-secreting plasma cells. All classes of antibody are produced with IgA predominating.

IgA is secreted into the lumen bound to a carbohydrate moiety which renders it resistant to proteolytic enzymes. This *secretory IgA* protects against pathogens before they breach the tissues. Secretory IgA also reaches the gut in bile being taken up from blood and secreted into bile in a similar fashion.

IgG and IgM are also secreted into the lamina propria to deal with organisms that elude the surface protective mechanisms. IgE is also produced and mediates release of histamine from mast cells which are present in large numbers in the lamina propria.

Considerable numbers of lymphocytes are also found within the epithelium of the small and large intestines and are present in particularly large numbers in the epithelium overlying Peyer's patches. These lymphocytes are almost exclusively T cells and the majority are of the suppressor/cytotoxic subset with most of the rest being natural killer cells.

The epithelium overlying all MALT aggregations is specialised for the sampling of luminal contents for antigen and acts as the equivalent of the afferent lymphatics of the lymph node. The lymphatics associated with MALT are all efferent, passing to regional lymph nodes (e.g. tonsillar, mesenteric, hilar), along with the lymphatics of the surrounding tract wall.

MALT is formed during fetal life but germinal centres do not develop until after exposure to antigen at birth. The amount of MALT is maximal during childhood undergoing progressive atrophy in adulthood.

The whole MALT organ probably acts as an integrated unit. When antigen is encountered, it is carried to local MALT tissue or regional lymph nodes where it evokes the relevant immunological response. Lymphocytes, antibodies and probably even plasma cells, then pass via the general circulation to the gastrointestinal and respiratory mucosae where lymphocytes and plasma cells await antigenic challenge. IgA is secreted either by diffusing directly through the lining epithelium or in specific secretions such as saliva, tears and in milk during lactation.

The lymphoid aggregates of the respiratory tract are similar though generally smaller than those of the gut and are covered by similar antigen sampling and transport cells. As in the gut there are no afferent lymphatics but efferent lymphatics drain lymph to the regional nodes and activated lymphocytes derived from the respiratory tract aggregations have a predilection for specifically homing to the respiratory mucosa.

Fig 11.19 Palatine tonsil *(H & E × 6)*

The palatine tonsils are large non-encapsulated masses of lymphoid tissue which along with the lingual, pharyngeal and tubal tonsils (adenoids) form *Waldeyer's ring*.

The luminal surface is covered by stratified squamous epithelium **E** which deeply invaginates the tonsil, forming blind-ended tonsillar crypts. The base of the tonsil is separated from underlying muscle by a dense collagenous hemi-capsule **Cap**. The tonsillar parenchyma contains numerous lymphoid follicles **F** dispersed just beneath the epithelium of the crypts and incorporating germinal centres similar to those found in lymph nodes. Tracer studies have demonstrated that particulate matter entering the crypts from the oropharynx is passed to the follicles, a process that appears to involve phagocytosis by the epithelial cells of the crypt lining. Likewise, bacteria applied to the tonsils of germ-free animals have been shown to enter the follicle in a similar manner inducing the formation of germinal centres. An immune response is initiated in a similar manner to that in Peyer's patches. Efferent lymphatics pass to the deep cervical chain of nodes and presumably there is a subsequent homing of lymphoblasts to the lamina propria of the oral and nasopharynx.

Antigen uptake occurs in a similar manner in the lingual, pharyngeal and tubal tonsils (adenoids), the latter being covered with respiratory type epithelium rather than stratified squamous epithelium.

(a)   (b)

Fig. 11.20 Peyer's patches and colonic lymphoid aggregations *(H & E (a) ×150 (b) ×64)*

Peyer's patches are large lymphoid aggregations found scattered in the small intestinal mucosa where they bulge dome-like into the gut lumen. Micrograph (a) illustrates a small Peyer's patch in the ileum. The usual mucosal form overlying these *dome areas* is more cuboidal, rather than the usual tall columnar form; goblet cells are absent and the epithelium contains large numbers of intraepithelial lymphocytes.

Some epithelial cells exhibit numerous surface microfolds instead of the usual microvilli and have been designated *M cells*; these migrate from the mucosal crypts and are responsible for antigen transfer from the gut lumen into the Peyer's patch.

Germinal centres **GC** containing large proliferating B lymphocytes are the dominant feature of the Peyer's patch; these are surrounded by a zone of small B lymphocytes which forms the dome on the luminal aspect of the germinal centre. The area between germinal centres is occupied by T lymphocytes and like its lymph node equivalent, the paracortex, contains high endothelial venules. The area immediately beneath the specialised surface epithelium is occupied by a mixture of T cells, B cells and plasma cells as well as a large number of macrophages.

Antigen entering the patch via the M cells is taken up by macrophages and presented to T lymphocytes, thus initiating the immune response. Peyer's patches are not a site of significant IgA secretion and it appears that IgA-committed B cell precursors and memory cells are stimulated in the Peyer's patches passing to mesenteric lymph nodes via efferent lymphatics where the

immunological response is greatly amplified. Activated lymphoblasts then enter the circulation via the thoracic duct subsequently homing on the lamina propria of the gut where they exhibit their major effector functions including final maturation into plasma cells and antibody secretion; unlike the Peyer's patches, the lamina propria does not contain high endothelial venules and the mechanism by which Peyer's patch derived lymphoblasts recognise and home in upon the gut lamina propria is unknown. During lactation, Peyer's patch derived B lymphocytes also migrate to the breast where they mature into plasma cells and secrete IgA into the milk; thus the newborn is protected from the same potential ingested pathogens to which the mother is exposed. A special subset of T lymphocytes in the Peyer's patches controls the differentiation of IgA-committed B cell precursors and thus ultimately IgA secretion.

Micrograph (b) illustrates a small lymphoid aggregation in the wall of the colon. It does not contain a germinal centre and the distribution of lymphoid cells is more diffuse, spreading out into the lamina propria between the colonic glands.

Lymph nodes draining the skin receive little of their lymphocyte traffic via afferent lymphatics; however the mesenteric lymph nodes receive 30–50% of lymphocytes via lymphatics or lacteals draining the gut wall. The mesenteric node thus appears to be a meeting place for lymphocytes from Peyer's patches and the gut lamina propria with recirculating lymphocytes entering the node from the bloodstream.

(a)

(b)

(c)

Fig. 11.21 Appendix

(a) H & E × 20
(b) Immunoperoxidase method for B lymphocytes × 40
(c) Immunoperoxidase method for T lymphocytes × 40

The appendix is a blind-ended tubular sac attached to the caecum with a general structure conforming to that of the large intestine. In children it is characterised by a large mass of lymphoid tissue forming numerous follicles which undergo progressive atrophy from early adulthood.

Micrograph (a) shows the typical appearance of an appendicular lymphoid follicle which is similar in form to that of Peyer's patches. Micrographs (b) and (c) employ markers for B and T cells respectively showing that the follicle is dominated by B lymphocytes with only a relatively small proportion of T cells mainly at the follicular periphery and beneath the overlying epithelium.

Spleen

The spleen is a large lymphoid organ situated in the left upper part of the abdomen; it receives a rich blood supply via a single artery, the *splenic artery*, and is drained by the *splenic vein* into the hepatic portal system.

In humans, the spleen has two main functions:

- production of immunological responses against blood-borne antigens
- removal of particulate matter and aged or defective blood cells, particularly erythrocytes, from the circulation.

In dogs and horses, the spleen also acts as a reservoir of blood which can be mobilised by contraction of the organ. In the human fetus, the spleen is an important site of haemopoiesis and this function may be resumed in adulthood in certain disease states.

Despite its large size and important functions, removal of the spleen appears to have few deleterious effects on the body as a whole and its functions are assumed to be taken over by the liver and bone marrow.

The manner in which the spleen performs its function, and many ultra-structural details, are still widely disputed; in many respects, however, the spleen may be considered analogous to a lymph node in which the lymphatic circulation is replaced by a blood circulation. The structure of the spleen provides for intimate contacts to be made between blood and immunologically active cells, just as the structure of the lymph node facilitates the interaction of afferent lymph and lymphoid cells. Although it is well established that the spleen is involved in removal of aged or defective blood cells from the circulation, it is still not clear whether this is a purely mechanical process or whether immunological recognition plays an important role.

Accounts of the histology of the spleen vary according to the animal models used, all being somewhat different from the human spleen and thus imposing certain inconsistencies in terminology; e.g. there are no periarteriolar lymphoid sheaths or marginal sinuses in the human spleen. This description is specific to the human spleen. A great deal remains to be discovered about the structure and function of the human spleen which is difficult to study for a number of reasons. Firstly, due to rapid autolysis, post-mortem specimens are unsuitable and surgical specimens are frequently abnormal due to alteration in physiological conditions in the body as a whole. Fresh specimens must be processed promptly and are best embedded in acrylic resin to avoid the shrinkage associated with paraffin embedding. Special staining techniques such as Methenamine silver/H & E yield more useful information than conventional H & E. Finally there is considerable variation in the normal between individuals and in the same individual under different physiological and immunological circumstances.

Fig. 11.22 Spleen *(H & E × 12)*

On macroscopic examination of the cut surface, the spleen appears to consist of discrete white nodules, the so-called *white pulp*, embedded in a red matrix called the *red pulp*. Microscopically, as seen in micrograph (a), the white pulp **WP** is seen to consist of lymphoid aggregations and the red pulp **RP**, making up the bulk of the organ, to be a highly vascular tissue.

The spleen has a thin but dense fibro-elastic outer capsule **C** from which short septa extend into the organ. The capsule is thickened at the hilum and is continuous with supporting tissue **T** which ensheaths the larger blood vessels entering and leaving the organ. In some mammals, these supporting tissues contain smooth muscle which exerts a rhythmic pumping action, clearing the spleen of blood and allowing the spleen to act as a reservoir. In humans only a few smooth muscle cells persist.

The splenic artery divides into several major branches which enter the splenic hilum giving rise to numerous arterioles which ramify into the splenic parenchyma.

Associated with the arterioles are masses of lymphoid tissue which in some species completely ensheathe the arterioles and are known as *periarteriolar lymphoid sheaths*. In humans, T lymphocyte masses are located around arterioles and B lymphocyte follicles lie adjacent to arterioles but without this regular sheath arrangement. This lymphoid tissue corresponds to the white pulp described above. As will be explained later, the white pulp as traditionally described is not the only significant site of splenic lymphoid tissue and these old terms are now of limited functional validity.

Fig. 11.23 Splenic supporting tissue

(Reticulin method/Neutral red × 42)

The staining technique employed demonstrates the reticular architecture of the spleen. The capsule **C** and perivascular supporting tissue sheaths **T** provide a robust framework which supports a fine reticulin meshwork ramifying throughout the organ in the red pulp. The reticular skeleton is almost absent in the centre of the white pulp nodules **WP** but is well developed at their margins and around the central arteriole **A**.

Fig. 11.24 Splenic vasculature and red pulp *(illustration opposite)*

Arterioles branch from the smaller arteries usually at right angles and then branch again into what have been traditionally termed the *penicillar arteries*. These in turn give rise to capillaries which also tend to leave the arterioles at right angles. The splenic capillaries of the red pulp have a standard endothelial cell structure which terminates abruptly in a cylindrical arrangement of mononuclear phagocytes, described as *sheathed capillaries*. Blood emanates from the ends of the sheathed capillaries into the splenic parenchyma proper. Sheathed capillaries are also present in the *perifollicular zones*; the capillaries of the white pulp are of standard conformation.

Splenic red pulp

The splenic parenchyma is permeated by an interconnected network of sinuses which drain into larger sinuses which in turn drain into tributaries of the splenic vein and thence the hepatic portal vein. The sinuses are lined by flattened endothelial cells resting upon a basement membrane which is interrupted by numerous narrow slits. The reticulin fibres of the sinusoidal basement membrane are disposed in a circular fashion and are continuous with the reticulin meshwork within the parenchyma.

Blood cells entering the parenchyma from the sheathed capillaries squeeze through the walls of the sinuses to drain out of the organ via the splenic vein, the rate of flow approximating that through capillaries elsewhere in the body.

The red pulp parenchyma consists of extremely loose tissue supported by reticulin fibres. Much of the parenchyma is permeated by capillaries terminating as sheathed capillaries and, as previously described, blood passes into the parenchyma and thence through the nearby sinusoidal walls into the sinusoidal lumen. There appears to be no direct opening of the arteriolar/capillary system into the sinusoidal system rendering the former concept of the 'closed' splenic circulation obsolete (at least in humans). Apart from the capillaries, the splenic parenchyma just described is mainly populated by macrophages as well as a cuff of lymphocytes immediately surrounding the capillaries. Such parenchyma is believed to perform the function of removing particulate matter and aged or abnormal erythrocytes from the bloodstream, the defective cells being less deformable and thus unable to negotiate the narrow slits in the sinusoidal basement membrane. Trapped cells are removed by the mononuclear phagocytes of the sheathed capillaries and other parenchymal macrophages. The mechanism of recognition of effete red cells is probably based on diminished deformability but it is known that aged red cells non-specifically accumulate immunoglobulin and this may mediate phagocytosis via Fc receptors on the macrophages.

In disorders where the number of abnormal erythrocytes is high, the sheathed capillaries appear to disaggregate, the phagocytes becoming disseminated through the parenchyma which undergoes hypertrophy; some phagocytes may also enter the sinuses and pass to the liver via the portal vein.

Numerous small patches of the red pulp parenchyma (comprising in total a volume comparable to that of the white pulp) are devoid of capillaries, the parenchyma being mainly occupied by T and B lymphocytes and mononuclear phagocytes. Adjacent sinuses are blind-ended and bulb-shaped and their endothelial lining cells have been shown to bind monoclonal antibodies raised against high endothelial venules of lymph nodes. It is thus proposed that lymphocytes may exit these sinuses to enter these *non-filtering parts of the red pulp parenchyma* in which case this part of the parenchyma should be considered as a functional part of the splenic lymphoid tissue.

Perilymphoid (perifollicular) zones

The zone of red pulp immediately surrounding the T and B lymphoid masses differs from that of the red pulp as a whole, being devoid of sinuses, having only a sparse reticulin meshwork and containing a large number of red and white blood cells in the same proportion as that of blood. About 10% of blood entering the spleen is believed to pass into perilymphoid parenchyma from which it passes much more slowly into the surrounding more widely spaced sinuses than in the rest of the red pulp. The function of these *perilymphoid (perifollicular) zones* is unclear but the sluggish blood flow may be a means for enhancing interaction of blood cells, antigens and antibodies.

Red pulp sinus

Red pulp sinus

NFA

SC

C

SC

Red pulp sinus

SC

Red pulp sinus

Mantle zone

Follicle with germinal centre

Marginal zone

Perilymphoid red pulp

A

Red pulp sinus

NFA

Red pulp sinus

NFA

SC

Red pulp sinus

SC

C

SC

Red pulp sinus

Red pulp sinus

NFA

SC

SC

SC

SC

Red pulp sinus

Red pulp sinus

C

Red pulp sinus

C

SC

SC

C

SC	Sheathed capillary
C	Capillary
NFA	Non-filtering area
A	Arteriole
→	Direction of blood flow

(a)

Fig. 11.25 Red pulp

(a) H & E × 800 (b) Reticulin method/Neutral red × 400

Micrograph (a) illustrates the red pulp, its major constituent being the parenchyma **P** which is permeated by broad interconnected venous sinuses **VS**. Seen in section, the parenchymal tissue between the sinusoids is considerably thinner than the diameter of the sinusoids and the area occupied by sinuses is greater than that of the parenchyma; in three-dimensional terms however, the parenchyma makes up 70% of the volume and the sinuses only 30%. The two-dimensional view gave rise to the misleading term *cords (of Bilroth)* to describe the parenchymal tissue. Together the sinuses and intervening parenchyma make up the red pulp, its three-dimensional structure being analogous to a Swiss cheese, the holes representing the sinuses and the cheese representing the parenchyma.

The parenchyma mainly comprises sheathed capillaries composed of mononuclear phagocytic cells, other macrophages and blood cells which have emanated from the capillaries and not yet crossed into the sinuses. Non-filtering areas are devoid of sheathed capillaries and contain a greater proportion of lymphocytes. The phagocytic cells are responsible for destruction of aged or damaged blood cells. The different nucleated cell types of the parenchyma cannot be reliably distinguished in this type of preparation.

The venous sinuses are lined by elongated, spindle-shaped endothelial cells **E** which lie parallel to the long axes of the sinuses. The venous sinuses have thus been likened to tall wooden barrels with both ends open, the epithelial cells being represented by the wooden staves and hence being described as *stave cells*.

Slits occur between the endothelial cells, the endothelial basement membrane being discontinuous over the slits.

(b)

Blood cells, particularly viable erythrocytes, squeeze between the stave cells to reach the venous sinuses.

The venous sinuses drain into progressively larger vessels which converge to form the splenic vein.

Micrograph (b) shows red pulp stained by the reticulin method to demonstrate the supporting framework of the parenchyma **P**. The basement membranes of the venous sinuses **VS** show the greatest concentration of reticulin fibres which encircle the endothelium in a manner reminiscent of the steel bands holding together a wooden barrel. Fine reticular strands traverse the parenchyma linking the whole structure together and providing support for parenchymal macrophages and a small number of fibroblasts responsible for elaboration of the reticulin. In this preparation, nuclei are counterstained red, those of the sinus endothelial cells being particularly well demonstrated. As the sinusoid lumina contain mainly (anucleate) erythrocytes they appear as if empty.

(a)

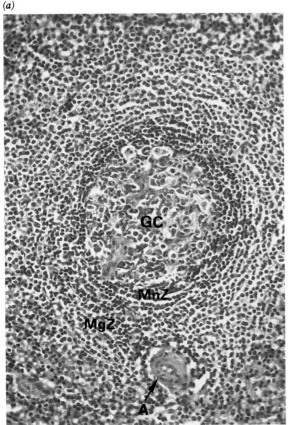

(b)

Fig. 11.26 Splenic lymphoid tissue

(H & E (a) ×160 (b) ×120)

The splenic lymphoid masses (white pulp) are of two types,
T cell and B cell, together making up 5 to 20% of the total
mass of the spleen. The functions of these areas appears to
be similar to those of the paracortex and superficial cortex of
lymph nodes respectively. The non-filtering areas of red
pulp parenchyma (see Fig. 11.24) should probably be
considered part of the splenic lymphoid tissue mass also but
its immunological function remains to be elucidated.

Micrograph (a) shows a T cell area typically forming an
irregular mass **T** around an arteriole **A** and containing small
lymphocytes mainly of the T helper subset. Note the way
the T cell mass merges with the surrounding red pulp
parenchyma **RP**. Small lymphatics arise in the T
lymphocyte areas forming a network around the arterioles
then continuing with the larger arteries to the hilum to drain
into a group of adjacent lymph nodes.

B cells form follicles usually located in the vicinity of an
arteriole as illustrated in micrograph (b). In young people,
many of the follicles exhibit germinal centres **GC** similar to
those of the lymph node although the proportion of follicles
with germinal centres diminishes with age. At the follicle
periphery is a narrow zone of small lymphocytes called the
mantle zone **MnZ** (*corona*) beyond which is a broader
marginal zone **MgZ** of less densely packed larger
lymphocytes supported by a framework of reticulin fibres.
In the rat, a marginal sinus is found between the mantle and
marginal zones but this is not present in the human spleen;
this may give rise to terminological confusion.

Also to be included in the lymphoid tissue of the spleen
are small areas around the arteries containing lymphocytes
and plasma cells; these *perivascular rims* may be analogous to
the medulla of the lymph node; their relationship to the
perivascular lymphatics, if any, is not known.

12. Respiratory system

Introduction
Respiration is a term used to describe two different but interrelated processes: cellular respiration and mechanical respiration. Cellular respiration is the process in which cells derive energy by degradation of organic molecules (see Ch. 1). Mechanical respiration is the process by which oxygen required for cellular respiration is absorbed from the atmosphere into the blood vascular system and the process by which carbon dioxide is excreted into the atmosphere. Mechanical respiration occurs within the respiratory system.

The respiratory system has two functional components: a conducting system for transport of inspired and expired gases between the atmosphere and the circulatory system and an interface for passive exchange of gases between the atmosphere and blood. The conducting system begins essentially as a single tube which divides repeatedly to form airways of ever decreasing diameter. The terminal branches of the conducting system open into blind-ended sacs called *alveoli*, which are the sites of gaseous exchange. The alveoli, which constitute the bulk of the lung tissue, are thin-walled structures enveloped by a rich network of capillaries, the *pulmonary capillaries*. This arrangement provides a vast interface of minimal thickness for gaseous exchange between the atmosphere and blood. The continuous process of gaseous diffusion requires appropriate gaseous pressure gradients to be maintained across the alveolar wall. This is achieved by rapid and continuous perfusion of the pulmonary capillaries by venous blood from the right side of the heart and regular replacement of alveolar gases by the process of breathing.

The respiratory system is divided anatomically into two parts, the *upper* and *lower respiratory tracts*, which are separated by the *pharynx*. The pharynx is best considered functionally and histologically as part of the gastrointestinal tract despite its important role as an airway.

Upper respiratory tract
The upper respiratory tract comprises a system of interconnected spaces, the *nasal cavity*, *paranasal sinuses* and the *nasopharynx*, and is principally involved in filtering, humidifying and adjusting the temperature of inspired air. In addition, the nasal cavity contains receptors for the sense of smell (see Ch. 21) whilst the paranasal sinuses act as resonance chambers for speech, as well as reducing the bony mass of the facial skeleton. The nasopharynx is connected via the *auditory (Eustachian) tubes* (see Fig. 21.23) to the middle ear cavities, an arrangement which permits equilibration of air pressure in the middle ear with that of the external environment.

The upper respiratory tract is lined by pseudostratified columnar epithelium with numerous goblet cells (respiratory epithelium, see Fig. 5.5) which is supported by a loose collagenous layer called the *lamina propria* containing numerous glands. Collectively, the epithelium and lamina propria are known as *respiratory mucous membrane* or *respiratory mucosa*. The terms *mucous membrane* and *mucosa* also have a common general use in describing the moist linings of other tracts such as the gastrointestinal tract and always refer to both the epithelium and its supporting lamina propria. A further supporting tissue layer called the *submucosa* separates the mucosa from underlying structures.

Lower respiratory tract
The lower respiratory tract begins at the *larynx* then continues into the thorax as the *trachea* before dividing into numerous orders of smaller airways to reach the alveoli; there are about twenty orders of branches in humans. The vocal cords of the larynx protect the lower respiratory tract against the entry of foreign bodies, in addition to performing a vital function in speech. The vocal cords are lined by stratified squamous epithelium which is better adapted than respiratory epithelium to withstand frictional stress.

The trachea first divides into left and right *primary* or *main bronchi* which supply the lungs. Each primary bronchus gives rise to *secondary* or *lobar bronchi* supplying the lobes of the lungs before dividing again to form *tertiary* or *segmental bronchi* which supply the segments of each lobe. The tertiary bronchi then ramify into numerous orders of progressively smaller airways called *bronchioles*, the smallest of which are called *terminal bronchioles* and mark the end of the purely conducting portion of the tract. The terminal bronchioles branch further into a series of transitional airways, the *respiratory bronchioles* and *alveolar ducts*, which become increasingly involved in gaseous exchange. These passages finally terminate in dilated spaces called *alveolar sacs* which open into the alveoli.

Each type of airway has its own characteristic structural features but there is a gradual, rather than abrupt, transition from one type of airway to the next along the whole length of the tract. In general terms, the airways are pliable tubes lined by respiratory mucosa and containing variable amounts of muscle and/or cartilage. The principal structural features of the lower respiratory tract are as follows:

- The respiratory epithelium undergoes progressive transition from a tall, pseudostratified columnar, ciliated form in the larynx and trachea to a simple, cuboidal, non-ciliated form in the smallest airways. Goblet cells are numerous in the trachea but decrease in number and are absent from the terminal bronchioles distally. Scattered throughout the respiratory tract epithelium are cells which contain electron-dense, secretory granules. These cells are known as *Kulchitsky* or *K* cells and constitute part of the diffuse neuroendocrine system (see Ch. 17); serotonin, bombesin and calcitonin are among the secretory products so far identified.

- The lamina propria consists of fibro-elastic tissue which contains lymphoid aggregations of variable size; these form part of the mucosa-associated lymphoid tissue (see Ch. 11). One of the functions of this immunological tissue is the production of antibodies of the IgA class which are secreted onto the mucosal surface as a defence against invading microorganisms.

- A layer of smooth muscle lies deep to the mucosa (except in the trachea) and becomes increasingly prominent as the airway diameter decreases. Smooth muscle tone controls the diameter of the conducting passages and thus controls resistance to air flow within the respiratory tree. Smooth muscle tone is modulated by the autonomic nervous system, adrenal medullary hormones and local factors. Sympathetic activity causes smooth muscle relaxation and thus dilatation of the airways which is a desirable response in the 'fight or flight' situation. Parasympathetic activity, on the other hand, causes airway constriction; the functional significance of this may be to reduce 'dead space' on expiration.

- The submucosal layer underlying the smooth muscle layer contains serous and mucous glands which become progressively less numerous in the narrower airways and are not present beyond the tertiary bronchi.

- Cartilage provides a supporting skeleton for the larynx, trachea and bronchi and prevents the collapse of these airways during respiration. The cartilage lies outside the submucosa, diminishing as the calibre of the airway decreases to be completely absent beyond the tertiary bronchi.

- The outermost layer of cartilage or smooth muscle, as the case may be, is surrounded by fibro-elastic tissue called the *adventitia* which merges with the surrounding lung parenchyma.

Blood supply of the lungs

The lungs have a dual blood supply, the *pulmonary system* and the *bronchial system*. The pulmonary supply conducts deoxygenated blood from the right side of the heart via a large pulmonary artery to each lung.

The *pulmonary arteries* enter the roots or *hila* of the lungs with the main bronchi and then divide and course in parallel with the branching airways to supply the pulmonary capillaries surrounding the alveoli. The pulmonary arterial system is structurally unusual in two respects. Firstly, the pulmonary arterial vessels are relatively thin-walled and of large calibre, their diameter approximating that of the accompanying airway. Secondly, the pulmonary arteries have the histological characteristics of elastic arteries rather than of muscular arteries. Elastic expansion and recoil of the vessels maintains the pulmonary arterial pressure at a relatively constant level throughout the cardiac cycle.

The bronchial arterial system constitutes the systemic circulation of the lower respiratory tract. It arises as small branches of the aorta and supplies oxygenated blood to the tissues of the airway walls and to the *pleura*, the layer which invests the outer surface of each lung. The bronchial vessels are of the usual type found in the rest of the systemic circulation.

A common venous system returns most of the blood to the left side of the heart via the *pulmonary veins* which are extremely thin-walled vessels of wide diameter. A small proportion of blood from the bronchial system drains to the right side of the heart via the *azygous venous system*.

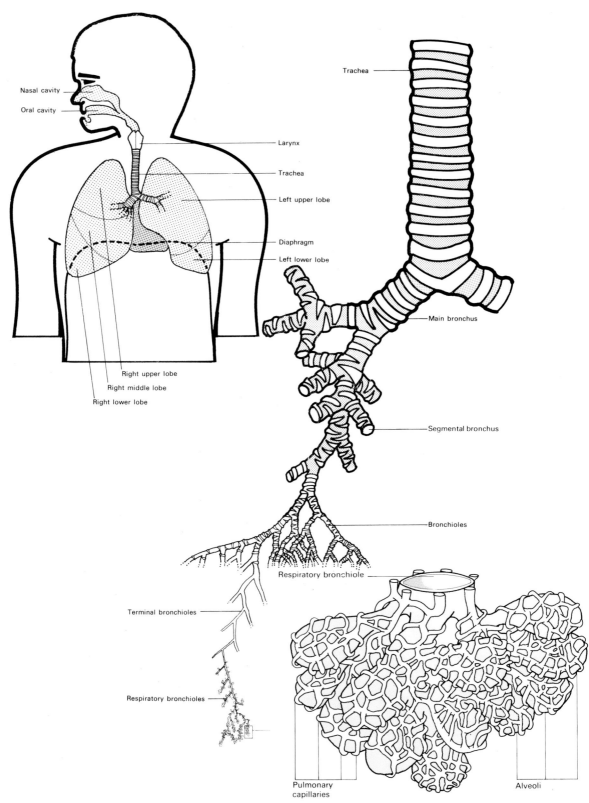

Fig. 12.1 Structure of the respiratory system

Fig. 12.2 Nasal cavity

(Kitten: coronal section, H & E/Alcian blue × 12)

The nose is subdivided into two nasal cavities **NC** by the cartilaginous *nasal septum* **NS**; cartilage is stained blue in this preparation.

The nasal cavities and paranasal sinuses **PS** are lined by respiratory mucosa, the major function of which is to filter particulate matter and to adjust the temperature and humidity of inspired air. These functions are enhanced by a large surface area provided by the turbinate system of bones **T** which project into the nasal cavities.

Part of the nasal mucosa, the *olfactory mucosa*, contains receptors for the sense of smell (see Fig. 21.2). Although the olfactory mucosa is extensive in lower mammals, in man it is confined to a relatively small area in the roof of the nasal cavities.

Note the close proximity of the nasal cavities to the orbital cavities **O** and the anterior cranial fossa **ACF**.

Fig. 12.3 Nasal mucosa *(H & E × 200)*

The nasal mucosa consists of a pseudostratified columnar ciliated epithelium **E** with numerous goblet cells supported by a richly vascular lamina propria containing serous and mucous glands. These features reflect the functions of the nasal mucosa, processes which begin in the nasal cavities and continue throughout the conducting portion of respiratory tract.

Particulate matter in inspired air is trapped in a thin layer of surface mucus secreted by the goblet cells of the surface epithelium and the mucous glands **M** of the lamina propria. Coordinated, wave-like beating of cilia propels mucus with trapped particles towards the pharynx where it is swallowed and inactivated in the stomach.

The entrance to each nasal cavity, the *nasal vestibule*, is lined by skin which has short, coarse hairs called *vibrissae* which trap the largest particles before they reach the nasal mucosa.

The temperature of inspired air is adjusted to that of the body by heat exchange between the air and blood flowing in a rich plexus of thin-walled venules **V** in the lamina propria. Inspired air is humidified by the watery secretions of serous glands **S** also located in the lamina propria.

A mucosa similar to that of the nasal cavities also lines the nasopharynx, paranasal sinuses and auditory tubes.

Fig. 12.4 Trachea

(H & E/Alcian blue × 9)

This specimen from a newborn child shows the general structure of the trachea. The trachea is a flexible tube of fibro-elastic tissue and cartilage which permits expansion in diameter and extension in length during inspiration, and passive recoil during expiration.

A series of C-shaped rings of hyaline cartilage **C** (stained blue) support the tracheal mucosa **M** and prevent its collapse during inspiration.

Bands of smooth muscle, called the *trachealis muscle* **T**, join the free ends of the rings posteriorly; contraction of the trachealis reduces tracheal diameter and thereby assists in raising intrathoracic pressure during coughing. A few strands of longitudinal muscle **L** can be seen disposed behind the trachealis muscle.

Fig. 12.5 Trachea *(H & E × 198)*

The layers of the tracheal wall are shown in this specimen from a young man.

The respiratory epithelium **E** of the trachea is tall, pseudostratified and ciliated and contains goblet cells. In response to the irritation of tobacco smoke, the epithelium commonly undergoes morphological change (metaplasia) to a stratified squamous form with consequent loss of ciliary action; ciliary activity is essential for continuous movement of glandular secretions towards the pharynx. The tracheal epithelium is supported by a particularly thick basement membrane (not visible at this magnification). Beneath the basement membrane, the lamina propria **LP** consists of loose, highly vascular supporting tissue which becomes more condensed at its deeper aspect to form a band of fibro-elastic tissue.

Underlying the lamina propria is the loose submucosa **SM** containing numerous mixed sero-mucous glands which decrease in number in the lower parts of the trachea; the serous cells stain strongly with H & E whilst the mucous cells remain poorly stained. The submucosa merges with the perichondrium of the underlying hyaline cartilage rings (not seen in this field) or, as here, with the dense fibro-elastic tissue **F** between the cartilage rings.

Fig. 12.6 Tracheal epithelium

(Scanning EM × 2000)

This micrograph illustrates the tracheal surface at high magnification; the film of surface mucus has been removed before fixation and processing.

The ciliated epithelial cells have an appearance reminiscent of clumps of seaweed, the cilia being several micrometres in length. The less numerous goblet cells are scattered amongst the ciliated cells being recognisable by their bulbous surface outline, lack of cilia and the presence of small surface projections associated with mucus secretion.

(a)

(b)

Fig. 12.7 Primary bronchus

(a) Elastic van Gieson/Alcian blue × 150
(b) H & E × 600 (c) Cytology, H & E × 900

The basic structure of the bronchi is similar to that of the trachea, but differs in several details as follows: The respiratory epithelium **E** is less tall and contains fewer goblet cells; the goblet cells have darkly stained, granular cytoplasm with the staining method used in micrograph (a). The lamina propria **LP** is more dense with a large quantity of elastin in its more superficial layers; elastic fibres are stained black in micrograph (a). The lamina propria is separated from the submucosa **S** by a discontinuous layer of smooth muscle **M** which becomes progressively more prominent in smaller airways. The submucosal layer contains fewer sero-mucous glands; none are seen in micrograph (a). The cartilage framework **C** is arranged into flattened, interconnected plates rather than discrete C-shaped rings as in the trachea.

Micrograph (c) is a cytology specimen obtained by bronchial brushing during bronchoscopic examination for suspected bronchogenic cancer. It well illustrates the tall columnar ciliated form of the epithelial cells with the nuclei located towards a tapered base.

(c)

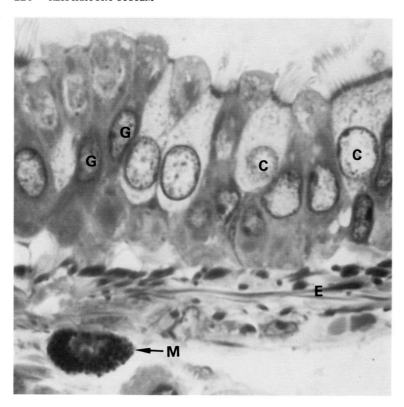

Fig. 12.8 Bronchial epithelium

(Rat: Thin section, toluidine blue × 800)

This micrograph illustrates the structure of the bronchial epithelium at the limit of resolution of the light microscope.

The epithelium is pseudostratified, the bases of all the cells extending down to the basement membrane, although not all the cells reach the luminal surface. The ciliated cells **C** have large nuclei and stain very poorly with this method. The goblet cells **G** stain most strongly due to their content of mucus, a mucopolysaccharide.

The underlying lamina propria contains a considerable amount of elastin **E** and mast cells **M** containing numerous darkly stained granules which contain histamine and the glycoprotein heparin which is responsible for the intense staining with this method (see also Fig. 4.14). The role of mast cells in normal function is unclear; however, when antigen-antibody complexes are formed on their cell membranes, they release large quantities of histamine causing smooth muscle constriction and vasodilatation leading to mucosal swelling. In the bronchioles, these phenomena are partly responsible for the clinical condition of *asthma*.

Fig. 12.9 Tertiary (segmental) bronchus

(Elastic van Gieson × 75)

As the bronchi diminish in diameter the structure progressively changes to more closely resemble that of large bronchioles. The respiratory epithelium, which cannot be seen at this magnification, is now tall columnar with little pseudostratification and goblet cell numbers are greatly diminished.

The lamina propria is thin, elastic and completely encircled by smooth muscle **M** which is disposed in a spiral manner. This arrangement of smooth muscle permits contraction of the bronchi in both length and diameter during expiration. Sero-mucous glands **G** are sparse in the submucosa; they are rarely found in smaller airways.

The cartilage framework **C** is reduced to a few irregular plates; cartilage also does not usually extend beyond the tertiary bronchi. Note that the submucosa **SM** merges with the surrounding adventitia and thence with the lung parenchyma. Small aggregations of lymphocytes **L** are seen in the adventitia representing part of the diffuse mucosa-associated lymphoid tissue.

Fig. 12.10 Bronchiole *(H & E × 160)*

Bronchioles are airways of less than one millimetre in diameter and have no cartilage support. The respiratory epithelium is simple, columnar and ciliated and contains few goblet cells, these being completely absent beyond the terminal bronchioles.

The smooth muscle layer **M** is the most prominent feature of bronchioles and is disposed in a spiral manner like that of the bronchi. The total cross-sectional area of all bronchioles combined is far greater than that of the rest of the conducting passages combined, thus the tone of the bronchiolar smooth muscle effectively controls resistance to air flow within the lungs.

Instability of the bronchiolar smooth muscle leading to contraction and consequent airway narrowing is a central feature of the disease asthma.

Fig. 12.11 Pulmonary artery

(Elastic van Gieson/Alcian blue × 75)

This micrograph shows a segmental branch of the pulmonary artery **A** adjacent to a segmental bronchus **B**. The airway can be identified as such by the absence of cartilage, the relatively thin muscular layer and occasional submucosal glands.

The pulmonary arterial vessels are described as elastic arteries (see Fig. 8.7) and contain relatively little smooth muscle; in this preparation, elastin is stained black and smooth muscle tan.

The walls of the pulmonary arteries are relatively thin in relation to their diameter, the pressures being much lower than that in the systemic circulation. Note the red-stained collagen in the supporting tissue of the vessel and airway.

Fig. 12.12 Terminal portion of the respiratory tree *(Elastic van Gieson × 40)*

Terminal bronchioles **T** are the smallest diameter passages of the purely conducting portion of the respiratory tree; beyond this, further branches become increasingly involved in gaseous exchange.

Each terminal bronchiole divides to form short, thinner-walled branches called *respiratory bronchioles* **R**, so named because their walls contain a small number of single alveoli **A**. The epithelium of the respiratory bronchioles is devoid of goblet cells and largely consists of ciliated cuboidal cells and smaller numbers of non-ciliated cells called *Clara cells*. In the most distal part of the respiratory bronchioles, the epithelium of respiratory bronchioles undergoes further transition from that of the terminal bronchioles, and Clara cells become the predominant cell type. Clara cells have the ultrastructural features of secretory cells, but the nature and function of their secretory product is not understood.

Each respiratory bronchiole divides further into several long, winding passages called *alveolar ducts* **AD** which open along their length into numerous *alveolar sacs* **AS** and alveoli **A**. In histological sections, all that can be seen of the walls of the alveolar ducts are small aggregations of smooth muscle cells and associated collagen and elastic fibres which

form rings surrounding the alveolar ducts and the openings of the alveolar sacs and alveoli. The smooth muscle of the respiratory bronchioles and alveolar ducts regulates alveolar air movements.

The alveolar ducts lead into alveolar sacs, each of which gives rise to several alveoli. Each alveolus consists of a pocket, open at one side and lined by flattened epithelial cells. Surrounding each alveolus is a rich network of pulmonary capillaries supplied by pulmonary vessels **V** which follow the general course of the airways. Between adjacent alveoli, the wall or *alveolar septum* consists of the flattened epithelial lining cells of each alveolus separated by capillaries and delicate collagen fibres and elastin, which condense around the opening of each alveolus and merge with those around the openings of adjacent alveoli to form a fine, three-dimensional supporting meshwork for the whole lung parenchyma.

The alveolar septa contain small openings about 8 nm in diameter, called *alveolar pores* which permit equalisation of pressure between alveoli, and provide a collateral air circulation should a bronchiole become obstructed.

(a)

(b)

Fig. 12.13 Alveoli

(a) H & E × 480 (b) Thin section, toluidine blue × 480

The conventional method of studying the structure of the alveolar wall in light microscopy has been to use relatively thick (5-8 μm) wax-embedded tissues, stained by routine methods as in micrograph (a); however the resolution obtained by such methods is limited. In contrast, thin resin sections, as shown in micrograph (b), reveal much greater structural detail since they permit better resolution.

In general terms, the alveolar wall consists of three tissue components: *surface epithelium, supporting tissue* and *blood vessels*.

Epithelium provides a continuous lining to each alveolus and consists of cells of two types. Most of the alveolar surface area is covered by large, flattened cells called *Type I pneumocytes (alveolar lining cells)*; since the cytoplasm of these cells covers such an extensive area, the characteristic densely stained nuclei of Type I pneumocytes P_1 are relatively infrequently seen in histological section. A second epithelial cell type, known as the *Type II pneumocyte*, represents some 60% of cells in the lining epithelium; these cells are rounded in shape and thus occupy a much smaller proportion (about 5%) of the alveolar surface area. Type II pneumocytes P_2 have large, rounded nuclei with a prominent nucleolus and vacuolated cytoplasm. Type I pneumocytes constitute part of the extremely thin gaseous diffusion barrier, whereas Type II pneumocytes secrete a surface-active material called *surfactant* which reduces surface tension within the alveoli preventing alveolar collapse during expiration. Clara cells of the respiratory bronchioles (see Fig. 12.12) may synthesise other components of surfactant. Type II pneumocytes retain the capacity for cell division and can differentiate into Type I pneumocytes in response to damage to the alveolar lining.

Supporting tissue forms an attenuated layer beneath the epithelium and surrounding the blood vessels of the alveolar wall. This layer primarily consists of fine reticular, collagenous and elastic fibres and occasional fibroblasts.

Blood vessels, mainly capillaries **C** (7–10 μm in diameter), form an extensive plexus around each alveolus. In most of the alveolar wall, the basement membrane which supports the capillary endothelium is directly applied to the basement membrane supporting the surface epithelium; in such sites the two basement membranes are fused and the supporting tissue layer is absent. This arrangement provides an interface of minimal thickness between alveolar air and blood. Note in these micrographs the nuclei of capillary endothelial cells **E** and the close proximity of the densely stained erythrocytes within these capillaries to the alveolar air spaces.

Although the defence mechanisms of the conducting passages filter most particulate matter from inspired air, small particles such as carbon reach the alveoli and are engulfed by large phagocytic cells (macrophages) found in the alveolar wall or free in the alveolar space. These phagocytes **M**, known as *alveolar macrophages* or *dust cells*, are derived from circulating blood monocytes and are usually recognisable by their content of engulfed, particulate material.

Fig. 12.14 Alveolar wall *(EM × 6 000)*

This micrograph shows the alveolar wall between three alveoli **A** at low magnification. Capillaries make up the bulk of the alveolar wall, branching and anastomosing to create a basket-like arrangement around each alveolus. This field shows parts of several capillaries, the uppermost one C_1 containing erythrocytes and a platelet. The plane of section has cut the lumen of a second capillary C_2 in three places and includes the nucleus of one of its lining endothelial cells E_2. The nucleus of an endothelial cell E_3 of another capillary is also included in this section. The cytoplasm of Type I pneumocytes P_1, which cover most of the alveolar surface,

and capillary endothelial cells **E** are both extremely attenuated and distinction between them is best made by tracing their basement membranes; alveolar lining cells lie outside the membrane whilst endothelial cells are enclosed.

A Type II pneumocyte P_2 is also seen, typically located at a branching point of the interalveolar septum; the cytoplasm is filled with vesicles containing phospholipid in the form of lamellar bodies **L**. These bodies are discharged into the alveolar air space where they contribute to a surfactant layer on the epithelium/air interface.

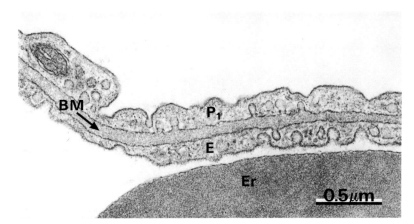

Fig. 12.15 Alveolar septum

(EM × 34 000)

This micrograph shows at high magnification the components of the gaseous diffusion barrier between blood and alveolar air. This consists of the attenuated cytoplasm of a Type I pneumocyte **P₁**, a common basement membrane **BM**, and the thin cytoplasm of a capillary endothelial cell **E**. Note the erythrocyte **Er** in the capillary lumen.

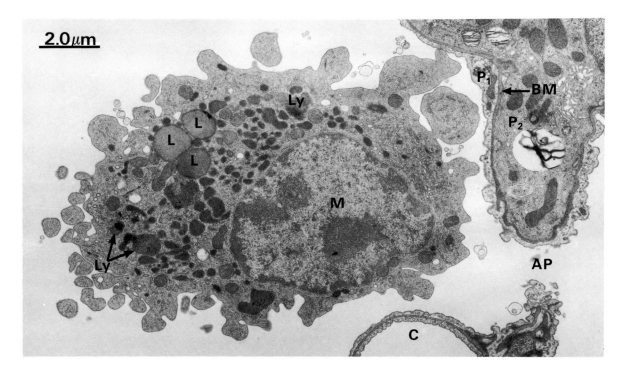

Fig. 12.16 Alveolar macrophage *(EM × 8 000)*

Macrophages are an important component of the defence system of the lungs being responsible for phagocytosis of microorganisms and other particulate matter evading the airway defences and reaching the alveoli. The macrophage population is essentially derived from circulating blood monocytes although some appear to arise from mitotic division of macrophages already resident in the lungs. Alveolar macrophages can be found on the surface of alveolar lining cells as well as in the supporting tissue of the alveolar septa. After engulfment of exogenous material, the majority appear to migrate into the airways where they are carried up on the mucociliary escalator and disposed of by coughing and swallowing. Others appear to be sequestered in the septa and account for the black discolouration of the

lung parenchyma in individuals chronically inhaling contaminated air, e.g. cigarette smoke.

The macrophage **M** in this micrograph lies within an alveolus adjacent to a septal capillary **C** and a Type II pneumocyte (surfactant cell) **P₂** between which is an alveolar pore **AP**. The aspect of the surfactant cell seen here is typically invested by the thin cytoplasm of a Type I pneumocyte (alveolar lining cell) **P₁**, the two being separated by a common basement membrane **BM** (see Fig. 12.17). The alveolar macrophage exhibits the typical features of macrophages elsewhere in the body (see Fig. 4.16) but in particular contains numerous secondary lysosomes **Ly** and lipid droplets **L**.

(a)

(c)

0.5μm

2.0μm

(b)

Fig. 12.17 Surfactant cells *(illustrations opposite; (a) H & E × 400 (b) EM × 9 000 (c) EM × 35 000)*

Micrograph (a) shows the light microscope appearance of Type II pneumocytes **P₂**, the cells responsible for surfactant production; their nuclei are large and plump with dispersed chromatin and prominent nucleoli. The plentiful eosinophilic cytoplasm is filled with fine unstained vacuoles representing lamellar bodies, the phospholipid of which is dissolved out during tissue preparation. In comparison, the nuclei of Type I pneumocytes (alveolar lining cells) and capillary endothelial cells are small, dense and flattened.

Micrograph (b) shows a branching point in an alveolar wall typically containing a Type II pneumocyte **P₂** recognisable by its lamellar bodies **L**. Most of the Type II pneumocyte is surrounded by basement membrane **BM₂** and only a small proportion of its surface is exposed directly to the alveolar space **A** where it exhibits numerous small microvilli **Mv** associated with surfactant secretion. Elsewhere, the alveolar aspect of the Type II pneumocyte is invested by a thin layer of cytoplasm of Type I pneumocytes **P₁** but separated by a common basement membrane. At the top of the field, the Type II pneumocyte abuts a capillary **C**, its cytoplasm being separated from that of the capillary endothelium **E** by the basement membranes of each cell and a little intervening supporting tissue **S**. At the lower left of the field, the Type II cell rests upon a thin layer of septal supporting tissue containing a fibroblast **F**. Beyond this lies the flattened nucleus of a capillary endothelial cell **NE**, its attenuated cytoplasm spreading out to line the capillary lumen **C**. A tight junction **TJ** is seen where this endothelial cell abuts an adjacent cell. Basement membranes can be traced on both aspects of this alveolar supporting tissue. The surfactant cell contains rough ER, free ribosomes and moderate numbers of elongated mitochondria.

Micrograph (c) shows lamellar bodies at high magnification. These are membrane bound and the lamellae within them are composed mainly of phospholipids particularly palmitoyl phosphatidylcholine. Phospholipid is released by exocytosis spreading out over the alveolar surface where it combines with other carbohydrate and protein-containing secretory products (some possibly derived from Clara cells) to form a tubular lattice of lipoprotein described as *tubular myelin*. In the event of two alveolar surfaces coming together, this overcomes the effects of surface tension which would otherwise cause them to adhere. This allows for normal inflation of the alveoli at birth and for the reinflation of alveoli which collapse after airway obstruction.

(a)

(b)

M
J
En E
F
BM P₁ En E 0.5 µm

Fig. 12.18 Pulmonary elastic tissue

(a) Elastic van Gieson × 480
(b) EM × 26 000

The staining method used in micrograph (a) demonstrates the large amount of elastin (stained black) in the alveolar walls. At the margins of the openings into the alveoli, the elastin and septal collagen is condensed to form a supporting ring. These fibrous elements are then continuous with those of adjacent alveoli, forming a fibro-elastic supporting framework for the lung parenchyma as a whole.

Micrograph (b) shows part of an alveolar septum containing elements of the elastin meshwork. The septum consists of the thin cytoplasmic layers of a Type I pneumocyte **P₁** and two capillary endothelial cells **En** separated by a common basement membrane **BM**; note the marginal fold **M** of one endothelial cell overlapping the other creating a seal and reinforced by a tight junction **J**.

The elastin **E** is an amorphous moderately electron-dense mass insinuated between the two epithelial layers. This space also contains a fine cytoplasmic extension of a fibroblast **F**.

Fig. 12.19 Pulmonary capillaries *(Dye perfused preparation × 420)*

The pulmonary arterial system terminates at the alveolar ducts where arterioles ramify to form a widely interconnected capillary basket surrounding each alveolus; the capillaries are of relatively large diameter (7-10 µm). Control of blood flow in the pulmonary capillary bed is predominantly effected by the partial pressure of gases within the alveoli. In poorly ventilated alveoli, the partial pressure of oxygen is low and that of carbon dioxide high; this causes local vasoconstriction, thus directing blood away from the poorly ventilated alveoli.

The lung tissue illustrated in this micrograph was prepared by perfusion of the pulmonary vasculature with a blue dye. This procedure outlines the pulmonary capillary bed; no other histological detail can be seen. In the centre of the field the richly anastomosing capillary network of part of an alveolar wall is included in the plane of section (see also Fig. 12.1). This type of technique, in combination with the study of very thick histological sections, provided early microscopists with valuable information about the structure, function and vascular system of the lungs.

Fig. 12.20 Visceral pleura *(H & E × 198)*

The cavities containing the lungs, the *pleural cavities*, are lined by a thin, flattened epithelium (mesothelium) called the *pleura* which is similar in structure to the pericardium surrounding the heart, and the peritoneum lining the abdominal cavity. The pleura lining the thoracic wall, called the *parietal pleura*, is reflected at the hilum of the lung so as to invest the outer surface of the lung, the *visceral pleura*. The visceral and parietal pleura are directly applied to one another but separated by a potential space (the *pleural space*) containing a minute amount of serous fluid. The two pleural layers adhere to one another by surface tension such that movements of the thoracic wall during ventilation result in corresponding expansion and contraction of the lungs.

This micrograph illustrates visceral pleura **P**. The outer surface is lined by a layer of flattened mesothelium **M** which is supported by a thin basement membrane. The underlying fibrous supporting tissue **F** is particularly prominent in the human lung and consists primarily of collagen and elastic fibres; smooth muscle cells are occasionally seen. The fibrous layer of visceral pleura extends into the lung as fibrous septa **S** which are continuous with the fibro-elastic framework of the lung parenchyma.

The visceral pleura contains a superficial plexus of lymph vessels which drain via the septa into a deep plexus surrounding the pulmonary blood vessels and airways. Lymph from the deep plexuses drains into the thoracic duct via lymph nodes in the hilar region. Lymph capillaries are not found in alveolar walls but they are present in the walls of respiratory bronchioles and all larger airways. Several lymph vessels **L** can be seen in the pleura in this micrograph. The visceral pleura also contains numerous small blood vessels and capillaries. Nerves are seen infrequently and are believed to originate from the parasympathetic and sympathetic systems supplying the airways and pulmonary vessels, and from pulmonary stretch receptors.

13. Oral tissues

Introduction

The digestive process commences in the oral cavity with the ingestion, fragmentation and moistening of food but, in addition to its digestive role, the oral cavity is involved in speech, facial expression, sensory reception and breathing. The major structures of the oral cavity, the *lips, teeth, tongue, oral mucosa* and the associated *salivary glands*, participate in all these functions.

Mastication is the process by which ingested food is made suitable for swallowing. Chewing not only involves coordinated movements of the mandible and the cutting and grinding action of the teeth but also activity of the lips and tongue, which continually redirect food between the *occlusal surfaces* of the teeth. The watery component of saliva moistens and lubricates the masticatory process whilst salivary mucus helps to bind the food bolus ready for swallowing.

The entire oral cavity is lined by a protective mucous membrane, the oral mucosa, which contains many sensory receptors, including the taste receptors of the tongue. The epithelium of the oral mucosa is of the stratified squamous type which tends to be keratinised in areas subject to considerable friction such as the palate. The oral epithelium is supported by dense collagenous tissue, the *lamina propria*. In highly mobile areas such as the soft palate and floor of the mouth, the lamina propria is connected to the underlying muscle by loose submucosal supporting tissue. In contrast, in areas where the oral mucosa overlies bone, such as the hard palate and tooth-bearing ridges, the lamina propria is tightly bound to the periosteum by a relatively thin dense fibrous submucosa. Throughout the oral mucosa, numerous small accessory salivary glands of both serous and mucous types are distributed in the submucosa.

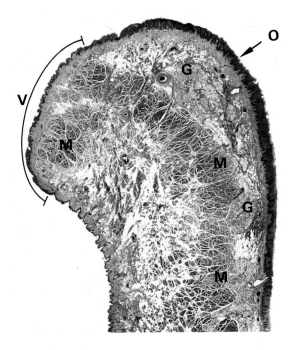

Fig. 13.1 Lip *(H & E × 6)*

This micrograph illustrates a midline section through a human lower lip, the bulk of which is made up of bundles of circumoral skeletal muscle **M** seen in transverse section.

The external surface of the lip is covered by hairy skin which passes through a transition zone to merge with the oral mucosa **O** of the inner surface. The transition zone constitutes the free vermilion border of the lip **V**, and derives its colour from the richly vascular dermis which here has only a thin, lightly keratinised epidermal covering. The free border is highly sensitive due to its rich sensory innervation. Since the vermilion border is devoid of sweat and sebaceous glands, it requires continuous moistening by saliva to prevent cracking.

The oral mucosa covering the inner surface of the lip has a thick stratified squamous epithelium and the underlying submucosa contains numerous accessory salivary glands **G** of serous, mucous and mixed sero-mucous types.

Fig. 13.2 Palatal mucosa *(H & E × 28)*

Like the rest of the mouth, the palate is covered by a thick stratified squamous epithelium **E** supported by a tough, densely collagenous dermis **D**. To assist mastication, the palatal mucosa is thrown up into transverse folds or *rugae*, one of which is shown in this micrograph.

The mucosa of the hard palate is bound down to the underlying bone **B** by relatively dense submucosal tissue **S** containing a few accessory salivary glands.

In rodents and many other mammals with a coarse diet, the surface epithelium of particularly exposed areas is keratinised for extra protection as in this specimen taken from a monkey.

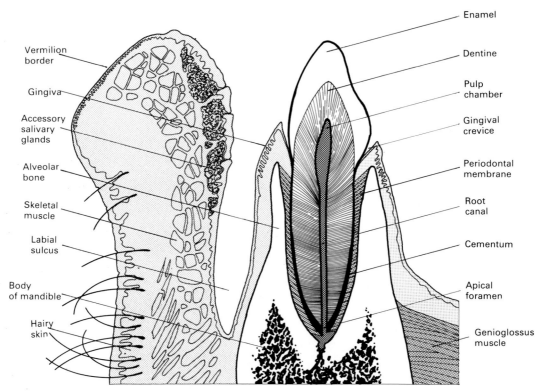

Fig. 13.3 Lip and tooth

This drawing of a section through the lower jaw near the midline illustrates the general arrangement of the lip and a tooth with its supporting structures.

Each tooth may be grossly divided into two segments, the *crown* and the *root*: the crown is that portion which projects into the oral cavity and is protected by a layer of highly mineralised *enamel* which covers it entirely. The bulk of the tooth is made up of *dentine*, a mineralised tissue which has a similar chemical composition to bone. The dentine has a central *pulp cavity* containing the *dental pulp* which consists of specialised supporting tissue containing many sensory nerve fibres. The tooth root is embedded in a bony ridge in the jaw called the *alveolar ridge*; the tooth socket is known as the *alveolus* and, at the lip or cheek aspect of the alveolus, the

bony plate is generally thinner than at the tongue or palatal aspect. The root of the tooth is invested by a thin layer of *cementum* which is connected to the bone of the socket by a thin fibrous layer called the *periodontal ligament* or *periodontal membrane*.

The oral mucosa covering the upper part of the alveolar ridge is called the *gingiva* and at the junction of the crown and root of the tooth (the *neck of the tooth*) the gingiva forms a tight protective cuff around the tooth. The potential space between the gingival cuff and the enamel of the crown is called the *gingival crevice*. All of the tissues which surround and support the tooth are collectively known as the *periodontium*.

(c)

(a)

(b)

Fig. 13.4 Tooth structure

(Undecalcified sections, unstained: (a) ×5 (b) ×5 (c) ×50)

These undecalcified sections cut with a diamond wheel demonstrate the arrangement of the calcified tissues of an upper central incisor tooth in micrograph (a) and a lower molar tooth in micrograph (b). Micrograph (c) demonstrates the tissues of the crown at high magnification.

The dentine **D** which forms the bulk of the crown and root is composed of a calcified organic matrix similar to that of bone. The inorganic component constitutes a somewhat larger proportion of the matrix of dentine than that of bone and exists mainly in the form of hydroxyapatite crystals. From the pulp cavity **P**, minute parallel tubules, called *dentine tubules*, radiate to the periphery of the dentine; in longitudinal sections of teeth, the tubules appear to follow an S-shaped course.

The crown of the tooth is covered by enamel **E**, an extremely hard, translucent substance composed of parallel rods or prisms of highly calcified material cemented together by an almost equally calcified interprismatic material.

The root is invested by a thin layer of cementum **C** which is generally thicker towards the apex of the root. The cementum is an amorphous calcified tissue into which the fibres of the periodontal membrane are anchored. Fragments of alveolar bone **B** have remained attached to the roots after extraction of these specimens.

The morphological form of the tooth crown and roots varies considerably in different parts of the mouth, nevertheless the basic arrangement of the dental tissues is the same in all teeth.

In humans, the *primary (deciduous) dentition* consists of 20 teeth comprising two *incisors*, one *canine* and two *molars* in each quadrant. These begin to be formed at the age of 6 weeks during fetal development and erupt between the ages of 6 and 30 months after birth. Between the ages of 6 and 12 years, the deciduous teeth are succeeded by permanent teeth, namely two incisors, one canine and two *premolars* in each arch. Distal to these will develop three permanent molars having no primary precursors; the first permanent molar erupts at age 6, the second at age 12 and the third (wisdom tooth) at age 17 to 21 years. The sharp points found on the posterior teeth are known as *cusps*.

(a)

(b)

(c)

(d)

Fig. 13.5 Tooth development *(illustrations opposite)*

(H & E (a) cap stage × 28 (b) bell stage × 96 (c) onset of root development × 45 (d) ameloblasts × 640)

This series of micrographs illustrate the important stages of tooth development.

The tissues of the teeth are derived from two embryological sources. The enamel is of epithelial (ectodermal) origin whilst the dentine, cementum, pulp and periodontal ligament are of mesenchymal (mesodermal) origin. The first evidence of tooth development in humans occurs at 6 weeks of fetal life with the proliferation of a horseshoe-shaped epithelial ridge from the basal layer of the primitive oral epithelium into the underlying mesoderm in the position of the future jaws; this is known as the *dental lamina*. In each quadrant of the mouth, the lamina then develops four globular swellings which will become the *enamel organs* of the future deciduous central and lateral incisors, canines and first molar teeth. Subsequently, the dental lamina proliferates backwards in each arch successively giving rise to the enamel organs of the future second deciduous molar and the three permanent molars. The permanent successors of the deciduous teeth will later develop from enamel organs which bud off from the inner aspect of the enamel organs of their deciduous predecessors.

The primitive mesenchyme immediately subjacent to the developing enamel organ proliferates to form a cellular mass whilst, at the same time, the enamel organ becomes progressively cap-shaped, as seen in micrograph (a), enveloping the mesenchymal mass which becomes known as the *dental papilla* DP. During the cap stage, the cells lining the concave face of the enamel organ in contact with the dental papilla begin to differentiate into tall columnar cells, the future *ameloblasts*, which will be responsible for the production of enamel. This, in turn, induces the differentiation of a layer of columnar *odontoblasts*, the future dentine-producing cells, in the apical region of the dental papilla. The interface between the differentiating ameloblast and odontoblast layers marks the position and shape of the future junction between enamel and dentine.

As the enamel organ develops further, it assumes a characteristic bell shape as seen in micrograph (b), the free edge of the 'bell' proliferating so as to determine the eventual shape of the tooth crown.

Meanwhile, the cells forming the main bulk of the enamel organ become large and star-shaped forming the *stellate reticulum* SR, the extracellular matrix of which is rich in glycosaminoglycans. Between the stellate reticulum and ameloblast layer, two or three layers of flattened cells form the *stratum intermedium* whilst the outer surface of the enamel organ consists of a simple cuboidal epithelium called the *external enamel epithelium*. By the cap stage of development, the dental lamina DL connecting the enamel organ with the oral mucosa has become fragmented and, around the whole developing bud, a condensation of mesenchyme forms the *dental follicle* DF which will eventually become the periodontal ligament.

As ameloblasts and odontoblasts differentiate at the tip of the crown, a layer of dentine matrix is progressively laid down between the ameloblast and odontoblast layers. As the odontoblasts retreat, each leaves a long cytoplasmic extension, the *odontoblastic process*, embedded within the dentine matrix thereby forming the dentine tubules. Dentine matrix has a similar biochemical composition to that of bone and undergoes calcification in a similar fashion. Deposition of dentine induces the production of enamel by the adjacent ameloblasts. Each retreating ameloblast lays down a column of enamel matrix which then undergoes mineralisation resulting in the formation of a dense

prismatic structure as described below. With the deposition of dentine and enamel, the overlying stellate reticulum atrophies and the enamel organ is much reduced in thickness. These changes are well demonstrated in micrograph (b). A thin layer of dentine D has been laid down by the underlying odontoblastic layer O of the highly cellular dental papilla DP. The ameloblastic layer A is about to lay down enamel in the area of the artefactual space E; note that in this area, the stellate reticulum has disappeared. Note also the surrounding dental follicle DF and early formation of cancellous bone B.

By the time that dentine and enamel formation is well under way at the incisal edge or tips of the cusps (as the case may be), the enamel organ will have fully outlined the shape of the whole tooth crown. This is the case in micrograph (c), the neck of the tooth N marking the junction of crown and root. A thin, densely-stained layer of poorly mineralised enamel E can be seen covered at its external surface by the now much thinner enamel organ EO. The unstained space S between this and the underlying dentine D represents fully mineralised enamel laid down earlier but dissolved away during tissue preparation. Although enamel production is confined to the crown, the rim of the 'bell' of the enamel organ nevertheless continues to proliferate, inducing dentine formation and thereby determining the shape of the tooth root. This part of the enamel organ, known as the *epithelial sheath of Hertwig* HS, disintegrates once the outline of the root is completed. The cementum which later forms on the root surface is derived from the dental follicle which, as previously stated, is of mesenchymal origin. As the dentine of the crown and root are progressively laid down, the dental papilla shrinks and eventually becomes the dental pulp contained within the pulp chamber and root canals.

Growth of the tooth root is one of the principal mechanisms of tooth eruption and root formation is not completed until some time after the crown has fully erupted into the oral cavity.

Micrograph (d) is taken from the same specimen as micrograph (c) at much higher magnification and illustrates the characteristic appearance of ameloblasts. Active ameloblasts A are tall columnar epithelial cells which form a single layer apposed to the forming surface of the enamel E. Each ameloblast elaborates a column of organic enamel matrix which undergoes progressive mineralisation by the deposition of calcium phosphate mainly in the form of hydroxyapatite crystals. Fully formed enamel contains less than 1% organic material and is the hardest and most dense tissue in the body.

The structure of mature enamel is not fully understood, but it appears that the process of mineralisation of the enamel matrix is not uniform and, as a result, mature enamel consists of highly calcified prisms separated by *interprismatic material* which may differ only in the orientation of its crystals. Each prism extends from the dentino-enamel junction to the enamel surface and may represent the enamel laid down by a single ameloblast.

Underlying the ameloblast layer are several layers of cells, also of epithelial origin, which constitute the remainder of the enamel organ EO. As enamel formation progresses, the enamel organ becomes much reduced in thickness compared with earlier stages of its development. At tooth eruption, the enamel organ, including the ameloblasts, degenerates leaving the enamel exposed to the hostile oral environment, completely incapable of regeneration.

(a)

(b)

Fig. 13.6 Odontoblasts and dentine

(Decalcified sections: H & E (a) × 200 (b) × 128)

Dentine, the dense calcified tissue which forms the bulk of the tooth, is broadly similar to bone in composition but is more highly mineralised and thus much harder than bone. The cells responsible for dentine formation, the odontoblasts, differentiate as a single layer of tall columnar cells on the surface of the dental papilla apposed to the ameloblast layer of the enamel organ. The odontoblasts initiate tooth formation by deposition of organic dentine matrix between the odontoblastic and ameloblastic layers; calcification of this dentine matrix then induces enamel formation by ameloblasts (see Fig. 13.5). Dentine formation proceeds by continuing odontoblastic deposition of dentine matrix and its subsequent calcification; unlike ameloblasts, each odontoblast leaves behind a slender cytoplasmic extension, the odontoblastic process, within a fine dentinal tubule. When dentine formation is complete, the dentine is thus pervaded by parallel odontoblastic processes radiating from the odontoblast layer on the dentinal surface of the reduced dental papilla which now constitutes the dental pulp. After tooth formation is complete, a small amount of less organised *secondary dentine* continues to be laid down resulting in the progressive obliteration of the pulp cavity with advancing age.

These micrographs illustrate active odontoblasts **O** forming a pseudostratified layer of columnar cells at the dentine surface. Parallel dentine tubules containing odontoblastic processes extend through a narrow pale-stained zone of uncalcified dentine matrix called *predentine* **P** into the mature dentine **D**; the dentine tubules are best seen in micrograph (b). Underlying the odontoblastic layer, a relatively acellular layer, called the *cell free zone of Weil* **W**, gives way to the highly cellular dental pulp **DP**.

Fig. 13.7 Dental pulp

(Decalcified section, H & E × 198)

The dental pulp consists of a delicate supporting/connective tissue resembling primitive mesenchyme (see Fig. 4.3); it contains numerous stellate fibroblasts, reticulin fibres, fine poorly organised collagen fibres and much ground substance. The pulp contains a rich network of thin-walled capillaries supplied by arterioles which enter the pulp canal from the periodontal membrane, usually via one foramen at each root apex. The pulp is also richly innervated by a plexus of myelinated nerve fibres from which fine, non-myelinated branches extend into the odontoblastic layer. Despite the acute sensitivity of dentine, nerve fibres are rarely demonstrable in dentine and the mechanism of sensory reception is unknown; it has been suggested that the odontoblastic processes may act as sensory receptors.

Fig. 13.8 Periodontal membrane and cementum *(Decalcified section, H & E × 200)*

The periodontal membrane **PM** forms a thin fibrous attachment between the tooth root and the alveolar bone. The dentine **D**, comprising the root, is covered by a thin layer of cementum **C** which is elaborated by cells called *cementocytes* lying on the surface of the cementum. Cementum consists of a dense, calcified organic material similar to the matrix of bone, and is generally acellular. Towards the root apex, the cementum layer becomes progressively thicker and irregular and cementocytes are often entrapped in lacunae within the cementum.

The periodontal membrane consists of dense collagenous tissue. The collagen fibres, known as *Sharpey's fibres*, run obliquely downwards from their attachment in the alveolar bone **B** to their anchorage in the cementum at a more apical position on the root surface. The periodontal membrane thus acts as a sling for the tooth within its socket, permitting slight movements which cushion the impact of masticatory forces. The points of attachment of the collagen fibres in both cementum and bone are in a constant state of reorganisation to accommodate changing functional stresses upon the teeth. Osteoclastic resorption is often seen at one aspect of a tooth socket and complementary osteoblastic deposition at the opposite side, thus indicating bodily movement of the tooth through the bone; this is the mechanism which permits tooth movement during orthodontic treatment.

The periodontal membrane is richly supplied by blood vessels and nerves from the surrounding alveolar bone, the apical region and the gingiva. Small clumps of epithelial cells are often found scattered throughout the periodontal membrane; these cells are remnants of Hertwig's sheath (see Fig. 13.5) and are known as *epithelial rests of Malassez* **M**.

Fig. 13.9 Gingival attachment *(Decalcified section, H & E × 320)*

This micrograph shows the relationship of the gingiva (gum) to the neck of the tooth. During tissue preparation the enamel has been completely dissolved from the surface of the crown, but the extent of the outer surface of the enamel can be visualised by shreds of remaining organic debris **Db** which had been adherent to the tooth surface.

The gingiva may be divided into the *attached gingiva*, which provides a protective covering to the upper alveolar bone **B**, and the *free gingiva* **FG**, which forms a cuff around the enamel at the neck of the tooth. Between the enamel and the free gingiva is a potential space, the gingival crevice, which extends from the tip of the free gingiva to the cemento-enamel junction **CEJ**.

The thick stratified squamous epithelium, which constitutes the oral aspect of the gingiva, undergoes abrupt transition at the tip of the free gingiva to form a thin layer of epithelial cells tapering to only two or three cells thick at the base of the gingival crevice. This *crevicular epithelium* **CE** is easily breached by pathogenic organisms and the underlying supporting tissue is thus frequently infiltrated by lymphoid cells.

Collagen fibres of the periodontal membrane **PM** radiate from the cementum **C** near the cemento-enamel junction into the dense supporting tissue of the free gingiva; these fibres, together with circular fibres surrounding the neck of the tooth, maintain the role of the gingiva as a protective cuff.

(a)   *(b)*

Fig. 13.10 Tongue *(H & E (a) ×6 (b) ×100)*

The tongue is a muscular organ covered by oral mucosa
which is specialised for manipulating food, general sensory
reception and the special sensory function of taste.

A V-shaped groove, the *sulcus terminalis*, demarcates the
anterior two-thirds of the tongue from the posterior one-
third. The mucosa of the anterior two-thirds is formed into
papillae of three types. The most numerous, the *filiform
papillae*, appear as short 'bristles' macroscopically. Among
them are scattered the small red globular *fungiform papillae*;
details of both types are shown in Figure 13.11. Twelve to
twenty large *circumvallate papillae* form a row immediately
anterior to the sulcus terminalis and these papillae contain
most of the taste buds (see Figs. 13.12 and 21.1); a
circumvallate papilla **C** and numerous filiform papillae **F** are
seen in micrograph (a).

The body of the tongue consists of a mass of interlacing
bundles of skeletal muscle fibres **M** which permit an
extensive range of tongue movements. The mucous
membrane covering the tongue is firmly bound to the
underlying muscle by a dense, collagenous lamina propria
LP which is continuous with the epimysium of the tongue
muscle.

Numerous small serous and mucous accessory salivary
glands are scattered throughout the muscle and lamina
propria of the tongue and are seen at higher magnification in
micrograph (b); in these preparations the serous glands **SG**
are stained strongly whereas the mucous glands **MG** are
poorly stained. Note bundles of skeletal muscle cut in both
transverse **T** and longitudinal **L** section.

Fig. 13.11 Filiform and fungiform papillae

(H & E × 30)

This micrograph illustrates several
filiform papillae **Fl** and a fungiform
papilla **Fg**. Filiform papillae are the
most numerous type and consist of a
dense supporting tissue core and a
heavily keratinised surface projection.
Fungiform papillae have a thin non-
keratinised epithelium and a richly
vascularised supporting tissue core
giving them a red appearance
macroscopically amongst the much
more numerous, whitish filiform
papillae.

(a) *(b)*

Fig. 13.12 Circumvallate papillae *(H & E (a) ×30 (b) ×100)*

Circumvallate papillae are the largest and least common type of papillae on the tongue. They are set into the tongue surface and encircled by a deep cleft **C** as seen at higher magnification in micrograph (b). The stratified epithelium lining the papillary wall of the cleft contains numerous taste buds **B**, the detail of which is shown in Figure 21.1.

Aggregations of serous glands, called *von Ebner's glands* **VE**, open into the base of the circumvallate clefts secreting a watery fluid which dissolves food constituents, thus facilitating taste reception.

Fig. 13.13 Lingual tonsil

(H & E ×30)

Apart from being of different embryological origin and having different sensory innervation to the anterior two-thirds, the posterior one-third of the tongue has a distinctly different mucosal surface. The posterior surface has a relatively smooth stratified squamous epithelium **E** under which lies masses of lymphoid tissue **L** containing typical lymphoid follicles **F**. This mass of lymphoid tissue is known as the lingual tonsil and with the palatine tonsils and adenoids completes a ring of lymphoid tissue guarding the entrance to the gastrointestinal and respiratory tracts. Like the palatine tonsils (see Fig. 11.19), the lingual lymphoid aggregations are penetrated by epithelial crypts **C** which function in a similar manner to those of the palatine tonsil.

Salivary glands

Saliva is produces by three pairs of major salivary glands, the *parotid*, *submandibular* and *sublingual glands*, and numerous minor *accessory glands* scattered throughout the oral mucosa. The minor salivary glands secrete continuously and are in general under local control whereas the major glands mainly secrete in response to parasympathetic activity which is induced by physical, chemical and psychological stimuli.

Saliva is a hypotonic watery secretion containing variable amounts of mucus, enzymes (principally *amylase* and the antibacterial enzyme *lysozyme*), antibodies and inorganic ions. Two types of secretory cells are found in the salivary glands: serous cells and mucous cells. The parotid glands consist almost exclusively of serous cells and produce a thin watery secretion rich in enzymes and antibodies. The sublingual glands have predominantly mucous secretory cells and produce a viscid secretion. The submandibular glands contain both serous and mucous secretory cells and produce a secretion of intermediate consistency. The overall composition of saliva varies according to the degree of activity of each of the major gland types.

Traditionally, the role of salivary amylase has been considered to be initiation of starch digestion in the oral cavity; its primary role, however, is more likely to be as a cleansing agent for starch debris retained around the teeth.

(a) *(b)*

Fig. 13.14 Salivary gland *(a) PAS/Iron haematoxylin × 10 (b) H & E × 120*

The general architecture of all the major salivary glands follows the pattern shown in micrograph (a). The glands are divided into numerous lobules **L** each containing many secretory units. Supporting tissue septa **S** radiate between the lobules from an outer capsule and convey blood vessels, nerves and large excretory ducts **E**.

Micrograph (b) shows part of an interlobular septum from a submandibular gland. It contains several excretory ducts **E** which have a stratified cuboidal epithelial lining. Small parasympathetic nerves **N** and a tiny parasympathetic ganglion **G** are also visible in this specimen.

The surrounding secretory lobules contain a mixture of serous and mucous secretory cells, the former staining strongly with H & E, the latter almost unstained.

Fig. 13.15 Parotid gland *(H & E × 42)*

The parotid gland is almost solely composed of serous secretory acini giving it a strongly stained appearance in H & E preparations.

Fig. 13.16 Sublingual gland *(H & E × 42)*

Mucous acini predominate in the sublingual glands making them stain very poorly with H & E; with methods such as PAS shown in Figure 13.14(a), the mucin stains strongly.

Striated duct

Mucous acinus

Myoepithelial cell

Serous demilune

Intercalated duct

Serous acinus

Fig. 13.17 Salivary secretory unit

The salivary secretory unit consists of a terminal branched tubulo-acinar structure composed exclusively of either serous or mucous secretory cells or a mixture of both types. In mixed secretory units where mucous cells predominate, serous cells often form semilunar caps called *serous demilunes* surrounding the terminal part of the mucous acini. Myoepithelial cells embrace the secretory units, their contraction helping to expel the secretory product.

The terminal secretory units merge to form larger *intercalated ducts* which are also lined by secretory cells. The intercalated ducts drain into larger ducts called *striated ducts* which are named for their striated appearance in light microscopy. The striations result from the presence of numerous deep infoldings of the basal plasma membranes of the large cuboidal cells which line these ducts.

In addition to the salivary proteins, the serous cells are involved in active secretion of a watery fluid containing a variety of inorganic ions; this secretion is isotonic with plasma. In the striated ducts, the ionic content of the secretion is modified by active reabsorption and further secretion of ions to produce saliva which is hypotonic with respect to plasma. The ionic composition of saliva varies at different flow rates but, in general, the concentrations of sodium and chloride ions are below that of plasma, and the concentrations of potassium and bicarbonate ions are above that of plasma. Transport processes in the striated ducts are facilitated by the large surface area offered by the basal infoldings of the lining cells and fuelled by their numerous associated mitochondria.

Fig. 13.18 Mixed sero-mucous secretory unit
(H & E × 480)

This micrograph of a mixed sero-mucous secretory unit shows several mucous acini **M** with serous demilunes **S**. In H & E stained preparations, mucigen granules within the mucous acini are poorly stained whereas the enzyme-containing (zymogen) granules of serous acini are strongly stained. The nuclei of mucous cells are characteristically condensed and flattened against the basement membrane whereas the nuclei of serous cells are rounded with dispersed chromatin, and usually occupy a more central position within the cell.

Fig. 13.19 Mucous acinus *(H & E × 800)*

Both serous and mucous acini are embraced by the processes of contractile cells called *myoepithelial cells* which, on contraction, force secretion from the acinar lumen into the duct system. Myoepithelial cells are located between the basal plasma membranes of secretory cells and the basement membrane. These cells are flattened and have long processes which extend around the secretory acinus but in section they can only be recognised by their large flattened nuclei lying within the basement membrane surrounding the acinus. This micrograph shows the typical appearance of a myoepithelial cell **M** embracing a mucous acinus.

Fig. 13.20 Striated ducts
(H & E × 600)

The striated ducts **S** are lined by large cuboidal cells with large nuclei located between the centre and luminal surface of the cell. The basal cytoplasm appears striated, reflecting the presence of deep basal infoldings of the plasma membrane and associated columns of mitochondria; the apical cytoplasm is uniformly stained and not striated. In predominantly serous salivary glands, the striated ducts are larger than in predominantly mucous glands, a feature associated with the role of the striated duct in modifying isotonic basic saliva to produce hypotonic saliva.

Note in this micrograph that the two striated ducts are surrounded by serous secretory units. The sparse supporting tissue between the secretory acini contains a rich network of capillaries **C**.

14. Gastrointestinal tract

Introduction

The gastrointestinal system is primarily involved in breaking down food for absorption into the body. This process occurs in five main phases: ingestion, fragmentation, digestion, absorption and elimination of waste products. The gastrointestinal system is essentially a muscular tract lined by a mucous membrane which exhibits regional variations reflecting the changing functions of the system from mouth to anus.

Ingestion and initial fragmentation of food occur in the oral cavity, resulting in the formation of a bolus of food; this is then conveyed to the *oesophagus* by the action of the tongue and pharyngeal muscles during swallowing (*deglutition*). Fragmentation and swallowing are facilitated by the secretion of saliva from three pairs of major *salivary glands* and numerous small *accessory glands* (see Ch. 13).

The oesophagus conducts food from the oral cavity to the *stomach* where fragmentation is completed and digestion initiated. Digestion is the process by which food is enzymatically broken down into molecules which are small enough to be absorbed into the circulation; e.g. ingested proteins are first reduced to polypeptides then further degraded to small peptides and amino acids which can then be absorbed. Initial digestion accompanied by intense muscular action of the stomach wall, reduces the stomach contents to a semi-digested liquid called *chyme*. Chyme is squirted through a muscular sphincter, the *pylorus*, into the *duodenum*, the short first part of the *small intestine*. Digestive enzymes from a large exocrine gland, the *pancreas*, enter the duodenum together with bile from the liver via the *common bile duct*. Bile contains excretory products of liver metabolism, some of which act as emulsifying agents necessary for fat digestion. The duodenal contents pass onwards along the small intestine where the process of digestion is completed and the main absorptive phase occurs. After the duodenum, the next segment of the small intestine is the *jejunum* which is responsible for the majority of the absorptive process. The distal part of the small intestine is called the *ileum*, but there is no distinct junction between these parts of the tract.

The liquid residue from the small intestine passes through a valve, the *ileo-caecal valve*, into the *large intestine*. Here, water is absorbed from the liquid residue which becomes progressively more solid as it passes towards the anus. The capacious first part of the large intestine is called the *caecum*, from which projects a blind-ended sac, the appendix. The next part of the large intestine, the colon, is divided anatomically into *ascending, transverse, descending* and *sigmoid* segments although histologically the segments are almost indistinguishable from one another. The terminal portion of the large intestine, the *rectum*, is a holding chamber for faeces prior to defaecation via the *anal canal*.

Food is propelled along the gastrointestinal tract by two main mechanisms: voluntary muscular action in the oral cavity, pharynx and upper third of the oesophagus is succeeded by involuntary waves of smooth muscle contraction called *peristalsis*. Peristalsis and the secretory activity of the entire gastrointestinal system are modulated by the autonomic nervous system and a variety of hormones, some of which are secreted by endocrine cells located within the gastrointestinal tract itself. These cells constitute a diffuse endocrine organ called the *gastrointestinal endocrine system* which not only regulates gastrointestinal function but also has a wide range of metabolic influences (see Ch. 17). Autonomic regulation of certain glandular secretions and smooth muscle of the gut and its blood vessels is mediated by the enteric nervous system comprising postganglionic sympathetic fibres, and ganglia and postganglionic fibres of the parasympathetic nervous system supplied by the vagus nerve.

Because of its continuity with the external environment, the gastrointestinal system is a potential portal of entry for pathogenic organisms. Thus the system incorporates a number of defence mechanisms which include prominent aggregations of lymphoid tissue (MALT) distributed throughout the tract (see Ch. 11).

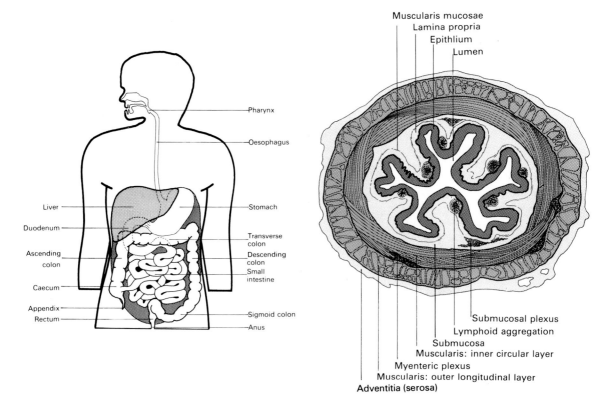

Fig. 14.1 Structure of the gastrointestinal tract

The structure of the gastrointestinal tract conforms to a general plan which is clearly evident from the oesophagus to the anus. The tract is essentially a muscular tube lined by a mucous membrane. The arrangement of the major muscular component remains relatively constant throughout the tract whereas the mucosa shows marked variations in the different regions of the tract.

The gastrointestinal tract has four distinct functional layers: *mucosa, submucosa, muscularis* and *adventitia*.

Mucosa. The mucosa is divided histologically into three layers: an epithelial lining, a supporting lamina propria and a thin smooth muscle layer, the *muscularis mucosae*, which produces local movement and folding of the mucosa. At four points along the tract the mucosa undergoes abrupt transition from one form to another: the oesophago-gastric junction, the gastro-duodenal junction, the ileo-caecal junction and the recto-anal junction.

Submucosa. This layer of loose collagenous tissue supports the mucosa and contains the larger blood vessels, lymphatics and nerves.

Muscularis propria. The muscular wall proper consists of smooth muscle which is usually dispersed as an inner circular layer and an outer longitudinal layer. The action of the two layers, at right angles to one another, is the basis of peristaltic contraction.

Adventitia. This outer layer of loose supporting tissue conducts the major vessels and nerves; in obese individuals it contains a large amount of adipose tissue. Where the gut lies within the abdominal cavity (peritoneal cavity), the adventitia is referred to as the *serosa (visceral peritoneum)* and is lined by a simple squamous epithelium (mesothelium). Elsewhere the adventitial layer merges with retroperitoneal tissues.

The smooth muscle of the bowel has its own inherent rhythmicity which is modulated by the autonomic nervous system, in particular the parasympathetic nervous system. As in other organs of the body, parasympathetic efferent fibres synapse with effector neurones in small ganglia located in or close to the organ involved. In the gastrointestinal tract, parasympathetic ganglia are concentrated in plexuses in the wall of the tract. In the submucosa, isolated or small clusters of parasympathetic ganglion cells give rise to postganglionic fibres which supply the mucosal glands and the smooth muscle of the muscularis mucosae; this submucosal plexus, sometimes referred to as *Meissner's plexus*, also contains postganglionic sympathetic fibres arising from the superior mesenteric plexus. Larger clusters of parasympathetic ganglion cells are found between the two layers of the muscularis, the postganglionic fibres mainly supplying the surrounding smooth muscle. This plexus is known as the *myenteric plexus* or *Auerbach's plexus*.

Glands are found throughout the tract at various levels in its wall. In some parts of the tract (i.e. stomach, small and large intestine), the mucosa is arranged into glands which have a variety of secretory functions. In the lower oesophagus and duodenum, glands penetrate the muscularis mucosa to lie in the submucosa. The pancreas and liver are large glands draining into the gastrointestinal lumen but lying entirely outside the tract wall.

Lymphoid tissue is distributed throughout the gastrointestinal tract both as diffusely scattered cells particularly in the lamina propria and as dense aggregations which may form follicles; in toto, this mass of lymphoid tissue constitutes the gut component of the mucosa-associated lymphoid tissue (MALT) described in Chapter 11.

Fig. 14.2 Basic mucosal forms in the gastrointestinal tract

(H & E (a) × 100 (b) × 100 (c) × 128 (d) × 128)

There are four basic mucosal types found in the gastrointestinal tract which can be classified according to their main function:

(a)

Protective. This type is found in the oral cavity, pharynx, oesophagus and anal canal. The surface epithelium is stratified squamous and may be keratinised in animals which have a coarse diet, e.g. rodents, herbivores.

(b)

Secretory. This type occurs only in the stomach. The mucosa consists of long closely packed tubular glands which are simple or branched depending on the region of stomach.

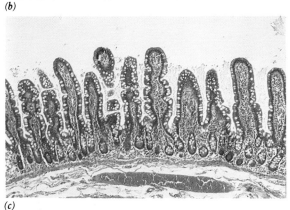

(c)

Absorptive. This mucosal form is typical of the entire small intestine. The mucosa is arranged into finger-like projections called villi (to increase surface area) with intervening short glands called crypts.
Note: in the duodenum, some crypts extend through the muscularis mucosae to form submucosal mucous glands.

(d)

Absorptive/protective. This form lines the whole of the large intestine. The mucosa is arranged into closely packed, straight tubular glands consisting of cells specialised for water absorption and mucus-secreting goblet cells which lubricate the passage of faeces.

(a)

(b)

Fig. 14.3 Components of the wall of the gastrointestinal tract

(H & E (a) × 480 (b) × 28 (c) × 320)

This series of micrographs illustrates the layers of the wall of the tract deep to the surface epithelium.

Micrograph (a) illustrates the deep part of the large bowel mucosa, the muscularis mucosae **MM** clearly demarcating the delicate lamina propria **LP** from the more robust underlying submucosa **SM**; this arrangement is typical of the whole of the gastrointestinal tract.

The *lamina propria* consists of loose areolar tissue which appears highly cellular due to the presence of considerable numbers of leucocytes and other cells of the general defence system (see Fig. 4.15) which deal with any microorganisms which might breach the intestinal epithelium. The lamina propria also contains numerous lymphocytes of the immune system (MALT) which in some areas form dense aggregations. The lamina propria is also typically rich in blood and lymphatic capillaries necessary to support the secretory and absorptive functions of the mucosa.

The *muscularis mucosae* consists of several layers of smooth muscle fibres, those in the deeper layers oriented parallel to the luminal surface. The more superficial fibres are oriented at right angles to the surface and extend up into the lamina propria between the glands; in the case of the small intestine, the fibres extend up into the villi as seen in Figure 14.22. Activity of the muscularis mucosae keeps the mucosal surface and glands in a constant state of gentle agitation which expels secretions from the deep glandular crypts, prevents clogging and enhances contact between epithelium and luminal contents for absorption.

The *submucosa* consists of fairly dense collagenous tissue which binds the mucosa to the main bulk of the muscular wall. The submucosa contains the larger blood vessels and lymphatics as well at the nerves supplying the mucosa. Tiny parasympathetic ganglia **PG** are scattered throughout the submucosa forming the submucosal (Meissner's) plexus from which postganglionic fibres supply the muscularis mucosae.

(c)

The typical arrangement of the two layers of the muscular wall proper is seen in micrograph (b) which shows a longitudinal section of the oesophagus. The *muscularis propria* **MP** is made up of an outer longitudinal layer and a somewhat broader inner circular layer; there has been some artefactual separation of the layers making them easier to visualise. The submucosa **SM** is separated from the lamina propria **LP** by the muscularis mucosae **MM**. In the oesophagus, where the function of the mucosa is to protect against friction, the lamina propria is more collagenous than elsewhere and the muscularis mucosae is more prominent.

Micrograph (c) illustrates, at high magnification, the junction of outer longitudinal **L** and inner circular **C** layers of the muscularis propria in the large intestine; between the layers are clumps of parasympathetic ganglion cells of the myenteric (Auerbach's) plexus. The two layers of the muscularis propria undergo synchronised rhythmic contractions which pass in peristaltic waves down the tract propelling the contents distally. Peristalsis is inherent in the smooth muscle itself but the level of activity is modulated by the autonomic nervous system, locally produced gastrointestinal tract hormones and other environmental factors. Parasympathetic activity enhances peristalsis whilst sympathetic activity slows gut motility.

(a)

Fig. 14.4 Oesophagus

(Masson's trichrome (a) ×9 (b) ×320)

The oesophagus is a strong muscular tube which conveys food from the oropharynx to the stomach. The initiation of swallowing is a voluntary act involving the skeletal musculature of the oropharynx which is then succeeded by a strong peristaltic reflex which conveys the bolus of food or fluid to the stomach. Food and fluid do not normally remain in the oesophagus for more than a few seconds and reflux and regurgitation are normally prevented by a physiological sphincter in the region of the oesophago-gastric junction. Below the diaphragm, the oesophagus passes a centimetre or so in the abdominal cavity before joining the stomach at an acute angle. Sphincter control appears to involve four complementary factors: diaphragmatic contraction, greater intra-abdominal pressure than intragastric pressure being exerted upon the abdominal part of the oesophagus, unidirectional peristalsis and maintenance of correct anatomical arrangements of the structures.

Micrograph (a) shows the lower third of the oesophagus. In the relaxed state, the oesophageal mucosa is deeply folded, an arrangement which permits marked distension during the passage of a food bolus.

The lumen of the oesophagus is lined by a thick protective stratified squamous epithelium **E** (see Fig. 14.2) which, in some animals with coarse diets (e.g. rodents) may be keratinised. The underlying lamina propria is relatively condensed and contains scattered lymphoid aggregations **Ly**; the underlying muscularis mucosae **MM** is barely visible at this magnification.

The submucosa **SM** is highly vascular and relatively loose, allowing for considerable distension during passage of

(b)

a food bolus. The submucosa also contains small mucous glands **G** which aid lubrication and are mainly confined to the lower third of the oesophagus.

The muscularis propria is thick and inner circular **CM** and outer longitudinal **LM** layers of smooth muscle are clearly distinguishable. Since the first part of swallowing is under voluntary control, fasciculi of skeletal muscle predominate in the muscularis of the upper third of the oesophagus.

Micrograph (b) shows part of the muscularis propria of the upper oesophagus at high magnification. A bundle of skeletal muscle fibres **Sk** is seen cut in transverse section. The longitudinal muscle here consists mainly of smooth muscle **Sm** with two skeletal muscle fibres **Sk** in their midst. The collagen of the endomysial supporting tissue stains green with this method.

Fig. 14.5 Oesophago-gastric junction (*H & E × 40*)

At the junction of the oesophagus with the stomach, the mucosa of the tract undergoes an abrupt transition from a protective stratified squamous epithelium **P** to a tightly packed glandular secretory mucosa **S**. The muscularis mucosae **MM** is continuous across the junction though it is less easily seen in the stomach where it lies immediately beneath the base of the gastric glands. The underlying submucosa **SM** and muscularis propria **M** continue uninterrupted beneath the mucosal junction. The muscularis propria does not form a thick anatomical sphincter but rather there is a physiological sphincter mechanism which is described with Figure 14.4.

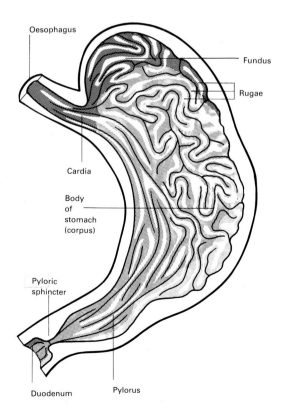

Fig. 14.6 Stomach

The stomach is a distensible organ which receives food from the oesophagus, retaining it for 2 hours or more during which time it undergoes mechanical and chemical breakdown to form chyme. Solid foods are broken up by a strong muscular churning action whilst chemical breakdown is produced by gastric juices secreted by the glands of the stomach mucosa. There is little absorption of most food products from the stomach, except for water, alcohol and some drugs. Once chyme formation is completed, the pyloric sphincter relaxes and allows the liquid chyme to be squirted into the duodenum.

In the non-distended state, the stomach mucosa is thrown into prominent longitudinal folds called *rugae* which permit great distension after eating. Anatomically the stomach is divided into four regions: the *cardia, fundus, body (corpus)* and *pylorus (pyloric antrum)*. The pylorus terminates in a strong muscular sphincter surrounding the gastroduodenal junction.

The mucosa of the entire stomach has a tubular glandular form but there are three distinctly different histological zones:

- The cardia is a small area of predominantly mucus-secreting glands surrounding the entrance of the oesophagus (see Fig. 14.5).
- The mucosa of the fundus and the body forms the major histological region and consists of glands which secrete acid-peptic gastric juices as well as some protective mucus.
- The glands of the pylorus secrete mucus of two different types and associated endocrine cells secrete the hormone *gastrin*.

(a)

(b)

Fig. 14.7 Body of the stomach

(H & E (a) × 12 (b) × 40 (c) × 120)

Micrograph (a) illustrates the body of the stomach in the non-distended state. The mucosa **M** is thrown into prominent folds or rugae and consists of *gastric glands* which extend from the level of the muscularis mucosae **MM** to open into the stomach lumen via *gastric pits* **GP**.

The muscularis comprises the usual inner circular **C** and outer longitudinal **L** layers but the inner circular layer is reinforced by a further inner oblique layer **O**. The submucosa **S** is relatively loose and distensible and contains the larger blood vessels. The serosal layer which covers the peritoneal surface is thin and barely visible at this magnification.

Micrograph (b) focuses on the mucosa at higher magnification and shows the muscularis mucosa **MM** lying immediately beneath the base of the gastric glands clearly demarcating them from the underlying submucosa **SM**. A small lymphoid aggregate **L** lies in the lamina propria.

The mucosa of the fundus and body of the stomach consists of straight tubular glands which synthesise and secrete gastric juice. Gastric juice is a watery secretion containing *hydrochloric acid* (pH 0.9–1.5) and the digestive enzyme *pepsin* which hydrolyses proteins into polypeptide fragments. The stomach mucosa is protected from self-digestion by a thick surface covering of mucus.

The gastric glands contain a mixed population of cells of three main types as seen in micrograph (c):

- **Mucus-secreting cells M** cover the luminal surface of the stomach and line the gastric pits **GP** into which the gastric glands open; the cytoplasmic mucigen granules which pack these cells are stained poorly by H & E. Another type of mucus-secreting cell, the neck mucous cell, is found in the necks of the glands.
- **Acid-secreting cells**, called *parietal* **Pl** or *oxyntic cells*, are distributed along the length of the glands but tend to be most numerous in the middle portion or isthmus of the glands. These large rounded cells have an extensive eosinophilic (oxyntic) cytoplasm and centrally located nucleus.
- **Pepsin-secreting cells**, called *peptic* **Pc**, *chief*, or *zymogenic cells*, are located towards the bases of the gastric

(c)

glands. Peptic cells are recognised by their condensed, basally located nuclei and strongly basophilic granular cytoplasm which reflects their large content of ribosomes.

Thin strands of the muscularis mucosae **MM** extend between the gastric glands from the base; contraction of this muscle expels gastric secretions into the stomach lumen.

(a)

(b)

(c)

Fig. 14.8 Gastric pit and neck mucous glands

(a) PAS/H & E × 150 (b) and (c) PAS/Haematoxylin/ Orange G (b) LS × 480 (c) TS × 200

The PAS method has been used in these preparations to highlight the mucus-secreting cells of the gastric mucosa; mucus is PAS-positive because it is a polysaccharide. The stomach surface is lined by a single layer of tall columnar mucus-secreting cells **M** which are shed continuously and replaced by cells which migrate from the gastric pits; the mucus-secreting cells of the stomach are not of the goblet form found in other parts of the body. Other mucus-secreting cells in the necks and isthmus portions of the gastric glands are less intensely stained by PAS; called *neck mucous cells* **N**, they secrete a less viscous mucus which may protect the gland duct from autodigestion.

Acid-secreting parietal cells **P** in the upper parts of the gastric glands can be recognised by their characteristic 'fried egg' appearance. With H & E as in micrograph (a), their large central nucleus stands out in the pale eosinophilic (pink) cytoplasm; in contrast, their acidophilic cytoplasm is stained quite strongly with Orange G as in micrograph (b).

In transverse section, as in micrograph (c), the tubular nature of the gastric pits is clearly evident. One or more gastric glands may open into each gastric pit. Note the loose richly vascularised tissue of the lamina propria **L** which supports the gastric pits and glands. The lightly PAS-positive basement membrane **BM** can be distinguished between the epithelium and lamina propria.

Fig. 14.9 Base of gastric gland *(H & E × 320)*

Peptic (chief) cells **Pc**, which synthesise and secrete the proteolytic enzyme pepsin, are the principal cell type in the basal third of the gastric glands, although some parietal cells **Pl** are also found at this level. Peptic cells have basally located nuclei and extensive granular cytoplasm packed with rough endoplasmic reticulum, the ribosomes accounting for the marked cytoplasmic basophilia. The inactive pepsin precursor, *pepsinogen* is synthesised by the ribosomes and stored in numerous secretory granules located towards the luminal surface. Pepsinogen remains inactive until it reaches the lumen of the stomach where it is activated by the gastric juices preventing autodigestion of the gastric glands.

The much larger parietal cells are round with large centrally located nuclei and eosinophilic (pink-stained) cytoplasm due to the numerous mitochondria which are a feature of highly metabolically-active cells.

The secretory activity of both parietal and peptic cells is controlled by the autonomic nervous system and the hormone gastrin secreted by endocrine cells mainly located in the pyloric region. A variety of other APUD cells of the gastrointestinal endocrine system are also scattered in the gastric mucosa and elsewhere in the gastrointestinal tract. Occasionally, the endocrine cells **E** can be identified in sections fixed with chromium containing fixatives as in this example. Note a fine extension of the muscularis mucosae **M** extending up between the glands.

Fig. 14.10 Peptic cell

(Rat: EM × 7200)

This electron micrograph illustrates a peptic cell at the base of a gastric gland. The ultrastructural features of peptic cells are those of protein secreting (zymogenic) cells in general; these features include an extensive rough endoplasmic reticulum **rER** and membrane bound secretory vesicles **ZG** (zymogen granules) crowded in the apical cytoplasm, thus restricting the nucleus to the base of the cell. The extensive rough endoplasmic reticulum accounts for the intense basophilia of peptic cells when seen with light microscopy.

Fig. 14.11 Parietal cell *(Rat: EM × 9600)*

This micrograph shows a parietal cell **P** within a gastric gland. The luminal plasma membrane of the parietal cell forms deep, branching canaliculi **C** which extend throughout the cytoplasm and between adjacent cells. Numerous short microvilli project into the lumina of the intracellular canaliculi greatly increasing the surface area.

The production of hydrochloric acid appears to involve the production of carbonic acid by the enzyme *carbonic anhydrase*, this then dissociating into hydrogen and bicarbonate ions. The hydrogen ions are actively transported accompanied by chloride ions across the canalicular membrane whilst bicarbonate diffuses into the intercellular space and is dissipated into the surrounding capillaries. Hydrogen ions are approximately one million times more concentrated in gastric juice than in plasma, the process requiring energy provided by the numerous mitochondria **M** which crowd the peripheral cytoplasm. Parietal cells also secrete a glycoprotein called *intrinsic factor* which is essential for the absorption of vitamin B_{12} in the terminal ileum.

Also seen in this micrograph are several endocrine cells **E** of the gastrointestinal endocrine system, recognised by their small electron-dense secretory granules. Special histochemical techniques must be used to identify the precise nature of their secretory product.

(a)

(b)

Fig. 14.12 Pyloric stomach

(a) H & E × 80 (b) PAS/H & E × 80

In contrast to the simple tubular glands of the fundus and body, the pyloric glands are branched, and are composed almost exclusively of mucus-secreting cells. These are similar to those of the neck region of the body and fundus of the stomach except that these cells also secrete some pepsinogen. A small number of acid-secreting parietal cells are also scattered amongst the pyloric glands which stain poorly with standard histological methods as in micrograph (a).

The PAS method which stains carbohydrates magenta has been used in specimen (b) to show better detail of glandular structure. In each micrograph, note the prominent muscularis mucosae **MM** separating the glands from underlying submucosa **SM**. The glands open into deep, irregularly shaped pits **P** giving the superficial mucosa a characteristic frond-like appearance in histological sections. The function of the mucus secreted by the pyloric glands is to protect the entrance to the duodenum from acid-pepsin attack and to lubricate the passage of chyme.

Some of the cells in the isthmus region of the glands in the pylorus and rest of the stomach are undifferentiated stem cells which replace effete or damaged glandular cells.

Scattered amongst the pyloric mucous cells are endocrine cells which secrete the peptide hormone gastrin and are thus called 'G' cells. Other representatives of the gastrointestinal endocrine system are also found in the pylorus; their secreting products include somatostatin which is involved in regulation of insulin, glucagon, gastrin and growth hormone secretion. Demonstration of such cells requires special histochemical methods as shown in Figure 14.13.

Fig. 14.13 Gastrin cells

(Frozen section, modified aldehyde fuchsin × 480)

Throughout the gastrointestinal mucosa are numerous APUD cells of the gastrointestinal endocrine system which is described in detail in Chapter 17. These cells secrete a variety of peptide hormones usually in response to local stimuli. Most of these hormones then act on the same or functionally related parts of the gastrointestinal tract.

Gastrin cells were amongst the earliest of the gastrointestinal endocrine cells to be recognised. Since they are found in fairly large numbers and their distribution is more or less restricted to the pyloric region of the stomach, their secretory product and its actions have been relatively easy to elucidate, unlike that of many of the new-found APUD cells.

The presence of food in the stomach stimulates the secretion of gastrin into the blood stream; gastrin then promotes secretion of pepsin and acid by the gastric glands of the fundus and body as well as enhancing gastric motility.

This empirical staining method demonstrates gastrin cells **G** in the pyloric mucosa, the cytoplasm of the gastrin cells being stained a dark purple colour. The cells are typically located in the basal region of the glands.

Note the difference in section quality between this and preceding sections. Many specialised staining techniques cannot be performed on standard formalin-fixed, paraffin-embedded tissue but require fresh tissue. This has to be snap frozen and cut on a *freezing microtome* which inevitably causes the section to break up a little as seen here.

Fig. 14.14 Gastroduodenal junction *(Monkey: H & E × 12)*

The pyloric sphincter **PS** marks a dramatic transition in the gastrointestinal mucosa from the glandular arrangement of the stomach **S** to the villous arrangement which characterises the duodenum **D** and the rest of the small intestine. In addition, the duodenum is characterised by the presence of numerous mucus-secreting glands **G** which lie in the submucosa. These submucosal glands, known as *Brunner's glands*, are not found elsewhere in the small intestine.

The pyloric sphincter consists of an extreme thickening of the circular layer of the muscularis at the gastroduodenal junction. Note the continuity of both the circular **CM** and longitudinal **LM** layers of the muscularis between the pylorus and duodenum. The inner oblique layer is found only in the body of the stomach.

Fig. 14.15 Duodenum *(Monkey: H & E × 20)*

The duodenum, which represents the first part of the small intestine, receives partly digested food in the form of acidic chyme from the stomach via the pyloric canal. The main function of the duodenum is to neutralise gastric acid and pepsin and to initiate further digestive processes.

This micrograph illustrates monkey duodenum, the wall of the human duodenum being too thick to be photographed in its entirety. The mucosa **M** has the characteristic villous form of the whole of the small intestine with glandular crypts between the villi extending down to the muscularis mucosae **MM**. The feature unique to the duodenum is the extensive mass of coiled branched tubular glands **G** in the submucosa **SM**. The ducts of these *Brunner's glands* pass up through the muscularis mucosae to open into the crypts between the mucosal villi **V**. Beneath the mass of submucosal glands, the smooth muscle wall consists of an inner circular layer **CM** and an outer longitudinal layer **LM** as in the rest of the small intestine.

The tall columnar cells of Brunner's glands have extensive poorly stained mucigen-filled cytoplasm and basally located nuclei. The presence of chyme in the duodenum stimulates Brunner's glands to secrete a thin alkaline mucus which helps to neutralise the acidic chyme and to protect the duodenal mucosa from autodigestion.

Chyme also stimulates the release of two peptide hormones, *secretin* and *cholecystokinin-pancreozymin* (*CCK*) from APUD cells of the gastrointestinal endocrine system scattered throughout the duodenal mucosa. Secretin and CCK promote pancreatic exocrine secretion into the duodenal lumen via the pancreatic duct; CCK also stimulates contraction of the gall bladder thus propelling bile into the common bile duct. The pancreatic and common bile ducts merge to empty their contents into the duodenum via a single short duct.

Pancreatic juice is alkaline due to a high content of bicarbonate ions and thus helps to neutralise the acidic gastric contents entering the duodenum. The pancreas also secretes a variety of digestive enzymes including the proteolytic enzymes *trypsin* and *chymotrypsin*; like pepsin in the stomach, these are secreted in an inactive pro-enzyme form. On entering the duodenal lumen, trypsin is activated by the enzyme *enterokinase* secreted by the duodenal mucosa; activated trypsin in turn activates chymotrypsin. The pancreatic enzymes, which also include *amylase* and *lipases*, initiate the processes of luminal digestion described with Fig. 14.17. The biliary secretions contain *bile acids* which act as emulsifying agents and are particularly important in the digestion of lipids.

(a)

(b)

(c)

Fig. 14.16 Duodenum *(a) H & E × 15*
(b) PAS/Haematoxylin × 150 (c) Alcian blue × 150

These micrographs of the human duodenum highlight the mucus-secreting glands. Micrograph (a) is stained by the standard H & E method which has little affinity for mucin. Nevertheless the extraordinary thickness of the Brunner's glands is evident, the main glandular mass lying in the submucosa **SM** deep to the muscularis mucosae **MM** with a small portion sometimes found in the lamina propria **LP**. The duodenal mucosa has the typical form found elsewhere in the small intestine, namely numerous elongated villi **V** between the bases of which are shorter crypts **C**.

At higher magnification, micrograph (b) focuses on the duodenal mucosa stained by the PAS method; this stains most complex carbohydrates, including all mucins, a strong magenta. Brunner's glands **B** are not the only mucus-secreting cells in the duodenum, mucus also being produced by goblet cells **G** scattered in the epithelium of the mucosal villi and crypts. The majority of the mucosal epithelial cells are not PAS-positive and are tall columnar absorptive cells. This piece of tissue was taken from close to the junction of pylorus and duodenum where the villous mucosal form is not as distinct as further distally.

Micrograph (c) shows a section from the same specimen stained by the Alcian blue method which is specific for the acid mucin typical of goblet cells **G** but which leaves the alkaline mucus of Brunner's glands **B** unstained. All goblet cell mucus is Alcian blue positive as in the respiratory tract (see Fig. 12.7) and colon (see Fig. 14.29). Such differential staining provides a useful tool in histopathology for distinguishing mucus-secreting glandular tumours of gastric origin from those arising from the small and large intestine.

Fig. 14.17 Small intestine

The small intestine, comprising the duodenum, jejunum and ileum, is the principal site for absorption of digestion products from the gastrointestinal tract. Digestion begins in the stomach and is completed in the small intestine in association with the absorptive process. Four factors combine to provide an enormous surface area:

- The small intestine is extremely long (4–6 metres in humans).
- The mucosa and submucosa are thrown up into circularly arranged folds called *plicae circulares* **PC** or *valves of Kerckring* which are particularly numerous in the jejunum.
- The mucosal surface is made up of numerous finger-like projections called *villi* **V** whilst the mucosa between the bases of the villi is formed into crypts, called *crypts of Lieberkuhn* **C**.
- Extensive microvilli **Mv** are present at the luminal surface of the *enterocytes* **E**, the columnar cells covering the villi and crypts; these cells are responsible for the processes of digestion and absorption.

The muscularis mucosae **MM** lies immediately beneath the mucosal crypts and separates the mucosa from the submucosa **S**. The vascular submucosa extends into, and forms the core of, the plicae circulares. Inner circular **CM** and outer longitudinal **LM** layers of the muscularis are responsible for continuous peristaltic activity of the small intestine. The peritoneal aspect of the muscularis is invested by the loose collagenous serosa **Se** which is lined on its peritoneal surface by mesothelium.

A prominent feature of the small intestine are two hundred or so lymphoid aggregations known as *Peyer's patches* **PP** within the lamina propria (see Fig. 11.20).

The mechanisms of digestion and absorption

Digestion occurs within the lumen or at the mucosal surface, the latter being linked with the process of absorption. *Luminal digestion* involves the mixing of chyme with pancreatic enzymes with subsequent molecular breakdown occurring within the intestinal lumen; the process is facilitated by adsorption of pancreatic enzymes onto the mucosal surface. *Membrane digestion* involves enzymes located within the luminal plasma membranes of the cells lining the small intestine. The principal means of digestion and absorption of the main food constituents are as follows:

Proteins are initially denatured by the acidic gastric juice before being hydrolysed to polypeptide fragments by the enzyme pepsin. In the duodenum, pancreatic enzymes including *trypsin, chymotrypsin, elastase* and *carboxypeptidases* mediate further luminal digestion to small peptide fragments. Membrane-bound *oligopeptidases* complete the process leading to amino acid absorption; this involves active transport with a different carrier system for each amino acid. In young infants, some proteins are absorbed without prior digestion by the process of endocytosis, colostrum having been shown to have some anti-digestive properties.

Carbohydrates occur in the diet mainly in the form of starches and the disaccharides, sucrose and lactose. *Pancreatic amylase* hydrolyses starch to glucose and the disaccharide maltose in the small intestinal lumen. This process is commenced by *salivary amylase* in the mouth though its contribution to digestion is probably insignificant. Membrane-bound disaccharidases and oligosaccharidases convert the sugars to monosaccharides, mainly glucose, galactose and fructose, which are actively absorbed against concentration gradients.

Lipids, predominantly triglycerides, are converted by the mechanical action of the stomach into a coarse emulsion which is converted to a fine emulsion in the duodenum by bile acids synthesised in the liver. Each triglyceride molecule is broken down into a monoglyceride and two free fatty acids by *pancreatic lipases* though some glycerol and diglycerides are also produced. These smaller lipid molecules are then absorbed and resynthesised back into triglycerides within the enterocytes in which form they are transported from the gut into the general circulation.

The products of protein and carbohydrate digestion, namely amino acids and monosaccharides respectively, enter the intestinal capillaries and pass via the portal vein to the liver. In contrast, the reconstituted triglycerides pass into intestinal lymphatics known as *lacteals*, and thence via the thoracic duct to the general circulation, bypassing the liver. For lymphatic transport, the triglycerides become coated with phospholipids and proteins to form fine globules known as *chylomicrons*. A minority of lipid digestion products, such as short-chain fatty acids and glycerol, pass in the portal system to the liver along with almost all the bile acids which are reabsorbed and recirculated.

(a)

Fig. 14.18 Small intestine

(a) H & E × 16 (b) Scanning EM × 100

Micrograph (a) shows a section of small intestine at very low magnification. The mucosa **M** is thrown into transverse folds, the plicae circulares **PC**, covered with villi **V**. The muscularis mucosae **MM** lies immediately beneath the basal crypts and is difficult to see at this magnification. The vascular submucosa **S** extends into the plicae circulares. Beneath it lie circular **CM** and longitudinal **LM** layers of the muscularis propria and the serosa **Sr**. Peyer's patches **P** dominate the mucosa at the left of the field.

Micrograph (b) shows villi **V** along the crest of a plica circularis. Surface openings of scattered goblet cells stud the villous surface.

(b)

Fig. 14.19 Intestinal villi and crypts

(H & E × 120)

The intestinal villi **V** are lined by a simple columnar epithelium which is continuous with that of the crypts **C**. The predominant cell type, the *enterocytes*, are tall columnar cells with basally located nuclei and are involved in membrane digestion and absorption. Mucus-secreting goblet cells are scattered among the enterocytes. Mitotic activity by stem cells at the base of the crypts produces a continuous supply of new cells which progress up the villi where they mature before degenerating and being shed; in this way the entire epithelial lining of the intestine is replaced every 3 to 5 days.

A third cell type is found in clusters at the base of the crypts. These *Paneth cells* **P** are packed with strongly eosinophilic granules and are a prominent feature of the small intestine in humans, although absent in some mammals. Paneth cells are a stable population of cells with the ultrastructural characteristics of exocrine protein-secreting cells; their secretory product remains to be fully characterised but includes the bactericidal enzyme *lysozyme*.

The lamina propria **L** extends between the crypts and into the core of each villus and contains a rich vascular and lymphatic network into which digestive products are absorbed. The muscularis mucosae **MM** lies immediately beneath the base of the crypts.

(a)

(b)

(c)

Fig 14.20 Crypts of Lieberkuhn *(H & E (a) TS × 400 (b) LS × 400 (c) Phloxine-tartrazine × 320)*

The majority of cells in the crypt bases are stem cells involved in replenishment of the enterocytes and goblet cells of the villi; immature goblet cells **G** are readily seen in micrograph (b). With such a high rate of cell turnover, it might be expected that mitotic figures would be very frequent; however, this is not the case as the mitotic phase only occupies a small proportion of the cell cycle. With

H & E staining, Paneth cells **P** exhibit intensely eosinophilic cytoplasmic granules; these are even more clearly demonstrated by the phloxine-tartrazine method which stains the granules scarlet.

In micrograph (a), a few large pale stained endocrine cells **E** can be seen; secretory products of such cells include secretin, somatostatin, enteroglucagon and serotonin.

(a)   *(b)*   *(c)*

Fig. 14.21 Intestinal villi *(LS: (a) H & E × 100 (b) PAS/Iron haematoxylin/Orange G × 320 (c) TS: H & E × 400)*

These micrographs illustrate the tall columnar nature of the enterocytes which invest the intestinal villi as well as the plump goblet cells scattered among them. The luminal surface of the enterocytes seen in micrograph (b) is strongly PAS-positive due to the presence of a particularly thick glycocalyx (see Fig. 1.2) and a surface layer of goblet cell-derived mucus; both protect against autodigestion. The glycocalyx may also be the site for adsorption of pancreatic digestive enzymes.

Lymphocytes **Ly** are scattered among the enterocytes; most appear to be cytotoxic T cells which may be responsible for destroying virus-infected enterocytes (see Ch. 11). Plasma cells **P** in the villous core secrete antibodies of the IgA class which pass into the intestinal lumen where they contribute to defence against invading pathogens.

The cores of the villi are extensions of the lamina propria and consist of loose supporting tissue containing numerous reticulin fibres. Capillaries **C** lie immediately beneath the layer of enterocytes and transport amino acids, monosaccharides and most other digestive products to the hepatic portal vein. Tiny lymphatic vessels drain into a single larger vessel called a *lacteal* **L** located in the centre of the core of the villus; being devoid of erythrocytes, these may be difficult to distinguish. The lacteals transport much of the absorbed lipid into the circulatory system via the thoracic duct, thus bypassing the liver. Strands of smooth muscle cells **M** are seen in the long axis of the villous core in micrograph (a) and represent extensions of the muscularis mucosae (see also Fig. 14.22).

Fig. 14.22 Tip of intestinal villus

(Thin section, toluidine blue × 320)

This method of tissue preparation shows several features of the intestinal villus which are not as well seen in thicker conventional paraffin wax-embedded sections.

Firstly, degenerating enterocytes and goblet cells are seen about to be shed from the tip of the villus. Secondly, a striated or brush border **SB** is identifiable at the luminal surface of the enterocytes representing the microvilli seen with electron microscopy. Thirdly, smooth muscle fibres **M** are seen in the long axis of the villous core where they are disposed around the central lacteal; these muscle cells are extensions of the muscularis mucosae. Contraction of the smooth muscle strands enhances drainage of lymph from the lacteals and probably also keeps the villi in a constant motile state reducing the prospect of clogging and enhancing contact of luminal contents with the villous surface.

Fig. 14.23 Intestinal villi

(Enzyme histochemical method for alkaline phosphatase × 128)

This frozen section from an intestinal biopsy has been stained for the enzyme *alkaline phosphatase* which is one of the many membrane-bound enzymes characteristic of enterocyte microvilli; enzyme activity is represented by a red deposit. Alkaline phosphatase is thought to be involved in the transport of calcium ions from the intestinal lumen. Other membrane enzymes are involved in the breakdown of peptides and disaccharides to amino acids and monosaccharides respectively. The enzymes of the striated border are an integral part of the plasma membrane and are synthesised by enterocytes, in contrast to those enzymes adsorbed on to the surface which are synthesised by the pancreas. Note that the relatively immature enterocytes in the intestinal crypts show little alkaline phosphatase activity.

Fig. 14.24 Intestinal villi *(Carmine perfused × 10)*

This specimen of small intestine has been perfused before fixation with a red dye and demonstrates the blood supply of the mucosa.

From a dense capillary network in the submucosa **SM**, long loops of branching capillaries extend up to the tips of the villi **V**. Note also the capillary network supplying the muscular wall **M**. Most of the absorbed food products, with the exception of triglycerides, enter the capillaries and pass via the portal vein to the liver.

Fig. 14.25 Intestinal villus *(Sudan black × 320)*

This frozen section from the intestine of a rat fed with milk has been stained to demonstrate the presence of absorbed lipids. Ingested triglycerides are emulsified by bile and hydrolysed by the pancreatic enzyme, *lipase*; the degradation products, mainly free fatty acids and monoglycerides, are absorbed by enterocytes where they are resynthesised into triglycerides in the smooth endoplasmic reticulum. Here, the triglycerides are reconstituted into small globules and form a lipoprotein complex incorporating protein, cholesterol and phospholipids. Membrane bound vesicles containing multiple droplets bud from the smooth endoplasmic reticulum and pass towards the base of the cell where they are released by exocytosis into the intercellular clefts; from here the small lipoprotein droplets, described as *chylomicrons*, pass into the lacteals from which they enter the general circulation. Note the high concentration of black-stained lipid in the enterocyte cytoplasm and in the chylomicrons within the central lacteal.

(a)

(b)

(c)

Fig. 14.26 Enterocytes *(illustrations (a) and (b) opposite; EM (a) × 4540 (b) × 56 000 (c) × 22 000)*

These micrographs illustrate the main ultrastructural features of the absorptive cells of the small intestine, the enterocytes. Micrograph (a) shows the enormous number of microvilli **Mv** (up to 3000 per cell) which increase the surface area of the plasma membrane exposed to the lumen by some 30 times. The microvilli are of uniform length, (approximately 1 μm), and constitute the striated border of light microscopy (see Fig. 14.22). Most absorption in the small intestine occurs by direct passage of low molecular weight digestion products across the luminal plasma membrane. Mitochondria **M** are particularly abundant within enterocytes reflecting the high energy demands of such processes. Between the bases of the enterocytes are intercellular clefts **IC** into which chylomicrons are first passed en route to the lacteals. From the clefts, the chylomicrons pass across the thin basement membrane **BM** to be preferentially absorbed into the lacteals. Lymphocytes **Ly** are commonly found in the intercellular clefts between enterocytes where they play an important part in the immunological defence of the tract. Note the close proximity of a blood capillary **C** to the enterocyte basement membrane.

As seen in micrograph (b), the glycocalyx **G** of the enterocyte microvilli is unusually prominent. It provides protection against autodigestion and acts as the site for adsorption of pancreatic digestive enzymes. This micrograph also shows the filamentous cytoskeleton of the microvilli extending into the superficial cytoplasm. Here, in the terminal web **TW**, it becomes integrated into the cytoskeleton of the body of the cell. Deeper in the cell, filaments **F** and microtubules **T** are readily identified. Enterocytes are tightly bound near their luminal surface by junctional complexes (see Fig. 5.10) which prevent direct

access of luminal contents into the intercellular spaces.

Endocytotic vesicles **EV** are often seen between the bases of microvilli and membranous vesicles **V** are common in the superficial cytoplasm. The importance of endocytosis as a mode of absorption in the small intestine is not well understood although it may be a minor pathway of lipid and in some cases protein absorption. Smooth endoplasmic reticulum **sER** is seen deeper in the cytoplasm.

Micrograph (c) illustrates the basal aspect of two enterocytes separated by an intercellular cleft **IC**. Their basement membrane is thin, the lamina densa **LD** appearing to be discontinuous. Close beneath the base of the enterocytes is a tiny lymphatic tributary of the central lacteal, its endothelial lining **En** being thin and fenestrated; note the junctional complex **J** binding adjacent endothelial cells and the thin discontinuous endothelial basement membrane **BM$_E$**. The delicate supporting tissue between the enterocytes and lymphatic contains fibroblasts **F** and fine collagen fibrils **Co**.

The main feature of the basal enterocytic cytoplasm is numerous free ribosomes **R**, scattered mitochondria **M** and membranous vesicles **V** containing lipoprotein droplets en route for exocytosis into the intercellular cleft. The cleft contains numerous small chylomicrons **Ch** which cluster near the lamina densa as if temporarily held up in their passage towards the lymphatic. In the lamina propria, the chylomicrons are larger, probably due to fusion of smaller ones coursing through from the intercellular cleft. Note that the chylomicrons in the extracellular environment are not membrane-bound but have a fine electron-dense limiting layer of protein.

Fig. 14.27 Ileo–caecal junction *(H & E × 5)*

Unabsorbed and indigestible food residues from the ileum are propelled by peristalsis into the distended first part of the large intestine, the caecum, through a simple cone-shaped valve which marks the ileo-caecal junction. There is an abrupt transition in the lining of the valve from the villiform pattern in the small intestine **S** to the glandular form in the large intestine **L**.

The ileo-caecal valve consists of a thickened extension of the muscularis **M** which provides robust support for the mucosa. Variable quantities of lymphoid tissue **Ly** are found in the mucosa.

(a)

(b)

Fig. 14.28 Colon *(H & E (a) × 4 (b) × 100)*

The principal functions of the large intestine are the recovery of water from the liquid residue of the contents of the small intestine and the propulsion of increasingly solid faeces to the rectum prior to defaecation.

As shown in micrograph (a), the muscular wall is consequently thick and capable of powerful peristaltic activity. As in the rest of the gastrointestinal tract, the muscularis propria of the large intestine consists of inner circular **CM** and outer longitudinal layers **LM** but, except in the rectum, the longitudinal layer does not completely surround the tract but forms three separate longitudinal bands called *taeniae coli*.

Consistent with its functions of water absorption and faecal lubrication, the mucosa consists of cells of two types, absorptive cells and mucus-secreting goblet cells. As seen in micrograph (b), these are arranged in closely packed straight tubular glands, an arrangement which greatly enhances the functional surface area. As faeces pass along the large intestine and become progressively dehydrated, the mucus becomes increasingly important in protecting the mucosa

from trauma. The glands are analogous to the crypts of Lieberkuhn of the small intestine and this term may also be applied to the glands of the large intestine. As in the stomach and small intestine, the epithelium undergoes continual turnover at the luminal surface, the cells being replaced by mitosis at the base of the glands. The thick glandular mucosa is folded in the non-distended state but it does not exhibit distinct plicae circulares like those of the small intestine. Immediately above the anal valves, the mucosa forms longitudinal folds called the *columns of Morgagni*. The muscularis mucosae **MM** is a prominent feature of the large intestinal mucosa; rhythmic contractions prevent clogging of the glands and enhance expulsion of mucus.

As protection from ingress of microorganisms, the large intestinal wall contains numerous leucocytes including lymphocytes which form large aggregations in the lamina propria and submucosa as seen in micrograph (a); these do not form domes projecting into the lumen as with the Peyer's patches of the small intestine (see Fig. 11.20).

(a)

(b)

(c)

Fig. 14.29 Colonic glands *(Alcian blue/van Gieson (a) LS × 80 (b) TS × 320 (c) H & E, TS × 320)*

The alcian blue staining method permits ready differentiation of the two major cell types which comprise the glands of the large intestine; goblet cell mucus is stained a greenish-blue colour whilst the absorptive cells remain poorly stained. As seen in micrograph (a), the simple tubular glands extend from the luminal surface to the muscularis mucosae **MM** and are separated from each other by thin plates of lamina propria, the collagen of which is stained red. Thin strands of the muscularis mucosae extend into the lamina propria between the glands, contraction facilitating the expulsion of mucus into the bowel lumen. Goblet cells predominate in the base of the glands whereas the luminal surface is almost entirely lined by columnar absorptive cells; the middle part of the glands represents the transition between the two.

Micrographs (b) and (c) show transverse sections through the upper part of large intestinal glands, highlighting the closely packed arrangement of the glands in the mucosa. The absorptive cells are tall columnar with large oval basally-located nuclei; in contrast, goblet cell nuclei are small and condensed. Lamina propria fills the space between the glands and contains numerous blood and lymphatic vessels into which water is absorbed by passive diffusion.

The large intestine is inhabited by a variety of commensal bacteria which further degrade food residues. Bacterial degradation is an important mechanism for the digestion of cellulose in ruminants but in humans this function is of less importance, most cellulose being excreted. Small quantities of fat-soluble vitamins derived from bacterial activity are absorbed in the large intestine.

Fig. 14.30 Recto-anal junction *(H & E × 60)*

The rectum is the short dilated terminal portion of the large intestine. The rectal mucosa **RM** is similar to that of the rest of the large bowel except that it has even more numerous goblet cells. At the recto-anal junction **J**, it undergoes an abrupt transition to become stratified squamous epithelium **SS** in the anal canal. Branched tubular *circumanal glands* **G** open at the recto-anal junction into small pits at the distal ends of the columns of Morgagni. The anal canal forms the last 2 or 3 cm of the gastrointestinal tract and is surrounded by voluntary muscle which forms the anal sphincter. Here, the stratified squamous epithelium undergoes a gradual transition to skin containing sebaceous glands and large apocrine sweat glands (see Fig. 9.16).

(a)

(b)

(c)

Fig. 14.31 Appendix

(H & E (a) ×5 (b) ×60 (c) ×42)

The appendix is a small blind-ended tubular sac extending from the caecum just distal to the ileo-caecal junction. The general structure of the appendix conforms to that of the rest of the large intestine. In some mammals, the appendix is capacious and involved in prolonged digestion of cellulose but in man it appears to have no significant digestive or absorptive function.

These specimens are taken from a young adult. Micrograph (a) illustrates the suspensory mesentery **M** which becomes continuous with the outer serosal layer and is a feature of all parts of the gastrointestinal tract which lie free in the peritoneal cavity. In this specimen, the serosa **S** contains a moderate amount of extravasated blood resulting from haemorrhage during surgical removal. The mesenteries conduct blood vessels, lymphatics and nerves to and from the gastrointestinal tract.

The most characteristic feature of the appendix, particularly in the young, is the presence of masses of lymphoid tissue in the mucosa and submucosa. As seen in micrographs (b) and (c), the lamina propria **LP** and upper submucosa **SM** are diffusely infiltrated with lymphocytes which are also seen to a lesser extent in the deeper submucosa and muscularis propria **M**. Note that the mucosal glands are much less closely packed than elsewhere in the large intestine. As seen in micrographs (a) and (b), the lymphoid tissue also forms follicles **F** often containing germinal centres (see also Fig. 11.21). These follicles bulge into the lumen and, like the follicles of Peyer's patches in the small intestine, are invested by a simple epithelium of M cells which presumably facilitates sampling of antigen in the appendicular lumen.

Undoubtedly, the appendix contains a significant part of the gut-associated lymphoid tissue (described in Ch. 11) but no specific function has yet been ascribed to it.

15. Liver and pancreas

Liver and biliary system

The liver, like the pancreas, develops embryologically as a glandular outgrowth of the primitive gut. The major functions of the liver may be summarised as follows:

- Detoxification of metabolic waste products, e.g. deamination of amino acids to produce urea.
- Destruction of spent red cells and reclamation of their constituents (in conjunction with the spleen).
- Synthesis and secretion of bile; bile contains many of the end products of the above processes and is thus an excretory product and an exocrine secretion.
- Synthesis of the plasma proteins including the clotting factors.
- Synthesis of plasma lipoproteins.
- Metabolic functions, e.g. glycogen synthesis, gluconeogenesis, storage of glycogen, some vitamins and lipid.

Many of these biosynthetic functions utilise the products of digestion. With the exception of most lipids, absorbed food products pass directly from the gut to the liver via the *hepatic portal vein*. Thus the liver is perfused by blood rich in amino acids, simple sugars and other products of digestion but relatively poor in oxygen. Oxygen required to support liver metabolism is supplied via the *hepatic artery*. The liver is thus unusual in having both arterial and venous blood supplies. Venous drainage of the liver occurs via the *hepatic vein*.

(a)

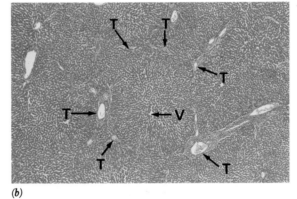

(b)

Fig. 15.1 Liver *(a) Pig: H & E × 20 (b) Human: H & E × 20*

Traditionally the liver parenchymal cells, the *hepatocytes*, are described as being arranged into *lobules*. The lobules are bounded by thin septa of collagenous supporting tissue **C** which, as seen in micrograph (a), are particularly easily identified in pig liver. The hepatic lobules are roughly hexagonal in shape when seen in any section, reflecting their polyhedral three-dimensional shape. Terminal branches of the hepatic artery and hepatic portal vein are located at the angles of the lobule boundaries in *portal tracts* **T**. Blood from the portal tracts converges upon a *terminal hepatic venule (centrilobular venule)* **V** of each lobule via sinusoids which pass between plates of hepatocytes. The terminal hepatic venules drain to the hepatic vein.

The human liver has a similar lobular pattern to that of the pig but the interlobular septa are absent. As seen in

micrograph (b), portal tracts **T** define the angles of the lobule margins and a terminal hepatic venule **V** defines the centre of each lobule. Note that each portal tract supplies more than one lobule whereas each terminal hepatic venule drains only a single lobule.

A more modern approach is to consider the functional unit of the liver to be the territory supplied by each terminal branch of the hepatic artery and hepatic portal vein. The *hepatic acinus* thus described is also a polyhedral shape with a portal tract forming its central axis with plates of hepatocytes and intervening sinuses radiating towards a number of terminal hepatic venules marking the boundary angles. Bile from each hepatic acinus drains to a bile collecting duct located in the portal tract. Lymphatic capillaries also drain to the portal tracts.

Terminal hepatic venule

Hepatic vein

Portal tract

Bile duct

Hepatic portal vein

Hepatic artery

Lobule

Bile duct

Hepatic artery

Hepatic portal vein

Fig. 15.2 Hepatic vasculature and biliary system

This schematic diagram shows the gross arrangement of the hepatic vascular and the bile collecting systems.

The hepatic portal vein and hepatic artery branch repeatedly within the liver, their terminal branches running within the portal tracts. Blood from both systems then percolates between the branching plates of hepatocytes in the sinusoids which converge to drain into a terminal hepatic (centrilobular) venule. These drain to *intercalated veins* and thence to the hepatic vein which drains into the inferior vena cava.

Bile is secreted into a network of minute *bile canaliculi* situated between the plasma membranes of adjacent hepatocytes; the canaliculi are too small to be represented in this diagram. The canalicular network then drains into a system of bile collecting ducts located in the portal tracts but coursing in the opposite direction to the two blood supply systems. The bile collecting system then drains to the common bile duct and ultimately to the duodenum.

Fig. 15.3 Portal tract *(H & E × 150)*

This micrograph focuses on a typical portal tract containing three main structures. The largest is a terminal branch of the hepatic portal vein **PV** (*terminal portal venule*) which has a very thin wall lined by flattened endothelial cells. Smaller diameter thick-walled vessels with the typical structure of arterioles are terminal branches of the hepatic artery **A**.

Bile collecting ducts are of variable size and lined by simple cuboidal or columnar epithelium; these comprise the *canals of Hering*, short channels that drain the canaliculi into *bile ductules* **B** usually located at the periphery of the tract. These merge to form larger more centrally located *trabecular ducts* which drain via *intrahepatic ducts* into the *right and left hepatic ducts*, the *common hepatic duct* and thence to the duodenum via the *common bile duct*. Because these three structures are always found in the portal tracts, the tracts are often referred to as *portal triads*. Lymphatics **L** are also present in the portal tracts but since their walls are delicate and often collapsed they are often less easily identified.

Surrounding the portal tract are anastomosing plates of hepatocytes **H**. Between them are the hepatic sinusoids **S** receiving blood from both the hepatic portal and hepatic arterial systems. The layer of hepatocytes immediately bordering the portal tract is known as the *limiting plate*. A network of bile canaliculi is located within each plate of hepatocytes but these are far too small to be seen at this magnification.

Fig. 15.4 Liver *(Perfusion method × 20)*

This preparation shows one of the techniques used by early histologists in mapping hepatic blood flow. The hepatic portal vein (supplying the liver) has been perfused with a red dye and the hepatic vein (draining the liver) has been back-perfused with a blue dye. Thus it can be seen how a hepatic lobule is defined by a number of portal tracts peripherally (stained red) with blood draining to a single terminal hepatic venule (stained blue) at the centre. Alternatively, an hepatic acinus is centred around a portal tract with blood radiating outwards to drain into a number of terminal hepatic venules.

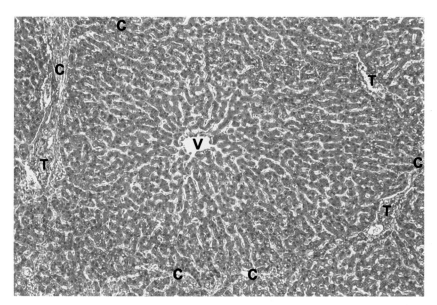

Fig. 15.5 Liver lobule
(H & E × 75)

This micrograph illustrates a single human liver lobule. The irregular hexagonal boundary of the lobule is defined by portal tracts **T** and sparse collagenous tissue **C**. Sinusoids originate at the lobule margin and course between plates of hepatocytes to converge upon the terminal hepatic venule **V**.

The plates of hepatocytes are usually only one cell thick and each hepatocyte is thus exposed to blood on at least two sides. The plates of hepatocytes branch and anastomose to form a three-dimensional structure like a sponge.

Fig. 15.6 Liver parenchyma
(H & E × 150)

The arrangement of hepatocytes within the liver parenchyma can be readily seen at this magnification. The hepatocytes form flat, anastomosing plates usually only one cell thick between which blood passes sluggishly towards the terminal hepatic venule **V**. The sinusoids are lined by a discontinuous layer of cells which do not rest on a basement membrane and which are separated from the hepatocytes by a narrow space (*space of Disse*); this drains into the lymphatics of the portal tracts.

(a)   (b)

Fig. 15.7 Hepatocytes *(a) H & E × 600 (b) PAS/Haematoxylin × 400*

Hepatocytes are large polyhedral cells with large round nuclei with peripherally dispersed chromatin and prominent nucleoli. The nuclei vary greatly in size, reflecting an unusual cellular feature; more than half the hepatocytes contain twice the normal (diploid) complement of chromosomes within a single nucleus (i.e. they are tetraploid) and some contain four or even eight times this amount (polyploid). Occasional binucleate cells are seen in section although up to 25% of all hepatocytes are actually binucleate.

The extensive cytoplasm has a variable appearance depending on the nutritional status of the individual. When well-nourished, hepatocytes store significant quantities of glycogen and process large quantities of lipid. Both these metabolites are partially removed during routine histological preparation leaving irregular unstained areas within the cytoplasm. The cytoplasm is otherwise strongly eosinophilic due to numerous mitochondria with a fine basophilic granularity due to extensive free ribosomes and rough ER. Fine brown granules of the 'wear and tear' pigment lipofuscin (see Fig. 1.3) are present in variable amounts, increasing with age. All these features are seen in micrograph (a).

Sinusoid lining cells **S** are readily distinguishable from hepatocytes by their flattened condensed nuclei and attenuated poorly stained cytoplasm.

Micrograph (b) demonstrates the presence within the hepatocytes of glycogen granules which, being polysaccharide, are PAS positive, i.e. stain magenta; the nuclei are counterstained blue.

Fig. 15.8 Sinusoid lining cells

(Perl's Prussian blue × 48)

The nature and function of the sinusoid lining cells has been in dispute ever since the liver was first studied. At least a proportion of these cells can be shown to be highly phagocytic when 'fed' either artificially or under pathological conditions with appropriate particulate matter. The animal used for this preparation was injected intravenously with a particulate iron-sugar compound which, with this staining method, is demonstrated as a dark deposit within the sinusoid lining cells.

The sinusoid lining cells include at least three cell types. The majority are endothelial cells **E** with flat darkly stained nuclei and attenuated cytoplasm. Scattered among the endothelial cells are large plump phagocytic cells with ovoid nuclei. Known as *Kupffer cells* **K**, these cells form part of the monocyte-macrophage defence system (see Chs. 3 and 4) and with the spleen, participate in the removal of spent erythrocytes and other particulate debris from the circulation. Occasional fibroblasts with the capacity to store lipid are found in the space of Disse between the sinusoid lining cells and the hepatocytes.

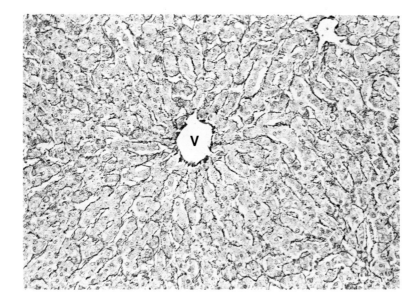

Fig. 15.9 Liver

(Reticulin method × 250)

Hepatocytes and sinusoid lining cells are supported by a fine meshwork of reticulin fibres (collagen type III, stained black in this preparation) which radiate from around the terminal hepatic (centrilobular) venules **V** to merge with a sparse collagenous framework in the supporting tissue of the portal tracts and lobule boundaries. At the periphery of the liver, the reticulin becomes continuous with a thin but tough collagenous capsule called *Glisson's capsule* which invests the external surface of the liver.

The reticulin architecture of the liver is distorted in a variety of liver diseases and this staining method is commonly used as an aid to diagnosis.

(a)

(b)

Fig. 15.10 Bile canaliculi *(a) Enzyme histochemical method for ATP-ase × 480 (b) Iron haematoxylin × 480*

Bile is synthesised by all hepatocytes and secreted into a system of minute canaliculi which form an anastomosing network within the plates of hepatocytes. The canaliculi have no discrete structure of their own but consist merely of fine channels formed by the plasma membranes of adjacent hepatocytes; the ultrastructural features are shown in Figure 15.11.

Bile canaliculi of adjacent hepatocyte plates merge to form canals of Hering before draining into the bile ductules of the portal tracts.

The hepatocyte plasma membranes forming the walls of

the canaliculi contain the enzyme ATP-ase which suggest that bile secretion is an energy-dependent process. A histochemical method for ATP-ase has been used in micrograph (a) to demonstrate bile canaliculi (stained brown) which are difficult to demonstrate with routine methods for light microscopy. Within each hepatocyte plate, the canaliculi form a regular hexagonal network reminiscent of chicken wire, each hexagon enclosing a single hepatocyte. In micrograph (b), iron has been deposited in the walls of the canaliculi **C**. Note two binucleate hepatocytes **B**.

(a)

Fig. 15.11 Liver *(a) EM × 4400 (b) EM × 15 200 (opposite)*

These micrographs demonstrate the main ultrastructural features of the liver. Hepatocytes **H** are exposed on each side to the sinusoids (filled with erythrocytes **E**) which are lined by a discontinuous layer of sinusoid lining cells **S**. These are supported by the fine reticulin framework of the liver (see Fig. 15.10) with the *space of Disse* **D** between the lining cells and the hepatocyte surface. Via the gaps in the sinusoid lining, the space of Disse is continuous with the sinusoid lumen, thus bathing the hepatocyte surface with plasma. Numerous irregular microvilli **Mv** extend from the hepatocyte surface into the space of Disse, greatly increasing the surface area for metabolic exchange. Between the bases of the microvilli are coated pits involved in endocytosis.

Reflecting the extraordinary range of biosynthetic and degradative activities, the hepatocyte cytoplasm is crowded with organelles, particularly rough endoplasmic reticulum **rER**, smooth endoplasmic reticulum **sER**, Golgi stacks, free ribosomes, mitochondria **M**, lysosomes **Ly** and peroxisomes. Lipid droplets **L** and glycogen rosettes are present in variable numbers depending on nutritional status.

Bile canaliculi **BC** are seen to be formed from the plasma membranes of adjacent hepatocytes, the plasma membranes being tightly bound by junctional complexes **J**; small microvilli project into the canaliculi. The subjacent cytoplasm contains a network of actin filaments, contraction of which reduces canalicular diameter, thus reducing flow rate.

(b)

(a)

(b)

Fig. 15.12 Gall bladder

(H & E (a) ×30 (b) ×480 (c) ×10)

The intrahepatic bile collecting system merges to form *right* and *left hepatic ducts* which join forming a single large duct, the *common hepatic duct*. On leaving the liver, this is joined by the *cystic duct* which drains the *gall bladder*. The *common bile duct* so formed joins the *pancreatic duct* to form the short *ampulla of Vater* before entering the duodenum. Bile draining down the common hepatic duct is shunted into the gall bladder where it is stored and concentrated.

The gall bladder is a muscular sac lined by a simple columnar epithelium; it has a capacity of about 100 ml in humans. The presence of lipid in the duodenum promotes the secretion of the hormone cholecystokinin-pancreozymin (CCK) by endocrine cells of the duodenal mucosa stimulating contraction of the gall bladder and forcing bile into the duodenum. Bile is an emulsifying agent facilitating the hydrolysis of dietary lipids by pancreatic lipases.

Micrograph (a) shows the wall of a gall bladder in the non-distended state in which the mucosa is thrown up into many folds. The relatively loose submucosa **S** is rich in elastic fibres, blood and lymphatic vessels which drain water reabsorbed from bile during the concentration process. The fibres of the muscular layer **M** are mainly disposed obliquely. Externally is a thick collagenous adventitia (serosal) coat **A** conveying the larger blood and lymphatic vessels. In the neck of the gall bladder, mucous glands are often found in the submucosa; mucus may provide a protective surface film for the biliary tract.

At high magnification in micrograph (b), the simple epithelial lining of the gall bladder is seen to consist of very tall columnar cells with basally located nuclei; numerous short irregular microvilli account for the unevenness of the

(c)

luminal surface. The lining cells concentrate bile 5- to 10-fold by an active process, water being passed into a rich capillary network in the lamina propria **LP**.

Micrograph (c) illustrates the wall of the cystic duct which is formed into a twisted mucosa-covered fold **F** known as the *spiral valve of Heister*.

Flow of bile into the duodenum is controlled by the smooth muscle *cholidochal sphincter* at the distal end of the common bile duct, closure of the sphincter directing bile from the liver into the cystic duct and protecting against reflux of pancreatic juice. A smooth muscle sphincter, the *sphincter of Oddi*, also surrounds the ampulla of Vater but this is probably mainly involved in control of flow of pancreatic juice. The ampulla passes obliquely through the duodenal wall and mucosa entering the duodenum via the *duodenal papilla* which projects into the duodenal lumen. This arrangement probably acts as a valve preventing reflux of duodenal contents into the ampulla.

Pancreas

The pancreas is a large gland which, like the liver, develops embryologically as an outgrowth of the primitive foregut. The pancreas has both exocrine and endocrine components; the endocrine pancreas is described in detail in Chapter 17. The exocrine pancreas, which forms the bulk of the gland, secretes an enzyme-rich alkaline fluid into the duodenum via the *pancreatic duct*. The high pH of pancreatic secretion is due to a high content of bicarbonate ions and serves to neutralise the acidic chyme as it enters the small intestine from the stomach. The pancreatic enzymes degrade proteins, carbohydrates, lipids and nucleic acids by the process of luminal digestion (see Fig. 14.17). Like pepsin in the stomach, the pancreatic proteolytic enzymes *trypsin* and *chymotrypsin* are secreted in an inactive form. *Enterokinase*, an enzyme secreted by the duodenal mucosa, activates protrypsin to form trypsin; trypsin then activates prochymotrypsin to form chymotrypsin. This mechanism prevents autodigestion of the pancreas. The other pancreatic enzymes are secreted in the active form.

Pancreatic secretion occurs continuously, the rate being modulated by hormonal and nervous influences. *Secretin*, a hormone released by endocrine cells scattered in the duodenum, promotes the secretion of copious watery fluid rich in bicarbonate. Cholecystokinin-pancreozymin (CCK), also derived from duodenal endocrine cells, stimulates the secretion of enzyme-rich pancreatic fluid. Gastrin, secreted by endocrine cells of the pyloric mucosa, has a similar action on the pancreas to that of CCK. The pancreas is richly innervated by the autonomic nervous system, but the significance of this on pancreatic secretion is not well understood.

Fig. 15.13 Pancreas *(H & E × 15)*

The pancreas is a highly lobulated gland invested by a thin loose collagenous capsule which extends as delicate septa **S** between the lobules. The exocrine component of the pancreas consists of closely packed secretory acini which drain into a highly branched duct system. Most of the secretion drains into the main *pancreatic duct* which joins the common bile duct to drain into the duodenum via the ampulla of Vater; a small, *accessory pancreatic duct* drains

into the duodenum more proximally. *Interlobular ducts* **D** of various sizes can be seen in this micrograph; their surrounding supporting tissue reinforces the septal framework.

The endocrine tissue of the pancreas forms *islets of Langerhans* **I** of various sizes scattered throughout the exocrine tissue.

(a)

(b)

Fig. 15.14 Exocrine pancreas *(a) H & E × 200 (b) H & E × 400 (c) EM × 8500 (opposite)*

Details of the pancreatic acini and duct system can be seen in these micrographs. Each acinus is made up of an irregular cluster of pyramid-shaped secretory cells, the apices of which surround a minute central lumen which represents the terminal end of the duct system. The smallest of the tributaries are known as *intercalated ducts*. Adjacent acini are separated by inconspicuous supporting tissue containing numerous capillaries. In histological section, the interacinar spaces tend to appear wider than in vivo due to a fixation artefact. The intercalated ducts then drain into small *intralobular ducts* which in turn drain into the *interlobular ducts* in the septa of the gland. The intercalated ducts are lined by simple low cuboidal epithelium which becomes stratified cuboidal in the larger ducts. With increasing size, the ducts are invested by a progressively thicker layer of dense collagenous supporting tissue; the wall of the main pancreatic duct contains smooth muscle.

Micrograph (a) shows the general arrangement of the glandular acini **A**.

An intralobular duct is seen in upper midfield and a larger interlobular duct in lower midfield, the latter with a much broader sheath of supporting tissue **S**.

As seen with further magnification in micrograph (b), the cells of each pancreatic acinus have a roughly triangular shape in section, their apices projecting towards a central lumen **L** of a minute duct. The acinar cells are typical protein-secreting (zymogenic) cells. The nuclei are basally located and surrounded by basophilic cytoplasm crammed with rough endoplasmic reticulum; the apices of the cells are

packed with eosinophilic zymogen secretory granules. The centres of the acini frequently contain one or more nuclei of *centroacinar cells* **C** with pale stained nuclei and sparse pale stained cytoplasm; these represent the terminal lining cells of intercalated ducts. Cells of similar appearance can be seen between the acini and are those of intercalated ducts **D** passing to join the larger intralobular ducts. The cells lining the intercalated ducts are responsible for elaborating the water and bicarbonate component of pancreatic secretion.

The electron micrograph (c) opposite illustrates part of a pancreatic acinus with its central lumen **L**. The pyramid-shaped secretory cells have round basally located nuclei with dispersed chromatin and prominent nucleoli **Nu**, both characteristic features of highly active cells. The basal cytoplasm is crammed with lamellar profiles of rough endoplasmic reticulum **rER** within which are scattered elongated mitochondria **M**. A large Golgi apparatus **G** is located in a supranuclear position and is responsible for packaging enzymes synthesised on the rough endoplasmic reticulum to form zymogen granules. Newly packed zymogen granules Z_1 are large and much less electron-dense than the smaller mature granules Z_2 which aggregate in the apical cytoplasm. Zymogen granules are released into the acinar lumen by exocytosis; small irregular microvilli associated with this process are seen projecting into the lumen. Note small capillaries **C**, a fibroblast **F** and collagen **Coll** in the fine supporting tissue which surrounds the acinus.

(c)

16. Urinary system

Introduction

The urinary system is the principal organ system responsible for water and electrolyte homeostasis. The maintenance of homeostasis requires that any input into a system is balanced by an equivalent output; the urinary system provides the mechanism by which excess water and electrolytes are eliminated from the body. A second major function of the urinary system is the excretion of many toxic metabolic waste products, particularly the nitrogenous compounds urea and creatinine; this function is intimately related to water and electrolyte elimination which provides an appropriate fluid vehicle. The end product of these processes is *urine*. Since all body fluids are maintained in dynamic equilibrium with one another via the circulatory system, any adjustment in the composition of the blood is reflected in complementary changes in the other fluid compartments of the body. Thus regulation of the osmotic concentration of blood plasma ensures the osmotic regulation of all other body fluids. This process which is primarily performed by the urinary system is called *osmoregulation*.

The functional units of the urinary system are long narrow tubes called *nephrons*, of which there are approximately one million in each human kidney. Nephrons perform the functions of osmoregulation and excretion by the following processes:

- Filtration of most small molecules from blood plasma to form a filtrate.
- Selective reabsorption of most of the water and some other molecules from the filtrate, leaving behind excess and waste materials to be excreted.
- Secretion of some excretory products directly from blood into the filtrate.

The kidney is also involved in two other homeostatic mechanisms which are mediated via hormones.

The *renin-angiotensin-aldosterone mechanism* contributes to the maintenance of normal blood pressure. The hormone *erythropoietin* stimulates erythrocyte production in bone marrow and hence contributes to the maintenance of the oxygen-carrying capacity of blood.

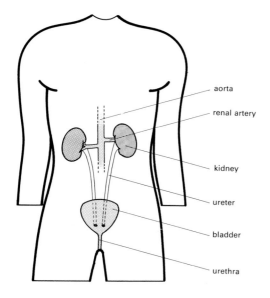

aorta

renal artery

kidney

ureter

bladder

urethra

Fig. 16.1 The urinary system

The urinary system comprises two *kidneys*, two *ureters*, a *bladder* and a *urethra*. Urine is produced in the kidneys and conducted by the ureters to the bladder where it is stored until voided via the urethra.

Blood is supplied to each kidney by *renal arteries* which arise from the aorta. One or more *renal veins* drains each kidney to the inferior vena cava. The total blood volume of the body is circulated through the kidneys about 300 times each day.

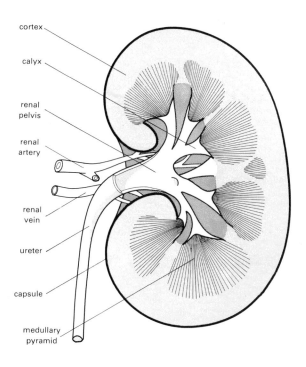

cortex

calyx

renal
pelvis

renal
artery

renal
vein

ureter

capsule

medullary
pyramid

Fig. 16.2 Kidney

The kidney is a bean-shaped organ lying in the upper retroperitoneal area and oriented with the hilum directed medially. The hilum is the site of entry and exit of the renal blood vessels and the ureter.

The archetypal kidney of lower mammals consists of a single lobe made up of a *medullary pyramid* (more accurately described as cone-shaped), the base of which is enveloped by a cortex containing the main bulk of the renal parenchyma. Nephrons arise in the cortex then loop down into the medulla for a variable distance returning again to the cortex. From here they drain into collecting ducts which descend again into the medulla to discharge urine from the apex of the medullary pyramid. The apical part of the pyramid is enveloped by a funnel-shaped *renal pelvis* which represents the dilated proximal part of the ureter; that part of the medullary pyramid surrounded by the pelvis is known as the *renal papilla*.

The human kidney is made up of multiple lobes, some 10–18 in all, its basic structure being outlined in this diagram. Each renal papilla is surrounded by an extension of the renal pelvis called a *calyx*, the whole urinary collecting system within the kidney being described as the *pelvicalyceal system*. The cortical components of the lobes fuse so that the outer zone of the convexity of the kidney forms the *renal cortex* which extends down between adjacent medullary pyramids. The *renal medulla* is made up of multiple medullary pyramids separated by medullary extensions of the cortex.

The kidney is invested by a tough fibrous capsule and usually surrounded by a thick layer of perinephric fat which provides some protection from trauma.

Fig. 16.3 Kidney *(H & E × 3)*

This micrograph of a kidney from a stillborn child illustrates the macroscopic features of the kidneys as described in Fig. 16.2. The kidney of a baby has been chosen as it is small enough to section and photograph as a whole. Furthermore its convex surface is irregular, reflecting the development of the many lobes making up the organ. In histological section, only a single plane through the pelvicalyceal system can be visualised; this plane of section includes the axis of three lobes, the papilla **P** of each one projecting into the central pelvicalyceal space; this drains into the ureter **U** which leaves the kidney via the hilum **H**.

The darker stained cortex **C** can be clearly differentiated from the paler stained medulla **M**. The cortex contains large numbers of tiny spheroidal structures, the developing renal corpuscles (see Fig. 16.4). The main feature of the medullary pyramids are numerous tubules converging towards the tips of the renal papillae. Note the continuity of the cortex throughout the outer zone of the kidney and the cortical extension between the two medullary pyramids at the top of the field. The fibrous capsule **Cp** of the kidney is continuous at the hilum with supporting tissue which packs the spaces between the hilar structures. In later life, the hilum often contains significant quantities of adipose tissue.

Cp

M

C

P

P

H

U

C

P

M

C

efferent arteriole

Bowman's capsule

Bowman's space

proximal convoluted tubule

pars recta

loop of Henle (thick limb)

loop of Henle (thin limb)

arcuate artery

interlobar artery

duct of Bellini

afferent arteriole

glomerulus

distal convoluted tubule

collecting tubule

collecting duct

cortical radial artery

cortico-medullary junction

CORTEX

MEDULLA

Fig. 16.4 Basic organisation of the nephron, collecting system and renal vasculature

The nephron and collecting system

The nephron, the functional unit of the kidney, consists of two major components, the *renal corpuscle* and the *renal tubule*.

Renal corpuscle. The renal corpuscle is responsible for the filtration of plasma and is a combination of two structures, Bowman's capsule and the glomerulus.

Bowman's capsule consists of a single layer of flattened cells resting on a basement membrane; it forms the distended, blind end of the renal tubule.

The *glomerulus* is a globular network of densely packed anastomosing capillaries which invaginates Bowman's capsule (see Fig. 16.8). Within the capsule, the glomerulus is invested by a layer of epithelial cells called *podocytes*, which constitute the *visceral layer of Bowman's capsule*; the visceral layer is reflected around the vascular stalk of the glomerulus to become continuous with the *parietal layer* which constitutes Bowman's capsule proper. The space between the visceral and parietal layers is known as *Bowman's space* and is continuous with the lumen of the renal tubule; the parietal epithelium of Bowman's capsule is continuous with the epithelium lining the renal tubule.

In the renal corpuscle, much of the water and small molecular weight constituents of plasma are filtered from the glomerular capillaries into Bowman's space, the *glomerular filtrate* then passing into the renal tubule. Thus the filtration barrier between the capillary lumen and Bowman's space consists of the capillary endothelium, the podocyte layer and their common basement membrane known as the *glomerular basement membrane* (see Fig. 16.12).

The afferent arteriole which supplies the glomerulus and the *efferent arteriole*, which drains the glomerulus, enter and leave the corpuscle at the *vascular pole* which is usually situated opposite the entrance to the renal tubule, the *urinary pole* (see Fig. 16.7).

Renal tubule. The renal tubule extends from Bowman's capsule to its junction with a *collecting duct*. The renal tubule is up to 55 mm long in humans and is lined by a single layer of epithelial cells. The primary function of the renal tubule is the selective reabsorption of water, inorganic ions and other molecules from the glomerular filtrate. In addition, some inorganic ions are secreted directly from blood into the lumen of the tubule. In humans, glomerular filtrate is produced at a steady rate of approximately 120 mL per minute; of this, all but about one mL is reabsorbed by the renal tubules. The renal tubule has a convoluted shape and has four distinct histo-physiological zones, each of which has a different role in tubular function.

1. *The proximal convoluted tubule (PCT)* is the longest, most convoluted section of the tubule and is responsible for the reabsorption of approximately 75% of the ions and water of the glomerular filtrate. PCTs are confined to the renal cortex and make up the greater part of its bulk. The last part of the PCT, the *pars recta*, is straight and descends towards the medulla before becoming the loop of Henle.

2. *The loop of Henle* arises from the PCT as a straight thin-walled tubule which descends from the cortex into the medulla as the *thin descending limb*; here it loops closely back upon itself as the *thin ascending limb*, abruptly becoming thicker-walled (the *thick ascending limb*) as it returns to the renal cortex. The length of the loop of Henle varies from short to long depending on the location of the renal corpuscle of the particular nephron. The corpuscles of short-looped nephrons tend to be located in the superficial and mid-cortical regions, the loops extending very little beyond the cortico-medullary junction. Long-looped nephrons are mainly associated with juxtamedullary corpuscles; a small proportion of long loops almost reach the tips of the renal papillae but successively greater numbers turn back at higher levels as necessitated by the tapering shape of the medullary pyramids. The limbs of the loop of Henle are closely associated with parallel wide capillary loops, the *vasa recta* (not shown in this diagram) which arise from the efferent arterioles of glomeruli located near the cortico-medullary junction. The vasa recta descend into the medulla then loop back on themselves to drain into veins at the junction of the medulla and cortex. The main function of the loops of Henle is to generate a high osmotic pressure in the extracellular fluid of the renal medulla; the mechanism by which this is achieved is known as the *counter-current multiplier system* (see Fig. 16.17). In some animals the loop of Henle plays a major role in reabsorption of water from the glomerular filtrate back into the circulation via the vasa recta; however this function is of lesser importance in the human kidney.

3. *The distal convoluted tubule (DCT)* is a continuation of the thick limb of the loop of Henle after its return from the medulla. Shorter and less convoluted than the PCT, the DCT is responsible for reabsorption of sodium ions by an active process which is controlled by the adrenocortical hormone *aldosterone*. Sodium reabsorption is coupled with the secretion of hydrogen or potassium ions into the DCT.

4. *The collecting tubule* is the straight terminal portion of the nephron, several collecting tubules converging to form a *collecting duct*. The collecting ducts descend through the cortex in parallel bundles called *medullary rays* (see Fig. 16.5) progressively merging in the medulla to form the large *ducts of Bellini* which open at the tips of the renal papillae to discharge urine into the pelvicalyceal system. The collecting tubules and ducts are not normally permeable to water; however in the presence of antidiuretic hormone (ADH) secreted by the posterior pituitary, the collecting tubules and ducts become permeable to water which is then drawn out by the high osmotic pressure generated by the counter current multiplier system into the interstitial tissues of the medulla; from here water is returned to the general circulation via the vasa recta. The loops of Henle and ADH thus provide a mechanism for the production of urine which is hypertonic with respect to plasma.

The nephron arises embryologically from the *nephrogenic blastema* and the collecting ducts from the *ureteral bud* and there is some question as to which the collecting tubules are derived from.

Renal vasculature

Each kidney is supplied by a single renal artery which divides in the hilum into two main branches. Each of these gives rise to several *interlobar arteries* which ascend between the pyramids to the cortico-medullary junction. Here they branch to form the *arcuate arteries* which run in an arc-like course parallel to the capsule of the kidney. The arcuate arteries give rise to numerous *cortical radial (interlobular) arteries* which radiate towards the capsule branching to form the afferent arterioles of the glomeruli.

As previously described, the vasa recta form a continuation of the efferent arterioles of juxtamedullary glomeruli and form the microcirculation of the renal medulla. The efferent arterioles of the rest of the cortex divide to form the plexus of capillaries that surround the tubules of the renal cortex. The cortical and medullary capillaries drain via *cortical radial (interlobular) veins* to *arcuate veins* at the cortico-medullary junction and thence to the *renal vein*.

Fig. 16.5 Kidney

(Monkey: Jones' methenamine silver/. H & E × 12)

The basic geography of the kidney can be seen in this unilobular kidney which has been sectioned through the axis of the medullary pyramid. Note the calyx **C** surrounding the renal papilla **RP** and converging via the pelvis **P** onto the ureter **U**.

In the cortex **Cx**, numerous renal corpuscles **RC** (200 μm in diameter) are just visible at this magnification. The corpuscles tend to be arranged in parallel rows at right angles to the capsule, separated by cortical radial arteries from which they derive their blood supply. Cortical radial arteries are too narrow to be identified at this magnification but a number of their accompanying thin walled cortical radial veins **V** are easily seen.

Most of the cortical parenchyma surrounding the renal corpuscles consists of proximal and distal convoluted tubules. From the cortex, pale stained *medullary rays* **MR** radiate towards the medulla; they consist of collecting ducts draining nephrons located high in the cortex. The collecting ducts merge to form the larger ducts of Bellini which converge towards the tip of the renal papilla. Although not visible at this magnification, long loops of Henle dip into the medulla between, and parallel with, the collecting tubules and ducts. The vasa recta, the long, straight vessels into which water is absorbed from the loops of Henle, collecting tubules and ducts, also dip down into the medulla alongside the loops of Henle; these vessels are also too small to be seen at this magnification.

The cortico-medullary junction is marked by several arcuate arteries **AA** and their associated thin-walled arcuate veins **AV**. Note a large interlobar branch of the renal artery **Ai** in the hilar supporting tissue.

Fig. 16.6 Renal cortex *(H & E × 40)*

Further magnification reveals more details of the cortical parenchyma. Renal corpuscles **RC** appear as dense rounded structures, the glomeruli, surrounded by narrow Bowman's spaces. Even at this magnification, it is evident that the tubules making up the bulk of the parenchyma between the renal corpuscles differ from one another in diameter, shape and staining intensity. The cortical tubules mainly consist of proximal convoluted tubules with smaller numbers of distal convoluted tubules and collecting tubules.

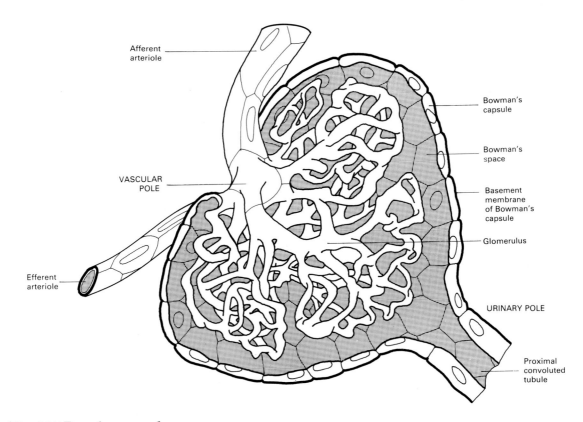

Fig. 16.7 Renal corpuscle

The main structural features of the renal corpuscle are demonstrated in this idealised diagram.

The relatively wide diameter afferent arteriole enters Bowman's capsule at the vascular pole of the renal corpuscle and then branches to form an anastomosing network of glomerular capillaries. The glomerulus is thus suspended in Bowman's space from the vascular pole. Although not shown in this diagram, the spaces between the capillary loops in each glomerular lobule are filled by specialised supporting tissue called *mesangium* extending into the glomerulus through the vascular pole. If the capillary loops are likened to the coils of the small bowel lying in the abdominal cavity, then the mesangium forms the equivalent of the mesenteries.

The efferent vessel which drains the glomerulus is unusual in that it has the structure of an arteriole and is thus called the efferent arteriole (rather than the efferent venule). The efferent arteriole is of smaller diameter than the afferent arteriole and a pressure gradient is thus maintained which drives the filtration of plasma into Bowman's space.

The layer of podocytes which invests the glomerular capillaries (visceral layer of Bowman's capsule) is not represented in this diagram. At the vascular pole, the podocyte layer is reflected to become continuous with the epithelium of Bowman's capsule proper which in turn becomes continuous with the first part of the renal tubule, the proximal convoluted tubule.

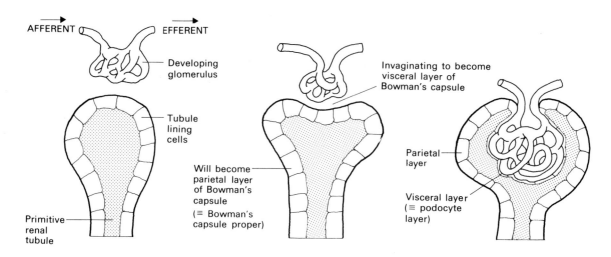

Fig. 16.8 Development of the renal corpuscle

This diagram illustrates in a highly schematic manner the mode of development of the renal corpuscle. The nephrons develop from the embryological *metanephros* as blind-ended tubules consisting of a single layer of cuboidal epithelium. The ends of the tubules dilate and become invaginated by a tiny mass of mesodermal tissue which differentiates to form the glomerulus. The layer of invaginated epithelium flattens and differentiates into podocytes which become closely applied to the surface of the knot of glomerular capillaries. The intervening tissue disappears so that the basement membrane of glomerular endothelial cells and podocytes

effectively fuse forming the glomerular basement membrane. A small amount of tissue nevertheless remains to support the capillary loops and differentiates to form the mesangium. Where the mesangium stretches between the capillary loops, its surface is invested by podocyte cytoplasm with podocyte basement membrane lying between the two. When examining ultra-thin light microscope specimens (e.g. Fig. 16.12) and electron micrographs (e.g. Fig. 16.15), the podocytes, endothelial cells and mesangium are identified most easily by tracing out the podocyte and endothelial cell basement membranes.

Fig. 16.9 Renal corpuscle *(H & E × 320)*

This renal corpuscle has been sectioned through the vascular pole and shows the afferent arteriole **Aa** cut transversely and the efferent arteriole **Ae** cut longitudinally. Glomerular capillaries are cut in transverse, longitudinal and oblique section but little detail can be resolved in such preparations. The numerous nuclei in the glomerulus are those of capillary endothelial cells, *mesangial cells* and podocytes.

Note the flattened nuclei of the squamous cells **S** lining Bowman's capsule. Due to shrinkage of the glomerulus which is inevitable in this type of tissue preparation, Bowman's space **BS** appears artefactually enlarged.

Fig. 16.10 Renal basement membranes

(Methenamine silver × 100)

This preparation employs a method which has strong affinity for basement membranes. Three renal corpuscles are seen, the two in midfield sectioned through the vascular pole. The basement membrane of Bowman's capsule **BC** is particularly well demarcated and is continuous at the vascular pole with the basement membranes within the glomeruli **G**. The basement membranes of surrounding renal tubules **T** are also stained as well as the endothelial basement membrane of a cortical radial artery **A**. Glomerular basement membranes are often damaged by disease processes and this technique is commonly employed in diagnostic histopathology.

Fig. 16.11 Blood supply of the glomerulus

(Carmine-gelatine perfused × 128)

This section is from a kidney which has been perfused with a red dye in order to demonstrate the renal blood supply; the nephrons remain unstained.

An interlobular artery **IA** can be seen branching to form the afferent arteriole **AA** of a glomerulus **G**. The efferent arteriole **EA** leaving the glomerulus is of much smaller diameter than the afferent arteriole, an arrangement which maintains pressure within glomerular capillaries necessary for blood plasma to be filtered into Bowman's space **BS**. Blood pressure within the glomerulus is controlled by variation of the diameter of the afferent and efferent arterioles.

In the superficial and mid-cortex as shown here, efferent arterioles gives rise to a network of capillaries which surround the renal tubules **RT**; towards the medulla, efferent arterioles give rise to the vasa recta. Molecules reabsorbed from glomerular filtrate are returned to the general circulation via this capillary network which drains into the renal venous system.

(a)

(b)

Fig. 16.12 Glomerulus *(a) Thin section, toluidine blue × 1200 (b) Explanatory diagram*

Using resin-embedding techniques it is possible to cut thin sections (approximately 0.5–1.0 µm thick) which permit much greater resolution at high magnification.

In this preparation, the glomerular capillaries **C**, some of which contain erythrocytes, are defined by the prominent glomerular basement membranes **BM**. Occasional capillary endothelial cell nuclei **E** are seen bulging into the capillary lumina. Mesangium, which consists of *mesangial cells* **M** and densely stained extracellular substance called *mesangial matrix* **MM**, provides support for the capillary loops particularly at their branching points. Mesangial cells contain contractile proteins suggesting a myoid origin, but also exhibit phagocytic properties. The mesangial matrix appears to resemble basement membrane in composition.

The surfaces of the glomerular capillary loops exposed to Bowman's space **BS** are invested by a continuous layer of podocytes **P** which have extensive branching pale stained cytoplasm and large round pale stained nuclei. Bowman's space is much less prominent in this type of preparation in which little glomerular shrinkage occurs. Note the nuclei of two squamous cells of Bowman's capsule **BC**, the outline of which may be traced by its prominent basement membrane.

Fig. 16.13 The glomerular filter

During filtration of plasma from glomerular capillaries into the renal tubule, the filtrate passes through three layers: the capillary endothelium, glomerular basement membrane and podocyte layer. All contribute to the filtration process.

- The capillary endothelium contains numerous large round fenestrations (50–100 nm in diameter) which occupy about 20% of the endothelial surface area. In adults the fenestrations do not exhibit diaphragms as in fenestrated capillaries elsewhere in the body (see Fig. 8.14). Another unusual feature is that the luminal surface of the endothelium has been shown to have a cell coat which exhibits a negative electric charge.
- The glomerular basement membrane (240–340 nm) is much thicker than other basement membranes and appears to be elaborated by both capillary endothelial cells and podocytes. As with basement membranes elsewhere (see Ch. 4), it consists of a feltwork of type IV collagen, structural glycoproteins (fibronectin and laminin) and proteoglycans rich in heparan sulfate, the interstices of this highly cross-linked structure being occupied by water molecules. By electron microscopy, the glomerular basement membrane consists of three layers, a *lamina rara interna* adjacent to the endothelium, central *lamina densa* and *lamina rara externa* in contact with the podocyte layer, although this layered appearance is difficult to discern in human adults. Both laminae rarae are negatively charged.
- The podocytes have long cytoplasmic extensions called *primary processes* which embrace the capillaries, giving rise to short *secondary foot processes (pedicels)* which interdigitate with those of other primary processes. The secondary foot processes are directly applied to the basement membrane and bound to it by fine filaments. The gaps between adjacent secondary foot processes, known as *filtration slits*, are of uniform width (25 nm) and bridged by a delicate electron-dense diaphragm 4 nm thick. A thick glycocalyx invests the outer surface of the podocytes including the filtration slits and exhibits a strong negative electric charge. Ultrastructural features of the podocyte cytoplasm suggest phagocytic and secretory functions.

As mentioned at the outset, all layers contribute to the selective filtration process. Clinical evidence demonstrates that free haemoglobin (mol. wt. 65 000) and smaller molecules pass through the glomerular filter whereas albumin (mol. wt. 68 000) and larger molecules are retained.

For macromolecules, three factors determine permeability, namely electrical charge, size and configuration. Negatively charged (cationic) molecules are blocked by the electronegative endothelial cell coat and laminae rarae of the basement membrane whilst the meshwork of the lamina densa of the basement membrane discriminates on the basis of molecular size and configuration. The filtration slit diaphragm restricts the passage of any large molecules but its main role is in controlling water flow which is also held back by the colloidal osmotic pressure of retained albumin and other large molecules. The phagocytic function of the podocytes is to remove any large molecules which become trapped in the outer layers of the filter. Molecules trapped on the endothelial side are phagocytosed by mesangial cells whilst their contractility appears to be involved in regulating blood flow within the glomerular capillaries.

(a)

(b)

Fig. 16.14 Glomerulus

(Scanning EM (a) ×1500 (b) ×6000)

Scanning electron microscopy readily
demonstrates the three-dimensional
relationships of podocytes and their
processes which extend like octopus
tentacles over the whole surface of the
glomerulus.

Micrograph (a) shows part of a
glomerular capillary tuft. The
capillaries are enveloped by podocytes
which have large flattened cell bodies
and bulging nuclei **N**. Each podocyte
has several long primary processes P_1
which embrace one or more capillaries.
Each primary process has numerous
secondary foot processes.

With further magnification in
micrograph (b), the secondary foot
processes P_2 can be seen as extensions
of the large primary processes P_1. The
secondary foot processes interdigitate
with those of other primary processes
separated by filtration slits of uniform
width.

(a)

(b)

Fig. 16.15 Glomerulus *(illustration (a) opposite)*

(EM (a) × 4800 (b) × 14 000 (c) × 30 000)

Micrograph (a) shows several capillary loops **C** recognised by their content of erythrocytes and precipitated plasma proteins; the capillaries are lined by a thin layer of fenestrated endothelial cytoplasm and endothelial cell nuclei **E** can be seen bulging into the capillary lumina; capillary endothelial fenestrations **F** are better seen at higher magnification in micrograph (c). A branched mesangial stalk comprising mesangial cells **M** and dense mesangial matrix **MM** provides support for the capillary loops. The nuclei of several podocytes **P** can be seen, their primary processes P_1 giving rise to numerous secondary foot processes P_2 which rest on the glomerular basement membrane **BM**. At the right midfield, the mesangial stalk is exposed to Bowman's space as it traverses the space between two capillary loops; in this situation it is invested by a continuous layer of podocytic cytoplasm devoid of secondary foot processes and filtration slits. Note the continuity of the glomerular basement membrane and mesangial matrix where the mesangium comes into contact with a capillary loop. Part of Bowman's capsule **BC** is seen at the periphery consisting of a squamous epithelial cell and underlying basement membrane. Note the labyrinth of Bowman's space **BS** which pervades the glomerulus.

Micrograph (b), shows three glomerular capillaries **C** lined by attenuated endothelial cytoplasm **E** with wide fenestrations **F**. A podocyte **P** extends several primary foot processes P_1 onto the capillaries, these in turn giving rise to multiple secondary foot processes P_2 separated by filtration slits **FS**. A common basement membrane **BM** separates the podocytes and capillary endothelium; the thickness of the basement membrane appears to increase from one point to another; however, this is a product of some obliquity of the plane of section and the basement membranes are in fact of uniform width.

With further magnification in micrograph (c), the three components of the glomerular filter are seen. The fenestrated capillary endothelium **E** is closely applied to the luminal surface of the glomerular basement membrane **BM**; on the opposite side are podocyte secondary foot processes P_2, separated by filtration slits of approximately uniform width and bridged by fine electron-dense diaphragms. The basement membrane does not exhibit laminae rarae since this specimen is from an adult.

(c)

(a)

(b)

Fig. 16.16 Proximal convoluted tubule

(a) Azan × 480 (b) PAS/Haematoxylin × 800
(c) EM × 600 (opposite above), (d) EM × 8500 (opposite below)

The proximal convoluted tubule (PCT) is the longest part of the renal tubule and sections of PCT thus dominate the parenchyma of the renal cortex.

Approximately 75% of the glomerular filtrate is reabsorbed from the PCT, this function being reflected in the structure of the epithelial lining.

Micrograph (a) shows a proximal convoluted tubule **PCT** arising from a renal corpuscle; convolutions of the PCT are also seen in longitudinal, oblique and transverse section. The simple tall cuboidal epithelium has a prominent blue stained brush border of tall microvilli which almost completely fill the lumen. This increases the surface area of plasma membrane some 30–40-fold. The cytoplasm of PCT epithelial cells stains intensely due to a high content of organelles, principally mitochondria. The basement membrane of the tubules stains blue with this staining method as do the glomerular basement membranes and that of Bowman's capsule.

The PAS staining method has been used in micrograph (b) to demonstrate the prominent brush border **BB** projecting into the lumen of the PCT. The brush border is PAS-positive since the surfaces of the microvilli are coated with a particularly dense glycocalyx (see Fig. 1.2) which is thought to afford physical and chemical protection to the microvilli. Like those elsewhere, the basement membrane **BM** supporting the tubular epithelium is strongly PAS-positive due to its condensed ground substance. In both micrographs, note the round nuclei with prominent nucleoli.

A rich network of capillaries **C** arising from the efferent arteriole of the glomerulus (see Fig. 16.11) surrounds the proximal tubules and returns molecules reabsorbed from the glomerular filtrate back into the general circulation.

In micrograph (c), electron microscopy of the proximal tubule reveals profuse tall microvilli **Mv** constituting the brush border seen with light microscopy. The plasma membrane of the microvilli contains a variety of transport proteins and enzymes involved in selective reabsorption of solutes from the glomerular filtrate. The cytoplasm immediately beneath the brush border contains many pinocytotic vesicles **V** and lysosomes **L** which are involved in reabsorption and degradation of small amounts of protein which have leaked through the glomerular ultrafilter. Reabsorbed solutes are transported into surrounding capillaries **Cap**.

The basal plasma membranes of PCTs exhibit deep infoldings which are closely related to columns of elongated mitochondria **M** which supply ATP for active transport processes. This mitochondrial arrangement may give rise to the appearance of basal striations in light microscopy. The basal infoldings of the plasma membrane increase the surface area for transport of reabsorbed molecules from PCT cells into the extracellular fluid and thence into capillaries. Complex lateral interdigitations make the boundaries between adjacent cells difficult to define although junctional complexes **J** can be identified towards the luminal surface.

Micrograph (d) shows at high magnification the basal infoldings of the plasma membrane **P** separated by columns of cytoplasm containing elongated mitochondria **M**. Note the basement membrane **BM** of the tubule lining cell. In very close proximity is a peritubular capillary **Cap** with attenuated endothelium **E** resting on a very thin basement membrane **BM$_E$**; note the narrow intervening supporting tissue layer **S**.

(c)

(d)

(a)   *(b)*

Fig. 16.17 Loop of Henle *(H & E (a) TS × 198 (b) LS × 100)*

The loop of Henle is a continuation of the PCT and constitutes the second histo-physiological zone of the renal tubule (see Fig. 16.4). Each loop of Henle arises in the renal cortex, dips down for a variable distance into the medulla as the *descending limb*, then returns to the cortex as the *ascending limb* before becoming continuous with the distal convoluted tubule. Most of the loop of Henle is very thin-walled but the wall of the ascending limb becomes abruptly thick-walled during its ascent. From a functional viewpoint, the thick ascending limb should be considered as the first part of the distal convoluted tubule. Thus loops of Henle are best seen in sections of renal medulla. In addition to loops of Henle, the medulla also contains the vasa recta, collecting tubules and collecting ducts. All these structures are seen in these micrographs and may be distinguished by the following features.

The thin limbs **T** have a simple squamous epithelium but may be differentiated from the vasa recta **V** by the absence of erythrocytes and their regular rounded shape in transverse section. The thick ascending limbs **A** are lined by low cuboidal epithelium and are also round in cross-section. Neither thick or thin limbs of the loop of Henle have a brush border. Collecting tubules **CT** have a similar epithelial lining to the ascending limbs but are wider and less regular in shape. The collecting ducts **CD** are easily recognised by their large diameter and pale stained columnar epithelial lining.

The function of the loop of Henle is to produce an increasing osmotic gradient from the cortex to the tip of the renal papilla by the *countercurrent multiplier mechanism*. In brief, this involves the active transport of sodium and chloride ions into the medullary interstitium by the ascending thin limb which is impermeable to water. The thin descending limb which contains water and ions from the PCT at a lower osmotic concentration, is readily permeable so that sodium and chloride ions are drawn back into the tubular fluid. As this fluid passes distally into the ascending limb, the sodium and chloride ions are once more pumped out into the interstitium, thus multiplying the effect and creating an osmotic gradient in the interstitium which increases from cortico-medullary junction to tip of papilla. The fluid reaching the thick limb of the loop of Henle is hypotonic. The high osmotic pressure in medullary extracellular fluid provides the mechanism by which urine later undergoes concentration in the collecting tubules and ducts under the influence of ADH (see Fig. 16.20). The vasa recta take up water from the medullary interstitium and return it to the general circulation.

The interstitium of the inner medulla in some species contains unusual cells called *lipid laden interstitial cells* arranged at right angles to the tubules and vasa recta and bound tightly to one another so as to subdivide the interstitium into numerous compartments from deep to more superficial layers; they may thus act as diffusion barriers facilitating the maintenance of the osmotic gradient described above.

Fig. 16.18 Distal convoluted tubule *(a) Azan × 320 (b) PAS/Haematoxylin × 480 (c) EM × 3000*

The distal convoluted tubule (DCT) is a continuation of the thick ascending limb of the loop of Henle after its return to the cortex and forms the third histo-physiological zone of the renal tubule. DCTs are thus found within the cortex among the proximal convoluted tubules.

The DCT is mainly involved in reabsorption of sodium ions from the tubular fluid. The process is directly coupled to the secretion of hydrogen and potassium ions into the tubular fluid, one hydrogen ion or one potassium ion being secreted for every one sodium ion reabsorbed; in this way the DCT plays an important role in acid-base balance. This process is controlled by the hormone *aldosterone* secreted by the adrenal cortex.

As seen in micrograph (a), distal convoluted tubules **DCT** may be differentiated from proximal convoluted tubules **PCT** by the absence of a brush border, a larger more clearly defined lumen, more nuclei per cross-section (since DCT cells are smaller than PCT cells) and less affinity for cytoplasmic stains (due to a smaller content of organelles). In addition, sections of DCT are much less numerous than

sections of PCT since the DCT is a much shorter segment of the renal tubule than the PCT.

Micrograph (b) differentiates between proximal and distal convoluted tubules on the basis of the presence or absence of a brush border. The PCT has a profuse PAS-positive brush border (see Fig. 15.16) which is absent from the DCT.

The distal convoluted tubule has many ultrastructural features in common with the proximal convoluted tubule, in particular the lateral cell interdigitations, a large number of mitochondria **M** and infolding of the basal plasma membrane. The most striking difference is that the DCT lacks a brush border, having only a few irregular microvilli **Mv** at the luminal surface. The DCT cells have less cytoplasm than those of the PCT although the nucleus is of about the same size and consequently occupies much more of the cell. The nuclei of the DCT cells lie close to the luminal surface and tend to bulge into the lumen; the overlying cytoplasm is devoid of mitochondria but contains large numbers of tiny vesicles.

(a)

afferent arteriole

distal convoluted tubule

lacis cells

macula densa

juxtaglomerular cell

efferent arteriole

Bowman's capsule

Bowman's space

glomerulus

proximal convoluted tubule

(b)

Fig. 16.19 Juxtaglomerular apparatus

(a) Azan × 640 (opposite above) (b) Explanatory diagram (opposite below) (c) Blood pressure control system (below left)

The juxtaglomerular apparatus (JGA) is a specialisation of the glomerular afferent arteriole **AA** and the distal convoluted tubule **DCT** of the corresponding nephron and is involved in the regulation of systemic blood pressure via the *renin-angiotensin-aldosterone mechanism*.

The juxtaglomerular apparatus is made up of three components, the *macula densa* of the DCT, renin-secreting *juxtaglomerular cells* of the afferent arteriole and *extraglomerular mesangial cells*.

Macula densa. On returning to the cortex from the renal medulla, the ascending thick limb of the loop of Henle becomes the first part of the distal convoluted tubule and comes to lie in the angle between the afferent and efferent arterioles at the vascular pole of the glomerulus. The macula densa **MD** is an area of closely packed, specialised cells lining the DCT where it abuts onto the glomerular vascular pole. Compared with other DCT lining cells, the cells of the macula densa are taller and have larger more prominent nuclei which are situated towards the luminal surface, the basal cytoplasm being crammed with mitochondria. The basement membrane between the macula and underlying cells is extremely thin.

The cells of the macula densa are thought to be sensitive to the concentration of sodium ions in the fluid within the DCT; a decrease in systemic blood pressure results in decreased production of glomerular filtrate and hence decreased concentration of sodium ions in the distal tubular fluid.

Juxtaglomerular cells. Juxtaglomerular cells **J** are specialised smooth muscle cells of the wall of the afferent arteriole forming a cluster around it just before it enters the glomerulus. Juxtaglomerular cell cytoplasm contains immature and mature membrane-bound granules of the enzyme *renin*.

Extraglomerular mesangial cells. Also called *Goormaghtigh cells* or *lacis cells* **L**, these cells form a conical mass, the apex of which is continuous with the mesangium of the glomerulus; laterally it is bounded by the afferent and efferent arterioles and its base abuts onto the macula densa. The lacis cells are flat and elongated with extensive fine cytoplasmic processes extending from their ends and surrounded by a network ('lacis') of mesangial material. Despite their central location in the JGA, the function of the extraglomerular mesangial cells remains obscure. They have previously been attributed the function of secretion of the hormone erythropoietin which stimulates red cell production in the bone marrow.

Role of the JGA in control of blood pressure

The juxtaglomerular apparatus is believed to act both as a baroreceptor and chemoreceptor controlling systemic blood pressure by the secretion of renin by the juxtaglomerular cells.

The juxtaglomerular cells are suitably placed to monitor systemic blood pressure, with a fall in blood pressure resulting in renin secretion. Reduction in blood pressure results in reduced glomerular filtration and consequently a lower concentration of sodium ions in the DCT. Acting as chemoreceptors, the cells of the macula densa in some way then promote renin secretion.

Renin diffuses into the bloodstream catalysing the conversion of *angiotensinogen*, an alpha2-globulin synthesised by the liver, into the decapeptide *angiotensin I*. In the lungs, *angiotensin converting enzyme*, cleaves two amino acids from angiotensin I to form *angiotensin II* which is a potent vasoconstrictor.

Angiotensin II raises blood pressure in two ways: constriction of peripheral blood vessels and release of aldosterone from the adrenal cortex. Aldosterone promotes the reabsorption of sodium ions and therefore water from the DCT, thus expanding the plasma volume and hence increasing blood pressure.

(c)

(a)   *(b)*

Fig. 16.20 Collecting tubules and ducts *(Azan (a)* ×750 *(b)* ×480)

The collecting tubule is a continuation of the distal convoluted tubule and is generally considered to be the fourth histo-physiological zone of the nephron. Several collecting tubules merge to form a collecting duct. The collecting ducts descend in the medullary rays (see Fig. 16.5) towards the renal medulla where they progressively merge to form the large ducts of Bellini which drain urine from the tip of the renal papilla into the pelvicalyceal system.

The collecting tubules and ducts concentrate urine by passive reabsorption of water into the medullary interstitium following the osmotic gradient created by the countercurrent multiplier system of the loops of Henle (see Fig. 16.17). The vasa recta return this water to the general circulation. The process is known as the *countercurrent exchange system* and is controlled by antidiuretic hormone (ADH) secreted by the posterior pituitary in response to dehydration. ADH acts by increasing the permeability to water of the collecting tubule and ducts resulting in retention of water by the body and the production of hypertonic urine. Conversely, ADH secretion is inhibited by water overloading and an increased volume of hypotonic urine is thus produced.

The collecting tubules are lined by a simple cuboidal epithelium which becomes increasingly tall distally so as to become columnar in the collecting ducts. The predominant cell type in the collecting tubules and ducts tends to be poorly stained (often described as *clear cells*) with fine cytoplasmic organelles and a smooth luminal surface. Scattered among the clear cells are strongly stained *intercalated cells* crammed with mitochondria and with a microvillous surface; the number of intercalated cells is greatest in the proximal part of the collecting tubules, diminishing distally with few in the collecting ducts.

Micrograph (a) illustrates two collecting tubules in the renal cortex, the tubule on the left being more proximal and the tubule on the right more distal as shown by the flatter cuboidal lining of the former. The majority of the lining cells are relatively poorly stained with a small number of dark intercalated cells **IC** (with microvillous surface) scattered among them. Note the blue stained tubular basement membranes **BM** and narrow intervening supporting tissue **S** mainly occupied by capillaries.

Micrograph (b) is from the renal medulla and illustrates two collecting ducts **CD** surrounded by thin loops of Henle and vasa recta which cannot be readily distinguished from one another. Collecting ducts are characterised by tall columnar epithelium, well defined cellular outlines, pale stained cytoplasm and the absence of a brush border. In contrast to the clear cells of the collecting tubules, the main collecting duct cells have a single central cilium (not visible at this magnification).

Fig. 16.21 Renal medulla *(Rat: EM × 4000)*

This micrograph from the outer medulla illustrates the
ultrastructural features of a collecting tubule **CT**, thin loops
of Henle **H** and vasa recta **V**.

The collecting tubules consist of simple cuboidal cells
with relatively sparse organelles. The cells of the thin limbs
of loops of Henle are similar to capillary endothelial cells in
structure, most of the wall consisting of a thin irregular layer
of cytoplasm with a few very short luminal microvilli and the

nucleus bulging into the lumen; the epithelium is supported
by a thin basement membrane **BM**. The vasa recta can only
be readily distinguished from the thin limbs by their content
of erythrocytes, occasional leucocytes **L** and precipitated
plasma proteins.

Between vasa recta and nephrons is delicate interstitial
supporting tissue **S** containing a little collagen, scattered
fibroblasts **F** and their slender cytoplasmic processes.

Fig. 16.22 Renal papilla

(Monkey: Azan × 30)

The renal papilla forms the apex of the medullary pyramid where it projects into the pelvicalyceal space **PCS**. Ducts of Bellini **DB**, the largest of the collecting ducts, converge to drain urine through a number of holes (*cribriform area*) at the tip of the papilla. Between the ducts are the longest loops of Henle and vasa recta, not visible at this magnification.

The pelvicalyceal system represents the proximal end of the ureter **U** and as such is lined by typical urinary (transitional) epithelium **E**. The wall of the pelvis contains smooth muscle **SM** which is continuous with that of the ureter.

Fig. 16.23 Ureter

(Masson's trichrome × 18)

The ureters are muscular tubes which conduct urine from the kidneys to the bladder. Urine is conducted from the pelvicalyceal system as a bolus which is propelled by peristaltic action of the ureteric wall. The wall of the ureter contains two layers of smooth muscle arranged as an inner elongated spiral but traditionally known as the longitudinal layer **L** and an outer tight spiral traditionally described as the circular layer **C**. Another outer longitudinal layer is present in the lower third of the ureter.

The lumen of the ureter is lined by transitional epithelium which is thrown up into folds in the relaxed state allowing the ureter to dilate during the passage of a bolus of urine. Beneath the epithelium is a broad collagenous lamina propria **LP**, the collagen fibres of which are stained greenish-blue in this preparation. Surrounding the muscular wall is a loose collagenous adventitia **A** containing blood vessels **V**, lymphatics and nerves.

Fig. 16.24 Bladder

(Masson's trichrome × 12)

The general structure of the bladder wall resembles that of the lower third of the ureters. The wall of the bladder consists of three loosely arranged layers of smooth muscle and elastic fibres which contract during micturition. Note the inner longitudinal **IL**, outer circular **OC** and outermost longitudinal **OL** layers of smooth muscle. The transitional epithelium lining the bladder is thrown into many folds in the relaxed state. The outer adventitial coat **A** contains arteries, veins and lymphatics.

The urethra, the final conducting portion of the urinary tract, is discussed as part of the male reproductive tract in Chapter 18.

Fig. 16.25 Urinary epithelium *(H & E × 480)*

Transitional epithelium, also called urinary epithelium or urothelium, is found only within the conducting passages of the urinary system for which it is especially adapted. The epithelium is stratified comprising three to six layers of cells, the number of layers being greatest when the epithelium is least distended at the time of fixation. The specimen shown here is typical and is taken from a non-distended bladder.

The cells of the basal layer are compact and cuboidal or columnar in form, those of the intermediate layers are more polygonal whilst the surface cells are tall columnar with large round nuclei with prominent nucleoli; some surface cells are binucleate. The surface outline has a characteristic scalloped appearance and the superficial cytoplasm is fuzzy, indistinct and more intensely stained than the rest of the cytoplasm.

Ultrastructural studies have revealed that much of the surface plasma membrane consists of thickened inflexible *plaques* with narrow zones of normal membrane between acting as 'hinges', allowing sections of the membrane to fold inwards somewhat like a concertina, forming deep clefts and stacks of flattened *fusiform vesicles*. This structure renders the urinary epithelium impermeable to urine which is potentially toxic. The permeability barrier also prevents water from being drawn through the epithelium into hypertonic urine.

Urinary epithelium rests on a basement membrane which is often too thin to be resolved by light microscopy and was formerly thought to be absent. The basal layer is irregular and may be deeply indented by strands of underlying lamina propria **LP** containing capillaries. This unusual feature led early histologists to believe, mistakenly, that urinary epithelium contradicted the principle that epithelium never contains blood vessels.

17. The endocrine glands

Introduction

Endocrine glands are responsible for the synthesis and secretion of chemical messengers known as *hormones* which are disseminated throughout the body by the bloodstream where they act on specific *target organs*. In conjunction with the nervous system, hormones coordinate and integrate the functions of all the physiological systems.

As a general rule, endocrine glands are composed of islands of secretory cells of epithelial origin with intervening supporting tissue which is rich in blood and lymphatic capillaries. The secretory cells discharge their hormone product into the interstitial spaces from which they are rapidly absorbed into the circulatory system. Unlike exocrine glands (see Ch. 5), endocrine glands have no duct system and are therefore sometimes called the *ductless glands*.

Reflecting their active synthetic function, endocrine secretory cells are usually characterised by prominent nuclei and prolific cytoplasmic organelles especially mitochondria, endoplasmic reticulum, Golgi bodies and secretory vesicles.

Some endocrine glands exist in the form of discrete organs, e.g. pituitary, thyroid, parathyroid and adrenal glands. Other endocrine tissues are found in association with exocrine glands, e.g. pancreas, or within complex organs, e.g. kidney, testis, ovary, placenta, brain and the gastrointestinal tract. This chapter deals with the pituitary, thyroid, parathyroid, adrenal, endocrine pancreas, pineal and the gastrointestinal and respiratory endocrine systems; other endocrine tissues are discussed with the organs with which they are associated.

Pituitary gland

The *pituitary gland*, also known as the *hypophysis*, is a specialised appendage of the brain which secretes a variety of hormones. The hormones mediate non-neural mechanisms by which the central nervous system integrates and controls many body functions. The pituitary hormones fall into two functional groups:

- Hormones which act directly on non-endocrine tissues: growth hormone (GH), prolactin, antidiuretic hormone (ADH), oxytocin and melanocyte stimulating hormone (MSH).
- Hormones which modulate the secretory activity of other endocrine glands (*tropic hormones*): thyroid stimulating hormone (TSH), adrenocorticotrophic hormone (ACTH) and the gonadotrophic hormones, follicle stimulating hormone (FSH) and luteinising hormone (LH).

Thus the thyroid gland, adrenal cortex and gonads may be described as *pituitary-dependent endocrine glands*.

The secretion of all pituitary hormones is directly controlled by the hypothalamus which is under the influence of nervous stimuli from higher centres in the CNS and controlled by feedback from the levels of circulating hormones produced by the pituitary-dependent glands. Thus the pituitary gland plays a central role in integrating the nervous and endocrine systems.

The pituitary gland is a small, slightly elongated organ, approximately 1 cm in diameter, lying immediately beneath the third ventricle in a bony cavity in the base of the skull. The gland is divided into anterior and posterior parts having entirely different embryological origins, functions and control mechanisms.

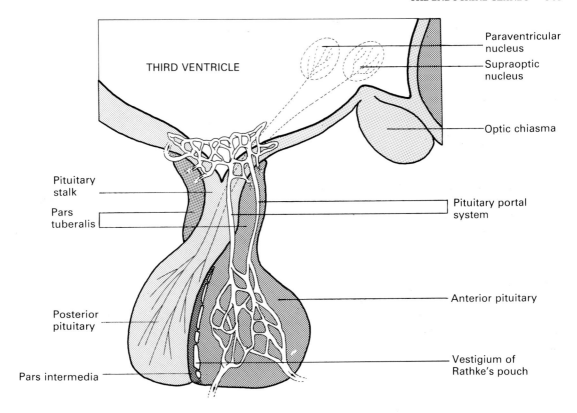

Paraventricular nucleus

Supraoptic nucleus

THIRD VENTRICLE

Optic chiasma

Pituitary stalk

Pars tuberalis

Pituitary portal system

Posterior pituitary

Anterior pituitary

Vestigium of Rathke's pouch

Pars intermedia

Fig. 17.1 Pituitary gland

The anterior and posterior parts of the pituitary originate from different embryological sources and this is reflected in their structure and function.

- **The posterior pituitary**, also called the *neurohypophysis* or *pars nervosa*, is derived from a downgrowth of nervous tissue from the hypothalamus to which it remains joined by the *pituitary stalk*.
- **The anterior pituitary** arises as an epithelial upgrowth from the roof of the primitive oral cavity, known as *Rathke's pouch*. This specialised glandular epithelium is wrapped around the anterior aspect of the posterior pituitary and is often called the *adenohypophysis*. The adenohypophysis may contain a cleft or group of cyst-like spaces which represent the vestigial lumen of Rathke's pouch. This vestigial cleft divides the major part of the anterior pituitary from a thin zone of tissue lying against the posterior pituitary and known as the *pars intermedia*. An extension of the adenohypophysis surrounds the neural stalk and is known as the *pars tuberalis*.

The type and mode of secretion of the posterior pituitary differs greatly from that of the anterior pituitary. The posterior pituitary secretes two hormones, *antidiuretic hormone* (ADH), also called *vasopressin*, and the hormone *oxytocin* both of which act directly on non-endocrine tissues. ADH is synthesised in the neurone cell bodies of the *supraoptic nucleus*, and oxytocin is synthesised in those of the *paraventricular nucleus* of the hypothalamus. Bound to glycoproteins, the hormones pass down the axons of the hypothalamo-pituitary tract through the pituitary stalk to the posterior pituitary where they are stored in the distended terminal parts of the axons. Release of posterior pituitary hormones is controlled directly by nervous impulses passing down the axons from the hypothalamus; this process is known as *neurosecretion*.

The anterior pituitary has the typical structure of epithelial-derived endocrine glands elsewhere in the body. It secretes both trophic and direct action hormones:

- *Trophic hormones*: thyroid stimulating hormone (TSH), adrenocorticotrophic hormone (ACTH), and the gonadotrophic hormones, follicle stimulating hormone (FSH) and luteinising hormone (LH).
- *Direct action hormones*: growth hormone (GH) and prolactin. (Recent evidence suggests that prolactin has a trophic action on the endocrine tissues of the ovary in some animals.)

Hypothalamic control of anterior pituitary secretion is mediated by specific hypothalamic releasing hormones, e.g. *thyroid stimulating hormone releasing hormone* (TSHRH); an exception to this is prolactin secretion which is under the inhibitory control of *dopamine*. These releasing hormones are conducted from the *median hypothalamic eminence* to the anterior pituitary by a unique system of *portal veins*.

The pars intermedia synthesises and secretes melanocyte-stimulating hormone (MSH); in humans, the pars intermedia is rudimentary and the physiological importance of MSH and the control of its secretion is poorly understood.

Fig. 17.2 Pituitary gland
(Monkey: H & E × 12)

This micrograph from a mid-line section through the brain and cranial floor illustrates the pituitary gland in situ. The pituitary is almost completely enclosed in a bony depression in the sphenoid bone, called the *sella turcica*. The two major components of the gland, the anterior pituitary **AP** and the posterior pituitary **PP**, are easily seen at this magnification. The posterior pituitary is connected to the hypothalamus **H** by the pituitary stalk **S** and like the hypothalamus is composed of nervous tissue. Note the close proximity of the third ventricle **V** above the hypothalamus and the relationship of the optic chiasma **O** which lies anteriorly.

Fig. 17.3 Anterior pituitary *(illustrations opposite: (a) H & E × 480 (b) Modified Azan × 480 (c) EM × 4270)*

The secretory cells of the anterior pituitary have been traditionally classified into two groups, *chromophils* and *chromophobes*, according to their affinities for histological dyes. The chromophils are subdivided into two groups, *acidophils* and *basophils* because of their staining properties with a variety of histological methods. For example in micrograph (b), acidophils **A** are stained orange and basophils **B** are stained blue. In H & E preparations, the distinction between basophils and acidophils is much less obvious.

The chromophobes **C** are the smallest cell type in the anterior pituitary and contain few cytoplasmic granules; they have little affinity for either acidic or basic dyes and probably represent resting or degranulated chromophil cells.

The secretory cells of the anterior pituitary form branching cords which are surrounded by a rich network of sinusoidal capillaries supported by a delicate stroma containing reticulin and fine collagen fibres. Reflecting their epithelial nature, the clumps of secretory cells are surrounded by basement membranes which stain blue in preparation (b).

Traditional histological methods of studying the pituitary have been superseded by specific immuno-histochemical techniques by which five types of cells are defined according to their secretory product.

- **Somatotrophs**, the cells responsible for growth hormone secretion, are the most numerous making up almost half of the bulk of the anterior pituitary.
- **Mammotrophs (lactotrophs)**, the prolactin secreting cells, comprise up to 20% of the anterior pituitary increasing in number during pregnancy; prolactin controls milk production during lactation.
- **Corticotrophs** secrete ACTH (corticotrophin) and constitute about 20% of the anterior pituitary mass.

ACTH is a polypeptide which becomes split from a much larger peptide molecule known as *pro-opiomelanocortin*. From the same molecule can be derived *lipotropins* (involved in regulation of lipid metabolism), *endorphins* (endogenous opioids) and various species of MSH; the last explains the hyperpigmentation associated with excessive ACTH secretion.

- **Thyrotrophs**, which secrete TSH (thyrotrophin), are much less numerous making up only about 5% of the gland.
- **Gonadotrophs**, the cells responsible for the secretion of FSH and LH, make up the remaining 5% of the anterior pituitary; there are probably two distinctive cell types, each responsible for one of the gonadotrophins.

The somatotrophs and mammotrophs represent the acidophils of traditional light microscopy, the basophils being the thyrotrophs, gonadotrophs and probably the corticotrophs (which were formerly thought to be chromophobic).

The secretory granules of each cell type have a characteristic size, shape and electron density by which the different cell types can be recognised with electron microscopy as in micrograph (c). Somatotrophs **S** are packed with secretory granules of moderate size. Thyrotrophs **T** have smaller granules which tend to be more peripherally located. Gonadotrophs **G** are large cells with secretory granules of moderate and variable size. Corticotrophs **C** have a pale cytoplasm and sparse secretory granules located at the extreme periphery of the cell.

The endothelial lining of capillary sinusoids in endocrine tissue is characteristically fenestrated (see Fig. 8.14) facilitating the passage of hormones into the sinusoids. Note the fenestrations **F** in the sinusoid seen in micrograph (c).

(a)

(b)

(c)

Fig. 17.4 Pituitary: pars intermedia

(Isamine blue/Eosin × 100)

The pars intermedia is a constituent of the anterior pituitary, being derived embryologically from the cells lining the cavity of Rathke's pouch; the cells are basophilic (stained blue in this preparation) and form irregular clumps lying between the pars anterior **PA** and pars posterior **PP** but tending to spill out into the neural tissue of the pars posterior.

Small cystic spaces filled with eosinophilic colloid may be seen representing the residuum of Rathke's pouch. The pars intermedia is poorly developed in humans (as in this specimen) but relatively well developed in other mammals and some lower species.

Ultrastructurally, the cells contain secretory granules similar to other anterior pituitary cells. Pro-opiomelanocortin, the same precursor peptide as found in corticotrophs, is synthesised in the pars intermedia where it can be broken into a number of fragments including two species of MSH, endorphins and lipotrophins. MSH promotes melanin synthesis by skin melanocytes thereby increasing skin pigmentation.

Fig. 17.5 Posterior pituitary

(H & E × 200)

The posterior pituitary contains the non-myelinated axons of neurosecretory cells, the cell bodies of which are located in the hypothalamus. The neurosecretory axons are supported by cells called *pituicytes* similar in structure and function to the neuroglial cells of the central nervous system (see Figs. 7.21 to 7.24). Most of the nuclei seen in this micrograph are those of pituicytes; the axons of the neurosecretory cells are indistinguishable from the cytoplasm of the pituicytes in H & E preparations. A rich network of small fenestrated capillaries pervades the posterior pituitary.

Thyroid gland

The thyroid gland is a lobulated endocrine gland lying in the neck in front of the upper part of the trachea. The thyroid gland produces hormones of two types:

- Iodine-containing hormones *tri-iodothyronine* (T_3) and *thyroxine (tetra-iodothyronine, T_4)*; T_4 is converted to T_3 in the general circulation by removal of one iodothyronine unit although a small amount of T_3 is secreted directly. T_3 is much more potent than T_4 and appears to be the metabolically active form of the hormone. Thyroid hormone regulates the basal metabolic rate and has an important influence on growth and maturation particularly of nervous tissue. The secretion of these hormones is regulated by TSH secreted by the anterior pituitary.

- The polypeptide hormone *calcitonin*; this hormone regulates blood calcium levels in conjunction with parathyroid hormone. Calcitonin lowers blood calcium levels by inhibiting the rate of decalcification of bone by osteoclastic resorption and by stimulating osteoblastic activity. Control of calcitonin secretion is dependent only on blood calcium levels and is independent of pituitary and parathyroid hormone levels.

The thyroid gland is unique among the human endocrine glands in that it stores large amounts of hormone in an inactive form within extracellular compartments called follicles; in contrast, other endocrine glands store only small quantities of hormones in intracellular sites.

The main bulk of the gland develops from an epithelial downgrowth from the fetal tongue whereas the calcitonin-secreting cells are derived from the ultimobranchial element of the fourth branchial pouch.

Fig. 17.6 Thyroid gland *(H & E × 12)*

The functional units of the thyroid gland are the *thyroid follicles*, irregular spheroidal structures composed of a single layer of cuboidal epithelial cells bounded by a basement membrane (see also Fig. 5.30). As seen in this micrograph of a normal active thyroid, the follicles **F** are variable in size and contain a homogeneous colloid material which is stained pink in this preparation.

The thyroid gland is enveloped by an outer capsule of loose supporting tissue and an inner capsule of fibro-elastic tissue. From the inner capsule, fine collagenous septa **S** extend into the gland dividing the gland into lobules and conveying a rich blood supply together with lymphatics and nerves; during histological preparation, the lobules tend to shrink as seen here leaving artefactual spaces in the septal planes.

(a)

(b)

(c)

Fig. 17.7 Thyroid gland

(H & E (a) Human × 240 (b) Human × 480 (c) Dog × 480)

Thyroid follicles are lined by a simple cuboidal epithelium which is responsible for the synthesis and secretion of the iodine-containing hormones T_3 and T_4. Thyroid follicles are filled with a glycoprotein complex called *thyroglobulin* (*thyroid colloid*) which stores the thyroid hormones prior to secretion. In actively secreting thyroid glands, as in these micrographs, the follicles tend to be small and the amount of colloid diminished; the cuboidal lining cells are relatively tall, reflecting active hormone synthesis and secretion. Conversely, the follicles of less active thyroid glands are distended by stored colloid and the lining cells appear flattened against the follicular basement membrane.

A second secretory cell type is found in the thyroid gland either as single cells scattered among the follicular cells or as small clumps in the interfollicular spaces. These *parafollicular cells* were first described in the dog in which they have an extensive unstained cytoplasm and were therefore also called '*C*' (*clear cells*) **C**; this characteristic feature is seen in micrograph (c). In other mammals, including humans, the cytological characteristics of parafollicular cells are similar to those of the dog but unusually much less distinctive. Parafollicular cells synthesise and secrete the hormone calcitonin in direct response to raised blood calcium levels.

Parafollicular cells have a different embryological origin from the follicular cells and in some species constitute a discrete endocrine organ called the ultimo-branchial body.

Fig. 17.8 Thyroid follicle *(Rat: EM × 6800)*

This micrograph demonstrates a thyroid follicle composed of cuboidal follicular cells **F** surrounding a lumen containing the homogeneous colloid, thyroglobulin **T**. A basement membrane **BM** bounds the follicle. Two portions of the cytoplasm of a parafollicular or 'C' cell **C** are seen within the follicular epithelium typically located on the basement membrane and not exposed to the follicular lumen. The cytoplasm contains numerous electron-dense secretory granules of the hormone, calcitonin. A fenestrated capillary **Cap** containing an erythrocyte is closely applied to the follicular basement membrane. Part of a mast cell **M** is seen in the interfollicular supporting tissue.

Follicular cells concentrate iodide from the blood by means of an iodide pump in the basal plasma membrane. Within the cell, iodide is oxidised to iodine and transported to the follicular plasma membrane where it is released into the follicular lumen. The glycoprotein thyroglobulin is synthesised in the rough endoplasmic reticulum, glycosylated and packaged by the Golgi apparatus, then released into the follicular lumen by exocytosis. Within the follicular lumen (not within the follicular cells), iodine combines with tyrosine residues of the thyroglobulin to form the hormones tri-iodothyronine (T_3) and tetra-iodothyronine (thyroxine, T_4) which remain bound to the glycoprotein in an inactive form.

Secretion of these hormones involves engulfment of the thyroglobulin-hormone complex to form cytoplasmic vacuoles; the vacuoles then fuse with lysosomes of the follicular cell cytoplasm and hydrolytic enzymes cleave the hormone from the thyroglobulin. The hormones are released in the basal cytoplasm from which they diffuse into the bloodstream. The synthetic and secretory activity of the thyroid gland is dependent on thyroid stimulating hormone (TSH) secreted by the anterior pituitary.

In this micrograph, rough endoplasmic reticulum **rER** is best demonstrated in the basal aspect of a secretory cell of an adjacent follicle. Mitochondria **Mi** are closely associated with the endoplasmic reticulum and are also scattered throughout the cytoplasm. Golgi complexes **G** are a prominent feature. Small microvilli **Mv** associated with the exocytosis of thyroglobulin and the endocytosis of thyroglobulin-hormone complex, protrude into the follicular lumen. In one cell a vacuole **V** of thyroglobulin-hormone is seen about to fuse with a large lysosome **L**. Electron-dense lysosomes are also seen scattered throughout the cytoplasm.

Parathyroid gland

The parathyroid glands are small oval endocrine glands closely associated with the thyroid gland. In mammals, there are usually two pairs of glands, one pair situated on the posterior surface of the thyroid gland on each side. The embryological origins of the parathyroid glands are the third and fourth branchial (pharyngeal) pouches. The parathyroid glands regulate serum calcium and phosphate levels via *parathyroid hormone (parathormone)*.

Parathyroid hormone raises serum calcium levels in three ways:

- Direct action on bone, increasing the rate of osteoclastic resorption and promoting breakdown of the bone matrix.
- Direct action on the kidney, increasing the renal tubular reabsorption of calcium ions and inhibiting the reabsorption of phosphate ions from the glomerular filtrate.
- Promotion of the absorption of calcium from the small intestine; this effect involves vitamin D.

Secretion of parathyroid hormone is stimulated by a decrease in blood calcium levels. In conjunction with calcitonin secreted by the parafollicular cells of the thyroid gland, blood calcium levels are maintained within narrow limits. Parathyroid hormone is the most important regulator of blood calcium levels and is essential to life whereas calcitonin appears to provide a complementary mechanism for fine adjustment and is not essential to life.

Fig. 17.9 Parathyroid gland *(H & E × 45)*

This micrograph shows a parathyroid gland **P** characteristically embedded in the capsule of a thyroid gland **T**. The thin fibrous capsule of the parathyroid gland gives rise to delicate septa **S** which divide the parenchyma into dense cord-like masses of secretory cells; as seen here they are very prone to shrinkage artefact during histological preparation. The septa carry blood vessels, lymphatics and nerves.

Note that in this specimen from a 55-year-old woman, there is some infiltration of the thyroid by lymphoid cells **L**; this is a normal feature of the ageing thyroid gland.

Fig. 17.10 Parathyroid gland *(H & E × 198)*

The parathyroid gland contains secretory cells of two types: *chief (principal) cells* and *oxyphil cells*.

Chief (principal) cells are the most abundant cells and are responsible for the secretion of parathyroid hormone. Chief cells have a prominent nucleus and relatively little cytoplasm which varies in staining intensity according to the degree of secretory activity of the cell. Actively secreting cells, which represent about 20% of the total in normocalcaemic adults, contain much rough endoplasmic reticulum and stain strongly; in contrast, inactive cells contain little rough endoplasmic reticulum and stain poorly.

Oxyphil cells are larger and much less numerous than chief cells and tend to occur in clumps. They have smaller densely stained nuclei and strongly eosinophilic (oxyphilic) cytoplasm containing fine granules. Few oxyphil cells are found in the human parathyroid gland until puberty after which they increase in number with age. Oxyphil cells do not secrete hormones except in certain pathological conditions and their function is poorly understood.

In this micrograph from a young adult, chief cells **C** predominate; note the range of staining intensity from strong to very pale. Oxyphil cells **O** mainly form clumps amongst the chief cells. Note the delicate septa **S** dividing the gland into small lobules and supporting a rich blood supply. With increasing age, adipocytes become characteristically scattered throughout the glandular tissue.

Adrenal gland

The adrenal (supra-renal) glands are small flattened endocrine glands which are closely applied to the upper pole of each kidney. In mammals, the adrenal gland contains two functionally different types of endocrine tissue which have distinctly different embryological origins; in some lower animals, these two components exist as separate endocrine glands. The two components of the adrenal gland are the *adrenal cortex* and *adrenal medulla*.

- **Adrenal cortex.** The adrenal cortex has a similar embryological origin to the gonads and like them secretes a variety of *steroid hormones* all structurally related to their common precursor, *cholesterol*. The adrenal steroids may be divided into three functional classes, *mineralocorticoids, glucocorticoids* and *sex hormones*. The mineralocorticoids are concerned with electrolyte and fluid homeostasis. The glucocorticoids have a wide range of effects on carbohydrate, protein and lipid metabolism. Small quantities of sex hormones are secreted by the adrenal cortex and supplement gonadal sex hormone secretion.

- **Adrenal medulla.** Embryologically, the adrenal medulla has a similar origin to that of the sympathetic nervous system and may be considered as a highly specialised adjunct of this system. The adrenal medulla secretes the catecholamine hormones, *adrenaline (epinephrine)* and *noradrenaline (norepinephrine)*.

The control of hormone secretion differs markedly between the cortex and medulla. Adrenocortical activity is mainly regulated by the pituitary trophic hormone ACTH, and release of each of the adrenal corticosteroid hormones is controlled by various other circulating hormones and metabolites. In contrast, the secretion of adrenal medullary catecholamines is directly controlled by the sympathetic nervous system. The function of the adrenal medulla is to reinforce the action of the sympathetic nervous system under conditions of stress, the direct nervous control of adrenal medullary secretion permitting a rapid response.

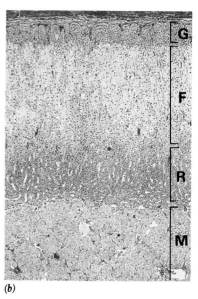

(a)   *(b)*

Fig. 17.11 Adrenal gland *(Azan (a) × 12 (b) × 20)*

At low magnification, the adrenal gland is seen to be divided into an outer cortex **C** and a pale stained inner medulla **M**. A dense fibrous tissue capsule, stained blue in this preparation, invests the gland and provides external support for a delicate collagenous framework supporting the secretory cells. A prominent vein is characteristically located in the centre of the medulla.

At higher magnification in micrograph (b), the adrenal cortex can be seen to consist of three histological zones which are named according to the arrangement of the secretory cells: *zona glomerulosa, zona fasciculata, zona reticularis.*

The zona glomerulosa **G** lying beneath the capsule contains secretory cells arranged in rounded clumps. The intermediate zona fasciculata **F** consists of parallel cords of secretory cells disposed at right angles to the capsule. The zona reticularis **R**, which lies adjacent to the medulla **M**, consists of small closely-packed cells arranged in irregular cords.

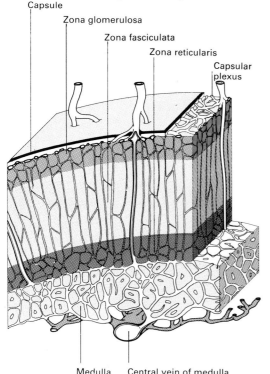

Capsule
Zona glomerulosa
Zona fasciculata
Zona reticularis
Capsular plexus

Medulla   Central vein of medulla

Fig. 17.12 Blood supply of the adrenal

The adrenal gland is supplied by three groups of arteries which form a plexus within the capsule of the gland.

The vascular system of the cortex consists of an anastomosing network of capillary sinusoids supplied by branches of the capsular plexus. The sinusoids descend between the cords of secretory cells in the zona fasciculata into a deep plexus in the zona reticularis before draining into small venules which converge upon the central vein of the medulla. The central medullary veins contain longitudinal bundles of smooth muscle between which the cortical venules enter; contraction of this smooth muscle is thought to dam back cortical blood and thus regulate flow.

The medulla is supplied by small arteries which descend from the capsular plexus through the cortex into the medulla where they ramify into a rich network of dilated capillaries surrounding the medullary secretory cells. The medullary capillaries also drain into the central vein of the medulla. Thus the secretory cells of the medulla are exposed to fresh arterial blood as well as blood rich in adrenocorticosteroids which are believed to have an important influence on the synthesis of adrenaline by the medulla.

Fig. 17.13 Adrenal cortex: zona glomerulosa *(Azan × 128)*

The secretory cells of the zona glomerulosa **G** are arranged in irregular ovoid clumps separated by delicate trabeculae containing wide diameter capillaries; the collagen of the capsule **C** and trabeculae **T** stains blue with Azan. The secretory cells have round strongly stained nuclei and relatively little cytoplasm giving rise to the moderately stained appearance of this zone when seen at lower magnification (see Fig. 17.11). The cytoplasm of the secretory cells contains much smooth endoplasmic reticulum, numerous mitochondria and triglyceride droplets which are the basic substrate for steroid synthesis. The abundance of smooth endoplasmic reticulum and small lipid droplets results in the relatively poor staining of the cytoplasm with routine staining methods.

The zona glomerulosa secretes the mineralocorticoid hormones, principally *aldosterone*. The major function of aldosterone is the regulation of body sodium and potassium ion levels by stimulating the sodium pump of cell membranes particularly in the renal tubules (see Ch. 16). Aldosterone also participates in blood pressure regulation via the renin-angiotensin-aldosterone hormone system controlled by the juxtaglomerular apparatus of the kidney (see Fig. 16.19). Aldosterone secretion is largely independent of ACTH.

Fig. 17.14 Adrenal cortex: zona fasciculata *(Azan × 128)*

The zona fasciculata is the intermediate and broadest of the three zones of the adrenal cortex. It consists of narrow cords of secretory cells, often only one cell thick, separated by fine strands of supporting tissue containing wide diameter capillaries. The secretory cells are large with an abundant poorly stained cytoplasm. The cytoplasm is even richer in smooth endoplasmic reticulum and lipid droplets than in the zona glomerulosa and this may confer a foamy appearance to the cells.

The zona fasciculata secretes glucocorticoid hormones principally *cortisol* which has numerous wide-ranging metabolic effects. Reflecting the name glucocorticoid, an important metabolic effect is to raise blood glucose levels and increase cellular synthesis of glycogen. These effects on carbohydrate metabolism are complemented by increased breakdown of proteins and liberation of lipid from tissue stores.

Control of cortisol secretion is maintained by the hypothalamus via the anterior pituitary hormone ACTH. By this means, many stimuli, including stress, promote secretion of glucocorticoids which adjust body metabolism appropriately.

The zona fasciculata is also the site of secretion of small amounts of androgenic sex hormones.

Fig. 17.15 Adrenal cortex: zona reticularis
(Azan × 128)

The zona reticularis is the thin innermost zone of the adrenal cortex. It consists of an irregular network of branching cords and clumps of glandular cells separated by numerous wide diameter capillaries. The glandular cells are much smaller than those of the adjacent zona fasciculata, and the cytoplasm, which contain few lipid droplets, stains more strongly. The brown wear and tear pigment lipofuscin (see Fig. 1.3) is a characteristic feature of H & E stained specimens.

The zona reticularis is probably responsible for the secretion of small quantities of androgens and glucocorticoids.

(a)

(b)

Fig. 17.16 Steroid–secreting cell

(EM (a) ×8500 (b) ×110 500)

These micrographs illustrate the typical ultrastructural features of steroid-secreting cells which are seen not only in the cells of the adrenal cortex but also in the steroid-secreting cells of the ovaries and testes (see Chs. 18 and 19). At low magnification in micrograph (a), a secretory cell is seen intimately associated with a fenestrated capillary **Cap**. Note the numerous irregular projections of the secretory cell plasma membrane subjacent to the capillary endothelium. The rounded secretory cell nucleus is characterised by more than one prominent nucleolus **Nu**.

The abundant cytoplasm contains many large triglyceride droplets **T**. A Golgi apparatus **G** is seen close to the nucleus. Numerous irregularly shaped mitochondria **M** crowd the cytoplasm. As seen in micrograph (b) at high magnification, the mitochondria **M** have unusual tubular cristae **C**. The cytoplasm contains a prolific system of tubular smooth endoplasmic reticulum **sER**.

Synthesis of steroids begins with the liberation of fatty acids from stored triglycerides. Mitochondrial oxidation of fatty acids provides acetate molecules for synthesis of cholesterol by the smooth endoplasmic reticulum. The basic steroid nucleus, cholesterol, is modified in the smooth endoplasmic reticulum or mitochondria depending on which steroid hormone is being synthesised.

Fig. 17.17 Adrenal medulla *(H & E × 198)*

The adrenal medulla **M** is composed of closely packed
clumps of secretory cells supported by a fine collagenous
network containing numerous wide diameter capillaries.
Many venous channels **V** draining blood from the sinusoids
of the cortex pass through the medulla towards the central
medullary vein (see Fig. 17.12).

The secretory cells of the adrenal medulla have large
granular nuclei and extensive strongly basophilic cytoplasm.
Note the contrasting eosinophilic cytoplasm of the cells of
the adjacent zona reticularis **ZR** of the cortex.

The adrenal medulla secretes the catecholamine hormones
noradrenaline and adrenaline under the direct control of the
sympathetic nervous system. Unlike most of the endocrine
glands, adrenal medullary hormones are not secreted
continuously but are stored in cytoplasmic granules and
released only in response to nervous stimulation in a manner
similar to the release of neurotransmitter substances from
nerve endings.

Recent investigations show that the adrenal medulla is
also responsible for the secretion of enkephalins, opioid
peptides which may be involved in control of pain.

Fig. 17.18 Adrenal medulla *(Chrome salt fixation, H & E × 800)*

When fixed in chrome salts, the stored catecholamine granules of adrenal
medullary cells are oxidised to a brown colour; consequently the name *chromaffin
cells* was often applied to the secretory cells of the adrenal medulla.

Some adrenal medullary cells synthesise noradrenaline; however, the majority
synthesise adrenaline by the addition of a further N-methyl group to
noradrenaline, the enzyme responsible being induced by the presence of cortisol
percolating down from the cortex. Those cells containing noradrenaline **N** exhibit a
much more strongly positive chromaffin reaction than adrenaline-secreting cells **A**.

Secretion of catecholamines by the adrenal medulla is controlled by
preganglionic neurones of the sympathetic nervous system; thus the secretory cells
of the adrenal medulla are functionally equivalent to the postganglionic neurones of
the sympathetic nervous system. Acute physical and psychological stresses initiate
release of adrenal medullary hormones; the released catecholamines act on
adrenergic receptors throughout the body particularly in the heart and blood
vessels, bronchioles, visceral muscle and skeletal muscle. Adrenaline also has
potent metabolic effects such as the promotion of glycogenolysis in liver and
skeletal muscle, thus releasing a readily available energy source during stress
situations.

Endocrine pancreas

The pancreas is not only a major exocrine gland (see Ch. 15) but also has important endocrine functions.

The embryonic epithelium of the pancreatic ducts consists of both potential exocrine and endocrine cells. During development, the endocrine cells migrate from the duct system and aggregate around capillaries to form isolated clumps of cells scattered throughout the exocrine glandular tissue. The clumps of endocrine tissue are known as *islets of Langerhans*. The islets vary in size and are most numerous in the tail of the pancreas. The islets contain a variety of cell types each responsible for secretion of one type of peptide hormone.

The main secretory products of the endocrine pancreas are *insulin* and *glucagon*, polypeptide hormones which play an important role in carbohydrate metabolism. Insulin promotes the uptake of glucose by most cells, particularly those of the liver, skeletal muscle and adipose tissue, thus lowering plasma glucose concentration. In general, glucagon has metabolic effects that oppose the actions of insulin. Apart from their role in carbohydrate metabolism, these hormones have a wide variety of other effects on energy metabolism, growth and development.

At least four other types of endocrine cells are present in the islets or else scattered singly or in small groups between the exocrine acini and along the ducts. Their secretory products include *somatostatin* (which has a wide variety of effects on gastrointestinal function and may also inhibit insulin and glucagon secretion), *vasoactive intestinal peptide (VIP)* and *pancreatic polypeptide (PP)*. Another cell type, the enterochromaffin (EC) cell, appears to secrete several different peptides including *motilin, serotonin* and *substance P*.

Fig. 17.19 Islet of Langerhans *(H & E × 480)*

The islets of Langerhans are composed of clumps of secretory cells supported by a fine collagenous network containing numerous fenestrated capillaries. A delicate capsule surrounds each islet. The endocrine cells are small with a poorly stained granular cytoplasm; in contrast, the large cells of the surrounding pancreatic acini stain strongly. This difference in staining intensity reflects the relatively greater amount of rough endoplasmic reticulum in the exocrine cells which secrete vast quantities of protein (see Figs. 15.13 and 15.14).

The endocrine pancreas contains secretory cells of several types; however, in H & E stained preparations, the cell types are indistinguishable from one another and special staining methods are required to differentiate between them. By tradition, the glucagon, insulin and somatostatin secreting cells have been designated as *alpha, beta* and *delta cells* respectively but with the discovery of further secretory products the most appropriate nomenclature is to employ the name of the secretory product.

Fig. 17.20 Islet of Langerhans

(Gomori's chrome alum haematoxylin/Phloxine method × 320)

This empirical staining method has traditionally been used to distinguish the glucagon and insulin-secreting cells of the endocrine pancreas. The glucagon-secreting cells, which constitute some 20% of the islet, are stained pink and are much less numerous than the blue-stained insulin-secreting cells which make up about 70% of the total. Generally, the glucagon-secreting cells tend to be distributed towards the periphery of the islets.

Fig. 17.21 Glucagon-secreting cells

(Immunoperoxidase method × 128)

Immunohistochemical techniques are now widely used to demonstrate the presence of specific molecules within cells; in this preparation, such a method has been used to demonstrate glucagon within cells of a pancreatic islet. The sites of glucagon localisation appear as brownish deposits; note the characteristic peripheral distribution of glucagon-secreting cells within the islet.

Fig. 17.22 Blood supply of the endocrine pancreas

(Carmine perfused/Haematoxylin × 128)

This specimen was perfused with a red dye before fixation to demonstrate the rich blood supply of the pancreatic islets. Each islet is supplied by as many as three arterioles which ramify into a highly branched network of fenestrated capillaries. The islet is drained by about six venules passing between the exocrine acini to the interlobular veins.

Pineal gland

The pineal gland is a small organ, 6–8 mm long, which represents an evagination from the posterior part of the roof of the third ventricle in the midline. The pineal is connected to the brain via a short stalk containing nerve fibres many of which communicate with the hypothalamus. In reptiles and other lower vertebrates, the pineal lies at or near the skin surface where it functions as a photoreceptor organ secreting the hormone *melatonin* which lightens skin colour by its action on melanophores, pigmented cells analogous to melanocytes in mammals.

Recent research has shown that melatonin is also secreted by the mammalian pineal as a derivative of serotonin. The pineal gland is at its greatest size in infancy and early childhood and involutes rapidly towards puberty. Melatonin appears to suppress production of gonadotrophin releasing hormone by the hypothalamus, thus suppressing pituitary gonadotrophin secretion and hence activation of gonadal growth and hormone secretion. In this way, the pineal gland controls the onset of puberty.

Fig. 17.23 Pineal gland *(H & E × 128)*

The pineal consists of two main cell types: *pinealocytes (pineal chief cells)* and *neuroglial cells*. Pinealocytes are highly modified neurones which are arranged in clumps and cords surrounded by a rich network of fenestrated capillaries. In H & E preparations, pinealocytes have round granular nuclei with prominent nucleoli and poorly stained cytoplasm. With special silver impregnation methods as used in neurohistology, pinealocytes appear to have many highly-branched processes, some of which terminate near or upon blood vessels. The cytoplasmic granules of pinealocytes contain a variety of indole compounds including melatonin and its precursor, serotonin.

The neuroglial cells, which are similar to the astrocytes of the rest of the CNS (see Fig. 7.21), are dispersed between the clumps of pinealocytes and in association with capillaries. Myelinated sympathetic nerve fibres enter the pineal where they ramify as unmyelinated axons throughout the substance of the gland.

A characteristic feature of the ageing pineal is the presence of basophilic extracellular bodies called *pineal sand* **S** consisting of concentric layers of calcium and magnesium phosphate within an organic matrix. The organic matrix may represent the remnants of carrier proteins for the pineal endocrine secretions. The calcified pineal can be seen on x-rays of the skull and its position can be a useful guide to pathological conditions causing the midline to be displaced to one side.

The gastrointestinal endocrine system

Scattered in the mucosa of the gastrointestinal tract and in the pancreas are a variety of endocrine cells which secrete peptide and amine hormones such as gastrin, secretin, CCK, serotonin and many more recently discovered substances including enteroglucagon, somatostatin, substance P, vasoactive intestinal peptide (VIP), bombesin, gastric inhibitory polypeptide (GIP), motilin and pancreatic polypeptide. These hormones constitute a balanced system of agonists and antagonists which collectively regulate and coordinate most aspects of gastrointestinal activity in concert with the autonomic nervous system.

The endocrine cells may be located at any level in the mucosa from the base of glands to the tips of villi. The cells which are exposed to the tract lumen may be receptive to gastrointestinal contents; these are termed the *open type*. Other endocrine cells are deep to the surface, the *closed type*, and may be receptive to changes in local tissue environment. The cells responsible for the secretion of a particular hormone tend to be located in a particular anatomical region in the tract but there is considerable overlap in distribution, e.g. gastrin-secreting cells are found in the body of the stomach, the duodenum and the pancreas.

The presence of endocrine cells in the gastrointestinal tract has long been demonstrable by staining with silver or chromium salts. Traditionally, the cells were divided into two types, *argentaffin cells* (silver reducing) and *argyrophil cells* (silver absorbing); furthermore, like the catecholamine-secreting 'chromaffin' cells of the adrenal medulla (see Fig. 17.18), both these cell types could be stained specifically with chromium salts and thus the gastrointestinal endocrine cells became collectively known as *enterochromaffin cells*. These classifications were subsequently found to be of little functional significance and currently the term enterochromaffin cell should only be applied to a specific cell type found throughout the tract in large numbers and which is responsible for the secretion of multiple amines including serotonin (5-hydroxytryptamine).

The various gastrointestinal endocrine cells have many ultrastructural features in common but they may be divided into at least 20 different types according to the shape, size and density of their secretory granules. On the basis of immunohistochemistry and other techniques, the various gastrointestinal hormones have been assigned to different ultrastructural cell types. Since gut hormones are a rapidly advancing field of research, there is considerable terminological confusion. It has been the practice for a cell type definitely known to produce a particular hormone to be known by the name of that hormone; for example gastrin-secreting cells are called *gastrin* or *G cells*. Difficulties have arisen where one cell type is found to produce more than one hormone.

Another major problem has been the lack of agreement about which secretory products should be classified as hormones since some of the known secretory products have only local activity. An example is serotonin, a potent local muscle constrictor, which is not generally recognised as a hormone since it does not normally have more distant effects. For such chemical messengers which appear to act principally on adjacent or nearby cells and tissues, the term *paracrine* may be applied.

A further problem has arisen with the discovery that some of the gastrointestinal endocrine secretory products such as gastrin, CCK, VIP, substance P, bombesin and serotonin are also found in the brain where they appear to act as neurotransmitters; indeed, this may be the mode of action of some of these substances in the gastrointestinal tract.

In summary, there is a mass of peptide and amine-secreting cells scattered throughout the gastrointestinal tract which may be considered as a diffuse endocrine organ. The substances produced by this organ have specific and overlapping activities which regulate and co-ordinate the function of the gastrointestinal system.

The respiratory endocrine system

The lower respiratory tract contains a system of scattered peptide and amine-secreting endocrine cells analogous to that in the gastrointestinal tract and which is probably involved in local and autonomically-mediated regulation of respiratory tract function particularly in early childhood. The endocrine cells are scattered individually in the epithelium or in clumps protruding into the airway and have a variety of secretory products including: serotonin, calcitonin, bombesin and lucine-enkephalin.

The APUD cell concept and diffuse neuroendocrine system

From comparative ultrastructural studies of endocrine tissues, it became evident that the diverse group of peptide or amine-secreting cells in the gastrointestinal tract and other endocrine organs have certain ultrastructural features in common. These cells have little rough endoplasmic reticulum, much smooth endoplasmic reticulum, numerous free ribosomes and small membrane-bound secretory granules. Subsequent histochemical investigations revealed that many of these cells share some common metabolic processes related to hormone synthesis. These processes include a high uptake of amine precursors and the ability to decarboxylate; on this basis, the descriptive term *APUD cell* (amine precursor uptake and decarboxylation) was applied and this group is now known to include at least the following diverse cells: adrenal medullary cells, thyroid 'C' cells, all pancreatic endocrine cells, all gastrointestinal hormone-secreting cells including enterochromaffin (serotonin) cells, ACTH and MSH cells of the pituitary, renin-secreting juxtaglomerular cells of the kidney, chemoreceptors of the carotid body and mast cells.

Further research has suggested that the APUD cells include an even more diverse group of cells which are derived embryologically from neural crest tissue and therefore may be considered as highly modified neurones. For this reason, the term *diffuse neuroendocrine system* has been applied to encompass all these cell types and the term *paraneurone* has been proposed to describe the cells.

In summary, the principal features of the diffuse neuroendocrine system are as follows:

- The cells produce amines or peptides with hormone-like activity and/or produce substances identical with, or related to, known or suspected neurotransmitters.
- The cells should possess synaptic vesicle-like structures or neurosecretory-type granules; the latter are round or ovoid membrane-bound secretory granules with an electron-dense core and surrounding electron-lucent halo giving rise to the term *dense-core vesicles*.
- The cells should exhibit both receptor and secretory functions.
- The cells should be of neuroectodermal origin.

Fig. 17.24 APUD cells in the large intestinal mucosa *(Alkaline diazo method × 320)*

This specimen of colonic mucosa has been stained by a histochemical method which demonstrates the presence of APUD cells **A**, the secretory granules of which are stained orange-brown. The endocrine cells are typically small and in this example are of the 'closed type' as they lie deep to the mucosal surface.

Fig. 17.25 Gastrointestinal endocrine cells *(EM × 8300)*

This micrograph shows two endocrine cells from the human pylorus, both of which exhibit the typical characteristics of open-type gastrointestinal APUD cells. The endocrine cell marked **G** is a gastrin-secreting cell recognised on the basis of its large moderately dense secretory granules. The adjacent endocrine cell marked **S** contains much smaller and more dense granules of the secretory product somatostatin which appears to have a broad range of actions including the inhibition of insulin and glucagon secretion and inhibition of the secretion of many gastrointestinal hormones. The open-type APUD cells are usually pyramidal in shape, the apex extending to the tract lumen and the base resting on the basement membrane **BM**. The apical surface forms a few microvilli **Mv** which may receive stimuli from the tract lumen. Secretory granules are aggregated in the basal cytoplasm from which they are released into the underlying extracellular space, diffusing into the capillaries of the lamina propria. Typically, the cytoplasm contains only a few short profiles of rough endoplasmic reticulum and numerous free ribosomes. The closed-type of APUD cells are usually rounded and lack the polarity of the open-type but otherwise have similar ultrastructural features.

18. Male reproductive system

Introduction
The male reproductive system may be divided into four major functional components:

- The *testes* or male gonads, paired organs lying in the scrotal sac, are responsible for production of the male gametes, *spermatozoa*, and secretion of male sex hormones.
- A paired system of ducts, each consisting of *ductuli efferentes, epididymis, ductus deferens* and *ejaculatory duct*, collect, store and conduct spermatozoa from each testis. The ejaculatory ducts converge on the *urethra* from which spermatozoa are expelled into the female reproductive tract during copulation.
- Two exocrine glands, the paired *seminal vesicles* and the single *prostate gland*, secrete a nutritive and lubricating fluid medium called *seminal fluid* in which spermatozoa are conveyed to the female reproductive tract. Seminal fluid, spermatozoa and cells desquamated from the lining of the duct system comprise *semen*.
- The *penis* is the organ of copulation. A pair of small accessory glands, the *bulbo-urethral glands of Cowper*, secrete a fluid which lubricates the urethra for the passage of semen during ejaculation.

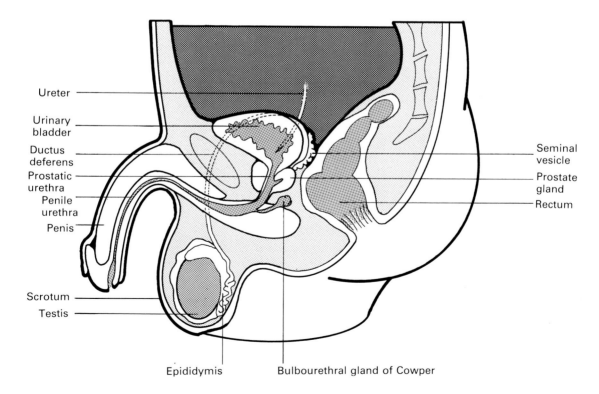

Fig. 18.1 Male reproductive system

Ductus deferens

Ductuli efferentes

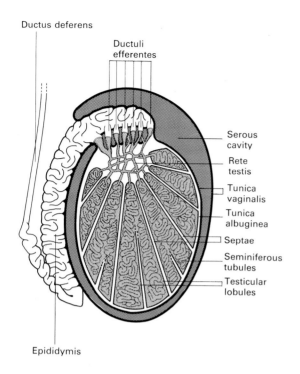

Serous cavity

Rete testis

Tunica vaginalis

Tunica albuginea

Septae

Seminiferous tubules

Testicular lobules

Epididymis

Fig. 18.2 Testis

During embryological development, each testis with the first part of its duct system, blood vessels, lymphatics and nerves, descends along a tortuous path from the posterior wall of the peritoneal cavity to the scrotum. During migration, the testis carries with it an investing layer of peritoneum so that in the scrotum the testis is almost completely surrounded by a serous space which represents an extension of the peritoneal cavity. The space around the testis becomes isolated from the peritoneum, its serosal lining being known as the *tunica vaginalis*. The tunica secretes a small amount of lubricant fluid and protects the testis by allowing it to move freely in the scrotal sac.

The testis is encapsulated by dense fibrous tissue, the *tunica albuginea*, which gives rise to numerous ill-defined collagenous septa which divide the testis into about 250 *testicular lobules*. Within each lobule are one to four highly convoluted tubes, the *seminiferous tubules*, in which spermatozoa are produced. The seminiferous tubules converge upon a plexus of spaces, the *rete testis*. From the rete testis, 15 to 20 small ducts, called the *ductuli efferentes*, conduct spermatozoa to the extremely tortuous first part of the *ductus deferens* which is known as the *epididymis*.

Fig. 18.3 Testis *(Monkey: H & E × 3)*

This micrograph illustrates the macroscopic features of a testis; cut in the sagittal plane, it shows the relationship of the epididymis **E** which lies on its posterior aspect. The testis is packed with coiled seminiferous tubules which can just be seen in various planes of section at this magnification. Groups of about four seminiferous tubules are segregated into testicular lobules; the interlobular septa are so delicate as to be barely seen at this magnification. The dense fibrous capsule which invests the testis, and which is continuous with many of the interlobular septa, is called the tunica albuginea **TA** since it appears white macroscopically. The tunica vaginalis contains fibroblasts and muscle-like cells (*myocytes*) particularly in the posterior aspect which subject the seminiferous tissue to rhythmic contractions. Beneath the tunica vaginalis is a loose supporting tissue layer containing blood and lymphatic vessels.

Spermatozoa pass from the seminiferous tubules into the rete testis **RT** which is connected to the epididymis via the ductuli efferentes at the upper posterior pole of the testis; the ductuli are not included in the plane of this section. The epididymis is a tightly coiled tube which forms a compact mass extending down the whole length of the posterior surface of the testis. The epididymis is the major site of storage of newly formed spermatozoa. At the lower pole of the testis, the epididymal tube becomes continuous with the relatively straight ductus (vas) deferens which is not seen in this section.

Blood supply to the testis is via the testicular artery which ramifies in the tunica albuginea giving rise to septal branches which pass inwards to the rete testis. From here, small arterial vessels radiate outwards to supply the rich capillary network around the tubules.

TA

E

RT

Gametogenesis

In all somatic cells, cell division (mitosis) results in the formation of two daughter cells each one genetically identical to the mother cell. Somatic cells contain a full complement of chromosomes (the diploid number) which function as homologous pairs (see Ch. 2). The process of sexual reproduction involves the fusion of specialised male and female cells called *gametes* to form a *zygote* which has the diploid number of chromosomes. Each gamete contains only half the diploid number of chromosomes; this half complement of chromosomes is known as the *haploid number*.

The production of haploid cells involves a unique form of cell division called *meiosis* which occurs only in the germ cells of the gonads during the formation of gametes; meiotic cell division is thus also called *gametogenesis*. Meiosis involves two cell division cycles of which only the first is preceded by duplication of chromosomes (see Ch. 2). Thus, meiotic cell division of a single diploid germ cell gives rise to four haploid gametes. In the male, each of the four gametes undergoes morphological development into a mature spermatozoon whereas in the female, unequal distribution of the cytoplasm during meiosis results in one gamete gaining almost all the cytoplasm from the mother cell, whilst the other three acquire almost no cytoplasm; the large gamete matures to form an ovum and the other three, called *polar bodies*, degenerate.

The primitive germ cells of the male, the *spermatogonia*, are present only in small numbers in the male gonads before sexual maturity. After puberty, spermatogonia multiply continuously by mitosis to provide a supply of cells which then undergo meiosis to form male gametes. In contrast, the germ cells of the female, called *oogonia*, multiply by mitosis only during early fetal development thereby producing a fixed complement of cells with the potential to undergo gametogenesis. Gametogenesis in the female is discussed more fully in Chapter 19. The production of male gametes is called *spermatogenesis* and the subsequent development of the male gamete into a motile spermatozoon is called *spermiogenesis*, the whole process taking approximately 70 days; both these processes occur within the testes although final maturation occurs in the epididymis.

Fig. 18.4 Seminiferous tubules *(H & E × 100)*

This micrograph illustrates seminiferous tubules cut in various planes of section. The seminiferous tubules are highly convoluted and lined by a stratified epithelium which consists of two distinct populations of cells:

- Cells in various stages of spermatogenesis and spermiogenesis are collectively referred to as the *spermatogenic series*.
- Non-spermatogenic cells called *Sertoli cells* support and nourish the developing spermatozoa.

In the interstitial spaces between the tubules, endocrine cells called *Leydig cells* are found either singly or in groups in the supporting tissue.

Fig. 18.5 Seminiferous tubule *(H & E × 640)*

This micrograph illustrates an active seminiferous tubule
cut in transverse section. The processes of spermatogenesis
and spermiogenesis are synchronised, with waves of activity
occurring sequentially along the length of each tubule. Thus
in any one histological section, all development phases will
not be represented.

   Spermatogonia, the germ cells, are found in the basal layer
of the seminiferous epithelium where they divide by mitosis
giving rise to further stem cells (designated as Type A
spermatogonia), and to spermatogonia committed to meiosis
(designated Type B). Spermatogonia Type A S_A are
characterised by a large round or oval nucleus with
condensed chromatin; nucleoli, which are associated with
the nuclear membrane, and a nuclear vacuole may be
prominent. Spermatogonia Type B S_B have dispersed
chromatin, centrally located nucleoli, and no nuclear
vacuole. Both types of spermatogonia have sparse poorly
stained cytoplasm.

   Spermatogonia Type B enter the first stages of meiotic
division when they become known as *primary spermatocytes*.
Primary spermatocytes S_1 are readily recognised by their
copious cytoplasm and large nuclei containing coarse clumps
or thin threads of chromatin; dividing cells may be seen. In
man, the first meiotic division cycle takes approximately 3
weeks to complete, after which time the daughter cells
become known as *secondary spermatocytes*. The smaller
secondary spermatocytes rapidly undergo the second

meiotic division and are therefore much less commonly seen.

   The gametes thus produced, called *spermatids* S_3, then
proceed through the long maturation process known as
spermiogenesis to become recognisable as spermatozoa.
During this process, the nuclei of the spermatids become
smaller, more condensed and less granular until they assume
the small pointed form of spermatozoa S_4 (see Fig. 18.7).
Examination of different sections of the tubules of a normal
testis shows about half the spermatogenic cells to be in the
late spermatid stage.

   During the developmental process, the cells of the
spermatogenic series are supported by Sertoli cells St, the
nuclei of which are usually found towards the basement
membrane of the seminiferous tubule. The Sertoli cell
nucleus is typically triangular or ovoid in shape with a
prominent nucleolus and dispersed chromatin. Although not
evident by light microscopy, Sertoli cells have an extensive
cytoplasm which ramifies throughout the whole germinal
epithelium enclosing all the cells of the spermatogenic series.

   The basal layer of germinal cells is supported by a
basement membrane which is surrounded by a lamina
propria containing several layers of spindle-shaped
fibromyocytes (myoid cells) M. These cells are responsible
for the production of collagen and elastin fibres in the lamina
propria whilst their contractile activity aids movement of
spermatozoa along the tubules.

Fig. 18.6 Sertoli cell *(EM × 3400)*

The intimate relationship of a Sertoli cell **St** to cells of the spermatogenic series is demonstrated in this electron micrograph.

The Sertoli cell rests on the basement membrane **BM** of the seminiferous tubule and its cytoplasm extends to the lumen of the tubule, filling the narrow spaces between the cells of the spermatogenic series. The cytoplasmic outline of the Sertoli cell is thus highly irregular and constantly changing to permit the progressive movement of developing spermatozoa towards the luminal surface. The oval nucleus of the Sertoli cell is characteristically orientated at right angles to the basement membrane and often exhibits a deep indentation. A prominent nucleolus **Nu** is a constant feature; dense chromatin bodies **C** are often associated with the nucleolus. The cytoplasm contains a moderate number of mitochondria, many lipid droplets and relatively little rough endoplasmic reticulum. The presence of a highly ordered smooth endoplasmic reticulum suggests that Sertoli cells synthesise lipid.

Sertoli cells are bound to one another by junctional complexes containing extensive tight junctions (see Ch. 5). The junctional complex is located towards the basal layer of the spermatogenic epithelium so as to divide the tubule into *basal* and *adluminal compartments*. The latter contains the spermatids which are thus isolated by a *blood-testis barrier*, the Sertoli cells mediating all metabolic exchange with the systemic compartment. The function of this barrier is to prevent exposure of gametes, which are antigenically different from somatic cells, to the immune system thus preventing an autoimmune response. Sertoli cells are postulated to act as 'nurse' cells, providing structural and metabolic support for the developing spermatogenic cells. During spermiogenesis, Sertoli cells phagocytose excess cytoplasm cast off by the spermatids.

A variety of cells of the spermatogenic series are seen in this micrograph. Spermatogonia **S** rest upon the basement membrane beneath which is a slender smooth muscle-like (myoid) cell **M**. Above the germ cell layer, primary spermatocytes S_1 are seen; secondary spermatocytes are short-lived and therefore rarely seen. Spermatids S_3 in different phases of spermiogenesis are seen in upper layers; these cells have developing acrosomal vesicles **AV** elaborated by a large Golgi apparatus **G** (see Fig. 18.7). At the luminal surface, the Sertoli cell envelops an almost fully formed spermatozoon S_4.

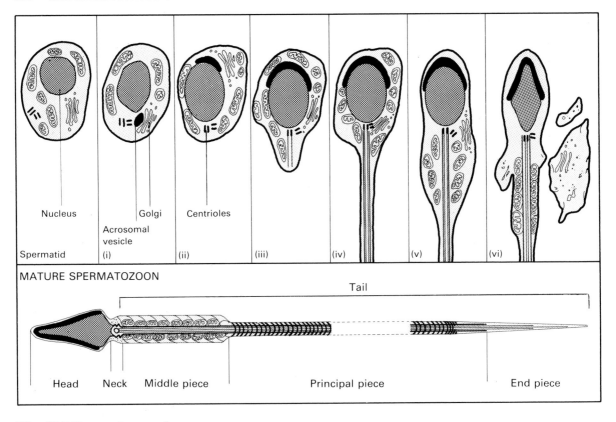

Fig. 18.7 Spermiogenesis

Spermiogenesis is the process by which spermatids, the gametes produced by meiotic division, are transformed into motile mature spermatozoa. This involves the following major stages:

1. The Golgi apparatus elaborates a large vesicle, the *acrosomal vesicle*, which accumulates carbohydrates and hydrolytic enzymes.
2. The acrosomal vesicle becomes applied to one pole of the progressively elongating nucleus to form a structure known as the *acrosomal head cap*.
3. Meanwhile, both centrioles migrate to the end of the cell opposite to the acrosomal head cap; the centriole aligned parallel to the long axis of the nucleus elongates to form a flagellum which has a basic structure similar to that of the cilium (see Fig. 5.15).
4. As the flagellum elongates, nine *coarse fibrils*, which may contain contractile proteins, become arranged longitudinally around the core of the flagellum. Further rib-like fibrils then become disposed circumferentially around the whole flagellum.
5. The cytoplasm migrates to surround the first part of the flagellum, with the remainder of the flagellum appearing to project from the cell but in fact remaining surrounded by plasma membrane. This migration of cytoplasm thus concentrates mitochondria in the flagellar region.
6. As the flagellum elongates, excess cytoplasm is phagocytosed by the enveloping Sertoli cell prior to release of the spermatid into the lumen. The

mitochondria become arranged in a helical manner around the fibrils which surround the first part of the flagellum.

The structure of fully formed spermatozoa varies in detail from species to species, but conforms to the basic structure seen in this diagram of a human spermatozoon.

Throughout the entire developmental process from spermatogonia to spermatozoa, hundreds of spermatids remain connected to one another by narrow cytoplasmic bridges which only break down upon release of spermatozoa into the lumen of the seminiferous tubule. This explains the synchronous development of spermatozoa at any one part of the tubule.

The control of spermatogenesis and spermiogenesis remains the subject of intense investigation; it is believed that Sertoli cells mediate some important regulatory mechanisms. It is well established that high concentrations of androgen hormones secreted by Leydig cells of the testicular interstitium (see Fig. 18.9) are essential for production and maturation of spermatogenic cells. Sertoli cells secrete an androgen-binding protein which transports testosterone and dihydrotestosterone to the lumen of the seminiferous tubule. These hormones are also necessary for function of the epithelium of the rete testis and epididymis; production of this binding protein is believed to be dependent on the pituitary gonadotrophin, follicle-stimulating hormone.

Fig. 18.8 Spermatozoa

(EM (a) Head: LS × 14 000 (b) Neck: middle piece and principal piece: LS × 17 000 (c) Middle piece: TS × 48 000)

The ultrastructural features of human spermatozoa are shown in these micrographs. The spermatozoon is an extremely elongated cell (about 65 μm long) consisting of three main components, the *head*, *neck* and *tail*. The tail is subdivided into three segments, the *middle piece*, *principal piece* and *end piece* (see Fig. 18.7).

The head is the most variable structure between different mammalian species. In man, the head is about 7 μm long and has a flattened pear shape. As seen in micrograph (a), the nucleus, which occupies most of the head, is composed of very condensed chromatin; in man, this contains a variable number of areas of dispersed chromatin called *nuclear vacuoles*. Surrounding the anterior two-thirds of the nucleus is the acrosomal cap **AC**, a flattened membrane-bound vesicle containing a range of glycoproteins and a variety of hydrolytic enzymes, principally *hyaluronidase*; the enzymes disaggregate the cells of the corona radiata and dissolve the zona pellucida during fertilisation (see Ch. 19). Note the plasma membrane **PM** which has become partially separated during preparation.

The neck is a very short segment connecting the head with the tail. It contains vestiges of the centrioles, one of which gives rise to the axoneme **Ax** of the flagellum which is seen in micrograph (c). The axoneme has the standard 'nine plus two' arrangement of microtubule doublets seen in cilia (see Fig. 5.15). The axoneme of the neck is surrounded by several condensed fibrous rings **Rn** seen in micrograph (b). In human spermatozoa, a significant amount of cytoplasm **C** often remains in the neck region.

The middle piece, the first part of the tail, is about the same length as the head and consists of the flagellar axoneme surrounded by nine *coarse (outer dense) fibres* **F** arranged longitudinally. External to this core, elongated mitochondria **Mi** are arranged in a tightly packed helix providing the energy required for flagellar movement. A fibrous thickening beneath the plasma membrane, called the *anulus* **An**, prevents the mitochondria from slipping into the principal piece. The principal piece, which constitutes most of the tail length, consists of a central core, comprising the axoneme and the nine coarse fibres continuing from the middle piece. Surrounding this core are numerous fibrous ribs **Rb** arranged in a circular manner and seen in micrograph (b). Two of the longitudinal fibrils of the core are fused with the surrounding ribs so as to form *dorsal* and *ventral columns* extending throughout the length of the principal piece (not illustrated). This arrangement divides the principal piece longitudinally into two functional compartments, one containing three coarse fibrils and the other containing four. Little is known of the mechanism of flagellar motion but this asymmetry may account for the more powerful stroke of the tail in one direction, the so-called 'power stroke'; this can easily be observed in fresh, live preparations of spermatozoa viewed with the light microscope. The end piece, not shown in these micrographs, is merely a short tapering portion of the tail containing the axoneme only.

Fig. 18.9 Interstitial (Leydig) cells of the testis *(H & E × 480)*

Leydig cells **L** synthesise and secrete the male sex hormones and are the principal cell type found in the interstitial supporting tissue between the seminiferous tubules. They occur singly or in clumps and are embedded in the rich plexus of blood and lymph capillaries which surrounds the seminiferous tubules. The nucleus is round with dispersed chromatin and one or two nucleoli at the periphery. The extensive eosinophilic cytoplasm contains variable numbers of lipid vacuoles and seen by electron microscopy closely resembles the steroid-secreting cells of the adrenal cortex (see Fig. 17.16). In man, but no other species, Leydig cells also contain elongated cytoplasmic *crystals of Reinke* which are large enough to be seen with light microscopy when suitably stained; these crystals become more numerous with age but their function is completely unknown.

Testosterone is the principal hormone secreted by Leydig cells. Testosterone is not only responsible for the development of male secondary sexual characteristics at puberty but is also essential for the continued function of the seminiferous epithelium. The secretory activity of Leydig cells is controlled by the pituitary gonadotrophic hormone, luteinising hormone, often referred to as *interstitial cell stimulating hormone (ICSH)* in the male.

Fig. 18.10 Rete testis *(H & E × 128)*

The seminiferous tubules converge upon the *mediastinum testis* which consists of a plexiform arrangement of spaces, the *rete testis*, surrounded by highly vascular collagenous supporting tissue containing myoid cells. The rete testis is lined by a single layer of cuboidal epithelial cells with surface microvilli and a single flagellum.

Myoid cell contraction helps to mix the spermatozoa and move them towards the epididymis. The lining epithelium is thought to secrete some constituents of seminal fluid. Flagellar activity is presumed to aid the progress of spermatozoa which do not become motile until after maturation is completed in the epididymis.

Fig. 18.11 Ductulus efferens *(H & E × 320)*

The rete testis drains into the head of the epididymis via some 15 to 20 convoluted ducts, the *ductuli efferentes*. The ductuli are lined by a single layer of epithelial cells, some of which are tall columnar and ciliated and others which are short and non-ciliated; both cell types often contain a brown pigment of unknown composition. Ciliary action in the ductuli propels the still non-motile spermatozoa towards the epididymis; the non-ciliated cells reabsorb some of the fluid produced by the testis. A thin band of circularly arranged smooth muscle **SM** surrounds each ductulus and aids propulsion of the spermatozoa towards the epididymis.

(a)

(b)

Fig. 18.12 Epididymis *(H & E (a) × 50 (b) × 320)*

The epididymis is a long extremely convoluted duct
extending down the posterior aspect of the testis to the lower
pole where it becomes the ductus deferens. The major
function of the epididymis is the accumulation, storage and
maturation of spermatozoa **S**; during this time the
spermatozoa develop motility.

The epididymis is a tube of smooth muscle lined by a
pseudostratified epithelium. From the proximal to the distal
end of the epididymis, the muscular wall increases from a
single circular layer as in these micrographs to three layers
organised in the same manner as in the ductus deferens (see
Fig. 18.13). Proximally, the smooth muscle exhibits slow
rhythmic contractility which gently moves spermatozoa
towards the ductus deferens. Distally, the smooth muscle is
richly innervated by the sympathetic nervous system which

produces intense contractions of the lower part of the
epididymis during ejaculation.

The epithelial lining of the epididymis exhibits a gradual
transition from a tall pseudostratified columnar form
proximally, as seen in micrograph (b), to a shorter
pseudostratified form distally. The principal cells of the
epididymal epithelium bear tufts of very long microvilli,
inappropriately called stereocilia (see Fig. 5.17), which are
thought to be involved in absorption of an excess of fluid
accompanying the spermatozoa from the testis. The
ultrastructure of the cells strongly suggests an additional
secretory function but the nature of epididymal secretory
products, if any, remains unknown. Occasional lymphocytes
L may be seen within the epithelium.

Fig. 18.13 Ductus deferens *(H & E × 30)*

The ductus (vas) deferens, which conducts spermatozoa
from the epididymis to the urethra, is a thick walled
muscular tube consisting of inner **I** and outer **O** longitudinal
layers and a thick intermediate circular layer **C**. Like the
distal part of the epididymis, the ductus deferens is
innervated by the sympathetic nervous system producing
strong peristaltic contractions to expel its contents into the
urethra during ejaculation.

The ductus deferens is lined by a pseudostratified
epithelium similar to that of the epididymis (see Fig. 18.12);
the epithelial lining and its supporting lamina propria are
thrown into longitudinal folds which permit expansion of
the duct during ejaculation. The dilated distal portion of
each ductus deferens, known as the *ampulla*, receives a short
duct draining the seminal vesicle, thus forming the short
ejaculatory duct; the ejaculatory ducts from each side
converge to join the urethra as it passes through the prostate
gland.

This specimen was obtained at operation for male
sterilisation (*vasectomy*).

(a)

(b)

Fig. 18.14 Seminal vesicle *(H & E (a) × 10 (b) × 320)*

Each seminal vesicle is a complex glandular diverticulum of the associated ductus deferens. Between them the seminal vesicles secrete about half of the total volume of seminal fluid, most of the rest being secreted by the prostate gland. The lumen of each seminal vesicle is highly irregular and recessed giving a honeycombed appearance at low magnification.

The epithelial lining is usually pseudostratified and consists of secretory cells which produce a yellowish viscid alkaline fluid containing fructose, fibrinogen, vitamin C and prostaglandins. The epithelial cells often contain brown lipofuscin granules. Although not thought to store spermatozoa, seminal vesicles are often seen to contain spermatozoa which have probably entered by reflux from the ampulla. The prominent muscular wall **M** is arranged into inner circular and outer longitudinal layers and supplied by the sympathetic nervous system; during ejaculation, muscle contraction forces secretions from the seminal vesicles into the urethra via the ampullae.

Fig. 18.15 Prostate gland *(Dog: H & E × 5)*

The prostate is a large gland which surrounds the bladder neck and the first part of the urethra **U** in the midline; the wall of the prostatic urethra is formed by the substance of the prostate gland. The ejaculatory ducts **ED** join the prostatic urethra just before its exit from the prostate gland.

The gland is invested by a fibro-elastic capsule **Cap** from which incomplete septa **Sp** extend in towards the central stroma **St** dividing the gland into 50 or so poorly defined lobules **L**. This supporting tissue contains numerous smooth muscle fibres which, like that of the seminal vesicles and the rest of the tract, are innervated by the sympathetic nervous system which stimulates powerful contractions during ejaculation.

The prostatic glandular tissue consists of three separate groups of compound tubulo-acinar glands arranged concentrically around the urethra. The *main prostatic glands* **M** which constitute the bulk of the organ occupy the peripheral two thirds of the gland and drain via about 20 long ducts into the distal urethra on either side of the *urethral crest* **C** which lies in the midline posteriorly; these ducts pursue an arching course approximately indicated by the dotted line on the micrograph. The inner third of the gland consists of the *submucosal (outer periurethral) glands* **SG** which drain via short ducts into the *urethral sinuses* **US** which lie on each side of the urethral crest. The innermost group of glands is very small and not visible at this magnification; these *mucosal (inner periurethral) glands* open directly into the urethra over its whole surface. With age, the mucosal and submucosal glands and their supporting tissue tend to become greatly enlarged leading to the condition of benign prostatic hyperplasia which may cause urinary outflow obstruction. In contrast, it is the main prostatic glands which give rise to prostatic cancer.

Fig. 18.16 Prostate gland *(H & E × 128)*

The prostatic glandular epithelium has a pseudostratified columnar form, the majority of cells being tall cuboidal or columnar with basally located nuclei and poorly stained foamy cytoplasm; a smaller number of flat basal cells with dark staining nuclei are located along the basement membrane. The epithelium forms branching folds **F** with a central core of lamina propria giving a characteristic papillary appearance. The secretory product of the prostate, which makes up about half of the seminal fluid volume, is thin and milky; it is rich in citric acid and hydrolytic enzymes, notably fibrinolysin, which liquefies coagulated semen after it has been deposited within the female genital tract. Lamellated glycoprotein masses called *corpora amylacea* **CA** are a feature of increasing age, becoming progressively calcified to form *prostatic concretions*.

Fig. 18.17 Penis *(H & E × 3)*

This transverse section through the penis of an adult human male demonstrates the general arrangement of the penile tissues. The penis consists of three cylindrical masses of erectile tissue: the paired *corpora cavernosa penis* **CCP** in the dorsal aspect, and the midline *corpus cavernosum urethrae* **CCU** (formerly called the *corpus spongiosum*) which surrounds and supports the penile urethra and distally forms the *glans penis*. Condensed fibro-elastic tissue, the *tunica albuginea*, invests the cavernous bodies, being thickest around the corpora cavernosa penis which are incompletely separated by a midline septum. This dense collagenous tissue is continuous with the very loose hypodermis **H** which allows the thin penile skin to move freely over the underlying structures. Note the prominent blood vessels of the hypodermis.

Fig. 18.18 Corpus cavernosum urethrae
(H & E × 20)

The erectile tissue of the penis consists of broad vascular lacunae or cavernous sinuses supported by trabeculae of fibro-elastic tissue containing smooth muscle fibres. The lacunae are lined by non-fenestrated vascular endothelium. The penile urethra **U** has an irregular outline due to the presence of deep outpocketings which are continuous with the ducts of simple acinar glands, the *paraurethral glands* **G**.

Fig. 18.19 Penile erectile tissue *(H & E × 128)*

The vascular sinuses **S** of the cavernous bodies of the penis are supplied by numerous anastomosing thick-walled arteries and arterioles called *helicine arteries* **HA** since they follow a spiral course in the flaccid state. Blood drains from the sinuses via veins which lie immediately beneath the dense fibro-elastic tissue investing the cavernous bodies. During erection, dilatation of the helicine arteries, mediated by the parasympathetic nervous system, results in engorgement of the vascular sinuses which enlarge, compressing and restricting venous outflow. The process is enhanced by relaxation of smooth muscle cells in the trabeculae of the cavernous bodies.

Fig. 18.20 Penile urethra

(H & E × 200)

Apart from the prostatic urethra which is lined by transitional epithelium, the male urethra is lined by stratified or pseudostratified columnar epithelium although small areas of stratified squamous epithelium may also be found in human adult males. The external opening (*urethral meatus*) is lined by stratified squamous epithelium which becomes continuous with the skin of the glans.

The urethra is lubricated by mucoid secretions from the paraurethral glands **P** and the *bulbo-urethral glands of Cowper* (see Fig. 18.1) which have a similar, but more discrete, organisation.

Fig. 18.21 Semen

(H & E × 1200)

Semen, the product of ejaculation, consists of spermatozoa and seminal fluid which is derived principally from the seminal vesicles and prostate gland. The volume of each human ejaculate is about 3.5 ml containing from 50–150 million spermatozoa per ml. In normal fertile human males, up to 25% of the ejaculated spermatozoa are abnormal or degenerate forms. By the time of ejaculation, spermatozoa have matured and acquired the property of motility; nevertheless, they remain incapable of fertilising an ovum until after undergoing a process called *capacitation* within the female genital tract. Metabolites for motility are provided in the form of fructose and citrate in the seminal fluid. Note that desquamated cells, prostatic concretions and other tract debris are normal constituents of semen.

19. Female reproductive system

Introduction

The female reproductive system has six major functions:

- Production of female gametes, the ova, by the process of *oogenesis*
- Reception of male gametes, the spermatozoa
- Reception of male gametes, the spermatozoa
- Provision of a suitable environment for the fertilisation of ova by spermatozoa
- Provision of an environment for the development of the fetus
- A means for the expulsion of the developed fetus to the external environment
- Nutrition of the newborn.

These functions are all integrated by an elegant system of hormonal and nervous mechanisms.

The female reproductive system may be divided into three structural units on the basis of function: the ovaries, the genital tract and the breasts.

The *ovaries*, which are the sites of oogenesis, are paired organs lying on either side of the uterus adjacent to the lateral wall of the pelvis. In sexually mature mammals, ova are released by the process of *ovulation* in a cyclical manner either seasonally or at regular intervals throughout the year. This cycle is suspended during pregnancy. The process of ovulation is controlled by the cyclical release of *gonadotrophic hormones* from the anterior pituitary. The ovaries themselves have an endocrine function, secreting the hormones *oestrogen* and *progesterone* which coordinate the activities of the genital tract and breasts with the ovulatory cycle.

The *genital tract* extends from near the ovaries to an opening at the external surface and provides an environment for reception of male gametes, fertilisation of ova, development of the fetus and expulsion of the fetus at birth. The genital tract begins with a pair of *uterine tubes*, also called *oviducts* or *Fallopian tubes*, which conduct ova from the ovaries to the uterus where fetal development occurs. Fertilisation of ova by spermatozoa occurs within the uterine tubes. The uterus is a muscular organ, the mucosal lining of which undergoes cyclical proliferation under the influence of ovarian hormones. This provides a suitable environment for implantation of the fertilised ovum and subsequent development of the placenta via which the developing fetus is nourished throughout gestation. At birth (*parturition*), strong contractions of the muscular uterine wall expel the fetus through the *cervix* into the birth canal or *vagina*. The vagina is an expansile muscular tube specialised for the passage of the fetus to the external environment and the reception of the penis during coitus. At the external opening of the vagina are thick folds of skin, the *labia*, which along with the *clitoris* constitute the *vulva*.

The breasts are highly modified apocrine sweat glands which, in the female, develop at puberty and regress at menopause. During pregnancy, the secretory components expand greatly in size and number in preparation for milk production (*lactation*).

In the non-pregnant state, the female reproductive system undergoes continuous cyclical changes from puberty to menopause. When ovulation is not followed by the implantation of a fertilised ovum, the thickened mucosal lining, the *endometrium*, regresses and a new ovulation cycle commences. In humans, the thickened endometrium is shed in a period of bleeding known as *menstruation*; the first day of bleeding marks the beginning of a new cycle of endometrial proliferation which is known as the *menstrual cycle*. In humans, the menstrual cycle is usually of 28 days duration and ovulation usually occurs at the midpoint of the cycle. The ovulatory and menstrual cycles are integrated by hormones secreted by the ovaries; these hormones also promote cyclical changes in all other parts of the female reproductive system.

In other mammals, the proliferated uterine mucosa is absorbed rather than shed and the female is receptive to the male only during the period of ovulation which is known as *oestrus* (or heat). The remaining part of the cycle is called the *dioestrus* and the whole cycle is known as the *oestrus cycle*.

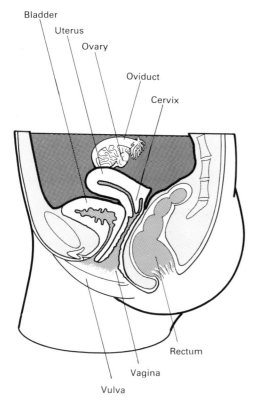

Fig. 19.1 Female reproductive system

(sagittal section)

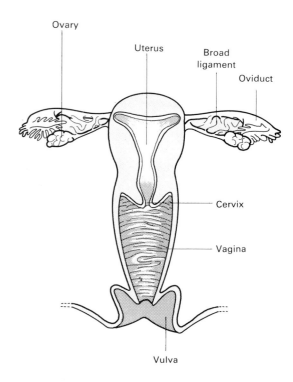

Fig. 19.2 Female reproductive system

(coronal view)

Fig. 19.3 Ovary *(illustrations opposite; (a) Monkey: Azan × 18 (b) Human: H & E × 8)*

The ovaries of all mammals have a similar basic structure. Their overall appearance however varies considerably in accordance with species differences in the pattern of the ovarian cycle and the state in the cycle at which the ovary is examined. These micrographs compare the ovarian appearance of the monkey with that of the human.

The ovaries, which are some 3–5 cm long in humans, have a flattened ovoid shape and are encapsulated by a fibrous tissue layer called the *tunica albuginea*, named for its white appearance on macroscopic examination.

The body of the ovary consists of spindle-shaped cells, fine collagen fibres and ground substance which together constitute the *ovarian stroma*. The stromal cells are mainly fibroblasts but also include bundles of smooth muscle cells. In the peripheral zone of the stroma, known as the *cortex*, are numerous *follicles* which contain female gametes in various stages of development. In addition, there may also be post-ovulatory follicles of various kinds namely corpora lutea (responsible for oestrogen and progesterone production, see Fig. 19.7), degenerate and former corpora lutea (corpora albicantes, see Fig. 19.9) and degenerate (atretic) follicles (see Fig. 19.10).

In the monkey ovary, numerous follicles **F** are seen in various sizes and states of development. In contrast,

developing follicles are difficult to see in the human ovary at this magnification; this human ovary is dominated by an active corpus luteum **CL** and several degenerating corpora lutea **D** and corpora albicantes **A**.

The central zone of the ovarian stroma, the medulla **M**, is highly vascular being supplied by the ovarian artery (a branch of the aorta) and ovarian branches of the uterine artery. These enter the hilum of the ovary from the *broad ligament* **L**, shown in micrograph (a), and branch and coil to become known as *helicine arteries* **H**. Smaller branches form a plexus at the cortico-medullary junction giving rise to straight cortical arterioles which radiate into the cortex. Here they branch and anastomose to form vascular arcades which give rise to a rich network of capillaries around the follicles. Venous drainage follows the course of the arterial system, the medullary veins being particularly large and tortuous. Lymphatics arise in the perifollicular stroma draining to larger vessels which coil around the medullary veins. Innervation of the ovary is by sympathetic fibres which not only supply blood vessels but also terminate on smooth muscle cells in the stroma around the follicles possibly playing some part in follicular maturation and ovulation. In micrograph (b), the nearby oviduct **O** is included in the plane of section.

(a)

(b)

Follicular development

During early fetal development, primordial germ cells called *oogonia* migrate into the ovarian cortex where they multiply by mitosis. By the fourth and fifth months of human fetal development, some oogonia enlarge and assume the potential for development into mature gametes. At this stage they become known as *primary oocytes* and commence the first stage of meiotic division (see Ch. 2). By the seventh month of fetal development, the primary oocytes become encapsulated by a single layer of flattened *follicular cells* of epithelial origin to form *primordial follicles* of which there are some four hundred thousand in the human ovary at birth. This encapsulation arrests the first meiotic division and no further development of primordial follicles then occurs until after the female reaches sexual maturity. The process of meiotic division is only completed during follicular maturation leading up to ovulation and fertilisation. Thus all the female germ cells are present at birth but the process of meiotic division is only completed some 15 to 50 years later! In contrast, in males, meiotic division of germ cells commences only after sexual maturity and formation and maturation of spermatozoa is accomplished within about 70 days (see Ch. 18). Female germ cells may undergo degeneration (*atresia*) at any stage of follicular maturation.

During each ovarian cycle, a cohort of up to 20 primordial follicles is in some way activated to begin the maturation process; nevertheless, usually only one follicle reaches full maturity and is ovulated whilst the remainder undergo atresia before this point. The reason for this apparent wastage is unclear; during maturation, however, the follicles have an endocrine function which may be far beyond the capacity of a single follicle and the primary purpose of the other follicles may be to act as an endocrine gland.

Follicular maturation involves changes in the oocyte, the follicular cells and the surrounding stromal tissue. Follicular maturation is stimulated by the gonadotrophic hormone FSH (follicle stimulating hormone) secreted by the anterior pituitary gland.

Fig. 19.4 Ovarian cortex *(Azan × 120)*

This micrograph, taken from a monkey, shows the typical appearance of follicles in the ovarian cortex and illustrates several stages in early follicular development.

In the mature ovary, undeveloped follicles exist as *primordial follicles* **PF** which are composed of a *primary oocyte* surrounded by a single layer of flattened *follicular cells*. The primary oocyte has a large nucleus with dispersed finely granular chromatin, a prominent nucleolus and little cytoplasm.

At the lower right of the field, a primordial follicle has been stimulated, increasing in size to form a *primary follicle*; its oocyte O_1 has greatly enlarged and the follicular cells **F** have multiplied by mitosis becoming cuboidal in shape; they are now also known as *granulosa cells*. A thick homogeneous layer of glycoprotein and acid proteoglycans, the *zona pellucida* **ZP**, develops between the oocyte and the follicular cells; both cell types probably contribute to its formation.

With further follicular development as seen in the large follicle at lower left, the surrounding stromal cells begin to form an organised layer around the follicle called the *theca folliculi* **TF** separated from the follicular cells by a basement membrane. The primary follicle continues to enlarge and the follicular cells proliferate to form a layer several cells thick called the *zona granulosa* **ZG**.

Note also in this micrograph, the fibrous tunica albuginea **TA** and the single layer of cuboidal or columnar epithelial cells **E** on the surface of the ovary. This epithelial layer is continuous with the mesothelial lining of the peritoneal cavity and was formerly known as the *germinal epithelium* from the mistaken belief that these cells were the origin of the female germ cells.

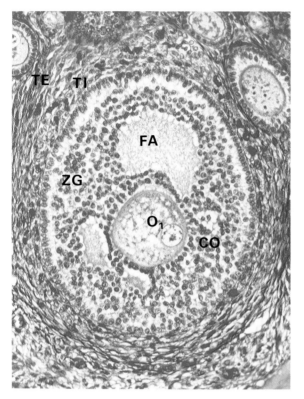

Fig. 19.5 Secondary follicle (*Azan* × 120)

Primary follicles continue to develop, acquiring the features seen in this micrograph and becoming known as *secondary follicles*; by now they are usually situated deeper in the ovarian cortex.

The zona granulosa **ZG** has proliferated greatly and within it appears a space, called the *follicular antrum* **FA**, in which follicular fluid accumulates. At this stage, the oocyte O_1 has almost reached its mature size and becomes situated eccentrically in a thickened area of the granulosa called the *cumulus oophorus* **CO**.

Externally, the former theca folliculi has differentiated into two layers, the *theca interna* **TI** comprising several layers of rounded cells and the less well defined *theca externa* **TE** consisting of spindle-shaped cells which merge with the surrounding stroma.

The cells of the theca interna have the features of typical steroid-secreting cells (see Fig. 17.16) and secrete oestrogen precursors (e.g. androstenedione), oestrogen and, in the preovulatory stage, progesterone. Follicular hormones promote proliferation of the uterine mucosa in readiness for the implantation of a fertilised ovum. The theca externa is composed of flattened stromal cells and has no endocrine function. The granulosa cells also have an endocrine function which begins at the stage of antral formation; oestrogen is produced from precursors secreted by the theca interna as well as small amounts of *intrafollicular FSH* and (at ovulation) the FSH inhibitor, *inhibin F*.

Fig. 19.6 Graafian follicle (*Azan* × 75)

Approaching maturity, further growth of the oocyte ceases and the first meiotic division is completed just before ovulation. At this stage, the oocyte becomes known as the secondary oocyte and commences the second meiotic division. The first polar body (see Ch. 2), containing very little cytoplasm, remains inconspicuously within the zona pellucida. The follicular antrum **FA** enlarges markedly and the zona granulosa **ZG** now forms a layer of even thickness around the periphery of the follicle. The cumulus oophorus diminishes leaving the oocyte O_2 surrounded by a layer several cells thick, the *corona radiata* **CR**, which remains attached to the zona granulosa by thin bridges of cells. Before ovulation, these bridges break down and the oocyte, surrounded by the corona radiata, floats free inside the follicle. Note the surrounding theca interna **TI** consisting of plump steroid-secreting cells. By this stage the follicle has reached between 1.5 and 2.5 centimetres in diameter and bulges under the ovarian surface. The overlying surface epithelial cells are flattened and atrophic and the thin intervening stroma becomes degenerate and avascular.

At ovulation, the mature follicle ruptures and the ovum, comprising the secondary oocyte, zona pellucida and corona radiata, is expelled into the peritoneal cavity near the entrance to the uterine tube. The second meiotic division of the oocyte is not completed until after penetration of the ovum by a spermatozoon.

DEVELOPMENTAL EVENTS

DEVELOPMENTAL STAGE

Migration to ovarian cortex
6th week of fetal development

Multiplication by mitosis

Some oogonia develop the potential
to become mature female gametes.
Encapsulation by follicular cells
First stage of meiotic division
arrested

BIRTH

No further follicular development until
sexual maturity

SEXUAL MATURITY

Secretion of pituitary gonadotrophins
FSH & LH
Some primordial follicles develop
towards maturity with each ovarian
cycle

Increasing secretion of oestrogen
progressively inhibits release
of FSH and promotes LH release

First meiotic division completed

Second meiotic division commences

High levels of oestrogen inhibit
FSH release and promotes large
release of LH

OVULATION

Progesterone secretion by
corpus luteum maintained by LH

Inhibition of LH secretion by progesterone

FERTILISATION

IMPLANTATION

Corpus luteum of pregnancy maintained
by HCG secreted by developing embryo

Primordial germ cells (oogonia)

Primordial follicles containing primary oocytes

Primordial follicle

Primary follicle

Early primary follicle

Secondary follicle

Graafian follicle
(now contains secondary
oocyte)

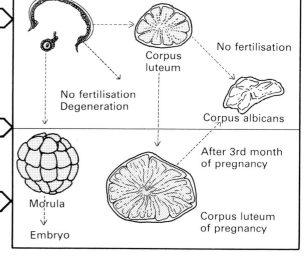

Corpus
luteum

No fertilisation

No fertilisation
Degeneration

Corpus albicans

After 3rd month
of pregnancy

Morula

Embryo

Corpus luteum
of pregnancy

Fig. 19.7 Follicular development

(a)

(b)

Fig. 19.8 Corpus luteum *(H & E (a) × 42 (b) × 3)*

Following ovulation, the ruptured follicle collapses and fills with a blood clot and the layers of the follicular wall become re-organised to form a temporary endocrine gland, the *corpus luteum of menstruation*; in size it approximates that of the antecedent ovulatory follicle, i.e. 1.5–2.5 cm. Under the influence of luteinising hormone (LH) secreted by the anterior pituitary, the cells of the former zona granulosa increase greatly in size and begin secretion of progesterone. The cytoplasm of these cells contains a bright yellow pigment (lutein) which gives rise to the name *granulosa lutein cells* and the name corpus luteum to the whole structure. Progesterone promotes exocrine secretion by glands in the uterine endometrium which have by now greatly proliferated under the influence of the oestrogens secreted by the follicle before ovulation. This provides a suitable environment for the implantation of a fertilised ovum.

The cells of the former theca interna also increase in size but to a lesser extent. Although interrupted by ovulation, these cells (as well as the granulosa cells) continue to secrete oestrogens, which are necessary to maintain the thickened uterine mucosa. These cells become known as *theca lutein cells*.

The blood clot, granulosa lutein and the theca lutein layers are invaded by capillaries and larger vessels from the former theca externa to form a rich vascular network characteristic of endocrine glands.

The corpus luteum is dependent on the secretion of LH from the anterior pituitary; however, rising levels of progesterone inhibit LH secretion. Without the continuing stimulus of LH, the corpus luteum cannot be maintained and 12–14 days after ovulation it regresses ultimately forming a functionless *corpus albicans* (see Fig. 19.11). Once

the corpus luteum regresses, secretion of both oestrogen and progesterone ceases. Without these hormones the endometrial lining of the uterus collapses resulting in the onset of menstruation.

Implantation of a fertilised ovum in the uterine wall interrupts the integrated ovarian and menstrual cycles. After implantation, a hormone called *human chorionic gonadotrophin (HCG)* is secreted into the maternal circulation by the developing placenta. HCG has an analogous function to that of LH and maintains the function of the corpus luteum in secreting oestrogen and progesterone until about the twelfth week of pregnancy. After this time, the *corpus luteum of pregnancy* slowly regresses to form a functionless corpus albicans and the placenta takes over the major role of oestrogen and progesterone secretion until parturition.

Micrograph (a) shows a corpus luteum of menstruation. In the centre, the remnant of the post-ovulatory blood clot **B** is seen surrounded by a broad zone of granulosa lutein cells **G** penetrated by septa **S** containing the larger blood vessels. Peripherally, a thin zone of theca lutein cells **T** can be seen. Externally, the corpus luteum is bounded by a zone of condensed stromal tissue representing the theca externa of the antecedent Graafian follicle.

The corpus luteum of pregnancy is a much larger structure than the corpus luteum of menstruation but has a similar basic organisation.

Micrograph (b) shows a human ovary during the first trimester of pregnancy. The corpus luteum **CL** is greatly enlarged compared with that of the second half of the menstrual cycle and by now occupies most of the ovary. Note the adjacent oviduct **O**.

(a)

(b)

Fig. 19.9 Corpus luteum *(H & E (a) × 100 (b) × 400)*

Micrograph (a) shows the margin of a corpus luteum at moderately high magnification. Most of the field is occupied by granulosa lutein cells **G**, the large polygonal cells containing abundant pale eosinophilic (pink stained) cytoplasm. At the periphery are the more intensely stained theca lutein cells **T** with a finger-like extension penetrating the granulosa forming a sheath **S** surrounding a small vascular septum.

At high magnification in micrograph (b), granulosa lutein cells **G** may be compared with theca lutein cells **T**. The pale stained cytoplasm of the granulosa lutein cells contains numerous small lipid droplets which give rise to the vacuolated appearance seen in this preparation; their large spherical nuclei contain one or two prominent nucleoli.

As previously described, the granulosa lutein cells secrete progesterone and the theca lutein cells secrete oestrogen. Theca lutein cells are smaller, with a more densely staining, less vacuolated cytoplasm; their irregular ovoid nucleus has a single large nucleolus. The ultrastructure of the endocrine cells of the corpus luteum is characteristic of all steroid secretory cells (see Fig. 17.16).

(a)

(b)

Fig. 19.10 Atretic follicles *(H & E (a) × 128 (b) × 128)*

The process of follicular atresia (degeneration) may occur at any stage in the development of the ovum. By the sixth month of development, the fetal ovary contains several million primordial follicles, yet by the time of birth less than half a million remain. Atresia continues until puberty and thereafter through the reproductive years.

In addition, with each ovarian cycle approximately 20 follicles begin to mature, usually all but one becoming atretic at some stage before complete maturity.

The histological appearance of *atretic follicles* varies enormously, depending on the stage of development reached and the progress of atresia. The atretic follicle seen in micrograph (a) is a secondary follicle in early atresia; the oocyte **O** has degenerated and the granulosa cells **G** have begun to disorganise. Advanced atresia, as seen in micrograph (b),is characterised by gross thickening of the basement membrane between the granulosa cells and the theca interna forming the so-called *glassy membrane* **GM**. Atretic follicles are ultimately replaced completely by collagenous tissue.

Fig. 19.11 Corpus albicans *(H & E × 20)*

The corpus albicans is the inactive fibrous tissue mass which forms following the involution of a corpus luteum. The secretory cells of the degenerate corpus luteum undergo autolysis and are phagocytosed by macrophages. The vascular supporting tissue regresses to form a relatively acellular collagenous scar which eventually merges with the surrounding ovarian stroma.

In the human ovary, corpora albicantes are a dominant feature, increasing in number with age and often appearing to occupy almost the whole ovarian stroma.

The genital tract

The genital tract consists of the oviducts, uterus and vagina, all of which have the same basic structure: a wall of smooth muscle, an inner mucosal lining and an outer layer of loose supporting tissue. The mucosal and muscular components vary greatly according to their location and functional requirements; the whole tract undergoes cyclical changes under the influence of ovarian hormones released during the ovarian cycle.

The cyclical changes in the genital tract facilitate the entry of ova into the oviduct, the passage of spermatozoa through the uterine cervix and up into the oviduct, the passage of the fertilised ovum into the uterus and the implantation and development of the fertilised ovum in the mucosal lining (endometrium) of the uterine wall. Implantation of a fertilised ovum results in the secretion of hormones which inhibit the ovarian cycle and produce the changes in the genital tract necessary for fetal development and parturition.

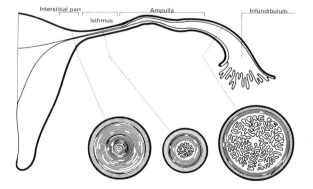

Fig. 19.12 Oviduct

The oviducts (also called uterine tubes or Fallopian tubes) conduct ova from the surface of the ovaries to the uterine cavity and are also the site of fertilisation by spermatozoa. The oviduct is shaped like an elongated funnel and is divided anatomically into four parts as shown in the diagram.

The *infundibulum* moves so as to overlie the site of rupture of the Graafian follicle at ovulation; finger-like projections called *fimbriae* extending from the end of the tube envelop the ovulation site and direct the ovum into the tube. Movement of the ovum down the tube is mediated by gentle peristaltic action of the longitudinal and circular smooth muscle layers of the oviduct wall; this is aided by a current of fluid propelled by the action of the ciliated epithelium lining the tube. Fertilisation usually occurs in the *ampulla*.

Fig. 19.13 Oviduct *(H & E (a) × 10 (b) × 150 (c) × 600 (d) Azan × 320)*

The mucosal lining of the oviduct is thrown into a labyrinth of branching, longitudinal folds which provide a suitable environment for fertilisation. This feature is most prominent in the ampullary part of the tube as shown in micrograph (a) which is from a specimen obtained during female sterilisation. Note also in this micrograph, the muscular wall **M** and the vascular supporting tissue of the serosa **S** which is continuous with the broad ligament **BL**.

Micrograph (b) focuses on one of the mucosal folds of the ampulla. These have a branching core of vascular supporting tissue **S** and are invested by a single layer of tall columnar epithelial cells **E**.

Micrograph (c) shows the tip of a mucosal fold at high magnification. The columnar cells of the epithelium are of two types, ciliated and non-ciliated. The non-ciliated cells produce a secretion which is propelled towards the uterus by the more numerous ciliated cells, carrying with it the ovum. This secretion probably also has a role in the nutrition and protection of the ovum. The ratio of ciliated to non-ciliated cells and the height of the cells undergo cyclical variations under the influence of ovarian hormones. The ciliated cells are generally shorter than the secretory cells making the epithelial surface somewhat irregular in outline. Micrograph (d) employs a method which stains the secretory cells blue. Note that the collagen of the core of lamina propria is also stained blue.

The human menstrual cycle

The uterus is a flattened pear-shaped organ approximately 7 cm long in the non-pregnant state. Its mucosal lining, the *endometrium*, provides the environment for fetal development; the thick smooth muscle wall, the *myometrium*, expands greatly during pregnancy and provides protection for the fetus and a mechanism for the expulsion of the fetus at parturition.

The endometrial lining of the uterine cavity consists of a simple columnar ciliated epithelium supported by a cellular stroma containing numerous simple tubular glands. Under the influence of oestrogen and progesterone secreted by follicles during the ovarian cycle, the endometrium undergoes regular cyclical changes so as to offer a suitable environment for implantation of a fertilised ovum. For successful implantation, the fertilised ovum requires an easily penetrable, highly vascular tissue and an abundant supply of glycogen for nutrition until vascular connections are established with the maternal environment.

The cycle of changes in the endometrium proceeds through two distinct phases, proliferation and secretion; these changes involve both the epithelium and supporting stroma.

- **The proliferative phase**: the endometrial stroma proliferates becoming deep and richly vascularised. The simple tubular glands proliferate to form numerous glands which begin secretion coincident with ovulation. The proliferative phase is initiated and sustained until ovulation by the increasing production of oestrogens from developing ovarian follicles.

- **The secretory phase**: release of progesterone from the corpus luteum after ovulation promotes production of copious thick glycogen-rich secretion by the endometrial glands.

Unless implantation of a fertilised ovum occurs, the continuing production of progesterone is inhibited by negative feedback upon the anterior pituitary, thus suppressing LH release leading to involution of the corpus luteum. In the absence of progesterone, the endometrium is unable to be maintained and most of it is shed during the period of bleeding known as menstruation. Activation of FSH secretion initiates a new cycle of follicular development and oestrogen secretion; this, in turn, initiates a new cycle of proliferation of the uterine mucosa from the remnants of the endometrium of the previous cycle. Although the process of menstruation represents the end-point of the cycle of endometrial changes, the first day of menstruation also marks the beginning of a new proliferative phase. Furthermore, being the most easily recognisable point it is usually taken to mark the first day of the 28-day menstrual cycle. Menstruation is usually completed by the fifth day; the proliferative phase continues until about the fourteenth day. Ovulation, which usually occurs at the fifteenth day, marks the beginning of the secretory phase which culminates in menstruation about the twenty-eighth day.

The endometrium is divided into three histologically and functionally distinct layers. The deepest or basal layer, the *stratum basalis*, adjacent to the myometrium, undergoes little change during the menstrual cycle and is not shed during menstruation. The broad intermediate layer is characterised by a stroma with a spongy appearance and is called the *stratum spongiosum*. The thinner superficial layer which has a compact stromal appearance is known as the *stratum compactum*. The compact and spongy layers exhibit dramatic changes throughout the cycle and are both shed during menstruation; hence they are jointly referred to as the *stratum functionalis*.

The arrangement of the arterial supply of the endometrium has important influences on the menstrual cycle. Branches of the uterine arteries pass through the myometrium and immediately divide into two different types of arteries, *straight arteries* and *spiral arteries*. Straight arteries are short and pass a small distance into the endometrium then bifurcate to form a plexus supplying the stratum basalis. Spiral arteries are long, coiled and thick walled and pass to the surface of the endometrium giving off numerous branches which give rise to a capillary plexus around the glands and in the stratum compactum. Unlike the straight arteries, the spiral arteries are responsive to the hormonal changes of the menstrual cycle. The withdrawal of progesterone secretion at the end of the cycle causes the spiral arteries to constrict and this precipitates an *ischaemic phase* which immediately precedes menstruation.

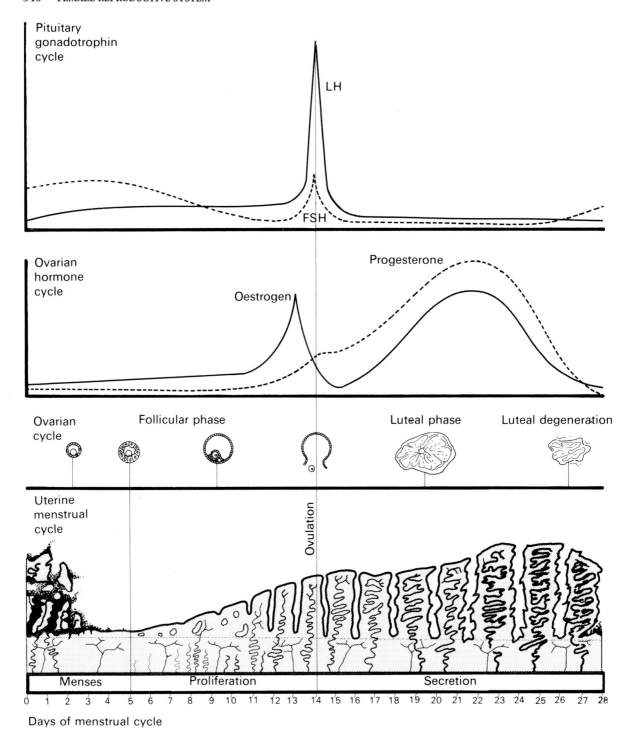

Fig. 19.14 The hormonal integration of the ovarian and menstrual cycles

Fig. 19.15 Proliferative endometrium
Early phase *(H & E (a) × 8 (b) × 100 (c) × 400)*; **Late phase** *(H & E (d) × 10 (e) × 100 (f) × 400)*

Micrograph (a) illustrates early proliferative endometrium at low magnification. At the bottom of the field is the muscular wall, the myometrium **M**. The relatively thin endometrium consists of the stratum basalis **B**, stratum spongiosum **S** and stratum compactum **C**. At this early proliferative stage, the stroma of the stratum functionalis (spongiosum and compactum) has proliferated but the simple tubular glands have as yet barely elongated into the stratum compactum.

At higher magnification in micrograph (b), the simple tubular form of the endometrial glands can be seen. At very high magnification in micrograph (c), the proliferating glandular epithelium is seen to consist of columnar cells with basally located nuclei exhibiting prominent nucleoli. Occasional mitotic figures **M** can be seen. Note the highly

cellular stroma almost devoid of collagen fibres.

By the late proliferative stage shown at low magnification in micrograph (d), the glands have extended to open onto the endometrial surface and the endometrium has doubled in thickness. Note that in contrast to the stratum functionalis **F**, the appearance of the stratum basalis **B** is little changed when compared with the early proliferative phase. With further magnification, micrograph (e) shows that the tubular glands are now becoming somewhat convoluted whilst, at very high magnification in micrograph (f), mitotic figures **M** are more prevalent in both the glandular epithelium and the supporting stroma. At this stage the glandular epithelium may have a pseudostratified appearance.

(a)   (b)   (c)

(d)   (e)   (f)

Fig. 19.16 Secretory endometrium

Early phase *(H & E (a) × 8 (b) × 100 (c) × 400);* **Late phase** *(H & E (d) × 8 (e) × 100 (f) × 400)*

Ovulation marks the onset of the secretory phase although endometrial proliferation continues for several days. At low magnification in micrograph (a), the glands are seen to have developed an irregular corkscrew configuration and the endometrium approaches its maximum thickness.

Under the influence of progesterone, the glandular epithelium is stimulated to synthesise glycogen. Initially the glycogen accumulates to form vacuoles in the basal aspect of the cells, thus displacing the nuclei towards the centre of the now tall columnar cells. This *basal vacuolation* of the cells is the characteristic feature of early secretory endometrium as seen at intermediate and high magnification in micrographs (b) and (c) respectively.

Glycogen is an important source of nutrition for the fertilised ovum.

As seen at low magnification in micrograph (d), the late secretory phase is characterised by a saw-tooth appearance of the glands which contain copious thick glycogen-rich secretions. This rather ragged, tortuous coiling is shown at higher magnification in micrograph (e).

At very high magnification in micrograph (f), basal vacuolation is not now evident in the glandular epithelium since active secretion is taking place and the cells are pale, irregular and bloated with glycogen. Mitotic figures are absent. The stroma is by now at its most vascular and interstitial fluid begins to accumulate between the stromal cells.

(a)

(b)

(c)

Fig. 19.17 Endometrium: onset of menstruation *(H & E (a) × 8 (b) × 100 (c) × 400)*

In the absence of implantation of a fertilised ovum, degeneration of the corpus luteum results in cessation of oestrogen and progesterone secretion which initiates phases of spasmodic constriction in the spiral arterioles of the endometrial stratum functionalis. The resulting ischaemia is initially manifest by degeneration of the superficial layers of the endometrium and leakage of blood into the stroma; this is seen in micrographs (a) and (b).

Further ischaemia leads to degeneration of the whole stratum functionalis which is progressively shed as *menses*. Menses is thus composed of blood, glandular epithelium and stromal elements. Normally, menses does not clot due to the local release of inhibitory (anticoagulant) factors. At high magnification in micrograph (c), the glandular and stromal cells are seen to be irregular and degenerate and neutrophils **N** have infiltrated both glands and stroma.

Fig. 19.18 Endometrial surface *(H & E × 600)*

This micrograph illustrates the surface epithelium of the endometrium which is tall columnar in form. Some of the cells bear cilia, the remainder having surface microvilli. The stroma is also well illustrated, the stromal cells being plump with cytoplasmic extensions similar to those of primitive mesenchymal cells. The specimen was obtained during the proliferative phase and mitotic figures **M** are frequent in the stroma.

(a)

(b)

(c)

(d)

Fig. 19.19 Post menopausal endometrium *(H & E (a) ×60 (b) ×60 (c) ×150 (d) ×400)*

After the menopause, the cyclical production of oestrogen and progesterone from the ovaries ceases and the whole genital tract undergoes atrophic changes. As seen in micrograph (a), the endometrium **E** is reduced to the former stratum basalis and the glands **G** are sparse and inactive. As shown in micrograph (b), in some women the glands become dilated to form cystic spaces **C** filled with fluid; the reason for this is unknown but this appearance is so common as to be considered a normal variant.

As shown at higher magnifications in micrographs (c) and (d), the glandular epithelial cells are cuboidal or near columnar with no features of proliferation (i.e. no mitotic figures) or secretory activity. The epithelium which lines cystically dilated glands **D**, as shown in micrograph (c), is often flattened. The stroma **S** is much less cellular than during the reproductive years and no mitotic activity is seen.

The myometrium also becomes atrophic after the menopause and the uterus shrinks to half its former size.

(a)

(b)

Fig. 19.20 Myometrium

(H & E (a) × 150 (b) × 400)

The main bulk of the uterus consists of smooth muscle, the myometrium, which is composed of interlacing bundles of long slender fibres arranged in ill-defined layers; this is readily seen in micrograph (a) which contains bundles of fibres in transverse **T**, longitudinal **L** and oblique section **O**. Within the muscle is a rich network of arteries and veins supported by dense collagenous tissue. Micrograph (b) shows detail of the smooth muscle cells at high magnification, highlighting the closeness with which the muscle fibres are packed.

During pregnancy, the myometrium increases greatly in size by both cell division (*hyperplasia*) and cell growth (*hypertrophy*).

At parturition, strong contractions of the myometrium are reinforced by the action of the hormone oxytocin secreted by the posterior pituitary. These contractions expel the fetus from the uterus and also constrict the blood supply to the placenta, thus precipitating its detachment from the uterine wall.

Fig. 19.21 Uterine cervix *(H & E × 200)*

The uterine cervix protrudes into the upper vagina and contains the *endocervical canal* linking the uterine cavity with the vagina. The function of the cervix is to admit spermatozoa to the genital tract at the time when fertilisation is possible, i.e. around the time of ovulation, but at other times, including pregnancy, to protect the uterus and upper tract from bacterial invasion. In addition, the cervix must be capable of great dilatation to permit the passage of the fetal head during parturition.

As seen in this micrograph, the endocervical canal **EC** is lined by a single layer of tall columnar mucus-secreting cells. Where the cervix is exposed to the more hostile environment of the vagina **V**, it is lined by thick stratified squamous epithelium as in the rest of the vagina. The cells of the *ectocervix* often have clear cytoplasm due to their high glycogen content (not apparent in this specimen). The junction **J** between the vaginal and endocervical epithelium is quite abrupt and is normally located at the external os, the point at which the endocervical canal opens into the vagina.

The main bulk of the cervix is composed of tough, collagenous tissue containing relatively little smooth muscle. Beneath the squamo-columnar junction, the cervical stroma is often infiltrated with leucocytes forming part of the defence against ingress of microorganisms.

Fig. 19.22 Cervical cytology *(Papanicolou method × 400)*

The cervical stroma is influenced by the ovarian hormones, particularly oestrogens, which soften the tissues by reducing collagenous cross-linkages and increasing uptake of water by the ground substance. At its most extreme, this provides the means by which the cervix stretches, thins and dilates in late pregnancy and during parturition. To a much lesser extent, similar changes occur during the normal menstrual cycle. One such effect is that the volume of the cervical stroma varies during each cycle causing eversion of the columnar epithelium near the squamo-columnar junction exposing it to the vaginal environment. This induces the growth of stratified squamous epithelium over the exposed area accounting for the red *ectropion* ('erosions') of the cervix often seen in normal women of reproductive age. The importance of this *transformation zone* is that it may undergo malignant change causing cancer of the cervix.

This area can be studied by scraping cells from the surface with a wooden spatula, smearing them on a glass slide, and staining them by the Papanicolou method (cervical smear or 'Pap test'); this technique is known as *exfoliative cytology* and is demonstrated here from a normal healthy cervix. The surface cells of the stratified squamous epithelium have contracted nuclei and are stained pink due to a small content of keratin; the deeper cells have plump nuclei of normal appearance and the cytoplasm is stained blue.

(a)   *(b)*

Fig. 19.23 Endocervical glands *(H & E (a) × 60 (b) × 100)*

As seen in micrograph (a), the mucus-secreting epithelial lining of the endocervical canal is thrown into deep furrows and tunnels giving the appearance of branched tubular glands and giving rise to the rather inaccurate term *endocervical glands*. The columnar mucus-secreting cells lining the 'glands' are shown at higher magnification in micrograph (b). Note the leucocytic infiltrate in the stroma and the presence of leucocytes in the endocervical mucus on the surface.

During the menstrual cycle, the endocervical glands

undergo cyclical changes in secretory activity. In the proliferative phase, rising levels of oestrogen promote secretion of thin watery mucus which permits the passage of spermatozoa into the uterus around the period of ovulation. Following ovulation, the cervical mucus becomes highly viscid forming a plug which inhibits the entry of microorganisms (and spermatozoa) from the vagina; this is particularly important should pregnancy occur. These changes in the quality of the cervical mucus form the basis for one of the 'natural' methods of contraception.

(a)

(b)

Fig. 19.24 Vagina *(Masson's trichrome (a) × 75 (b) × 128)*

The vagina is a fibromuscular canal and, as seen in micrograph (a), the wall consists of a mucosal layer lined by stratified squamous epithelium **E**, a layer of smooth muscle **SM** and an outer adventitial layer **A**. In the relaxed state, the vaginal wall collapses to obliterate the lumen and the vaginal epithelium is thrown up into folds. The dense lamina propria **LP** contains many elastic fibres, has a rich plexus of small veins and is devoid of glands. The vagina is lubricated by cervical mucus, a fluid transudate from the rich vascular network of the lamina propria and mucus secreted by glands of the labia minora. The smooth muscle bundles of the muscular layer are arranged in ill-defined circular and longitudinal layers; the longitudinal layers predominate especially in the outer region.

The combination of a muscular layer and a highly elastic lamina propria permits the gross distension which occurs during parturition. Conversely after coitus, involuntary contraction of the smooth muscle layer ensures that a pool of semen remains in the cervical region. Thick elastic fibres in the outer adventitial layer also facilitate these functions.

Micrograph (b) illustrates the stratified squamous epithelium which lines the vagina. During the menstrual cycle, this epithelium undergoes cyclical changes which includes slight keratinisation of the superficial cells; histological examination of cells scraped from the surface provides a useful means for estimation of the time of the last ovulation. Throughout the cycle, the superficial cells produce glycogen which is anaerobically metabolised by vaginal commensal bacteria to form lactic acid which inhibits the growth of pathogenic microorganisms.

The placenta

The placenta is formed from elements of the membranes which surround the developing fetus as well as the uterine endometrium and provides the means for physiological exchange between the fetal and maternal circulations. The structure of the placenta varies greatly from one species to another and the following discussion is thus necessarily confined to the human placenta. At various stages during fetal development, the placenta performs a remarkable range of functions until the fetal organs become functional. These include gaseous exchange, excretion, maintenance of homeostasis, hormone secretion, haemopoiesis and hepatic metabolic functions.

FERTILISED OVUM   MORULA (20-50 cells)   BLASTOCYST

Trophoblast
Inner cell mass
Polar trophoblast

Blastomere
Zona pellucida

Fig. 19.25 Fertilisation and implantation *(Diagram (a) above; (b) opposite)*

Within about 12 hours after ovulation, fertilisation of an ovum by a spermatozoon occurs in the ampulla of the oviduct with the formation of a *zygote*; the zona pellucida remains intact (see Fig. 19.4). Within 24 hours, the zygote undergoes its first mitotic cell division, the process continuing over the next 4 to 5 days until there are some 20 to 50 cells called *blastomeres*, each with a small portion of the original cytoplasm. The mass, now called a *morula* (for its resemblance to a mulberry), remains enclosed by the now thinning zona pellucida through which it is nourished by diffusion of oxygen and small molecular weight metabolites from oviduct secretions.

By now the morula has reached the uterus and begins to absorb uterine fluid forming a central cavity. The *blastocyst*, as it is now known, consists of a peripheral layer of blastomeres forming the *trophoblast*, with a mass of cells at one aspect, the *polar trophoblast*, bulging into the central lumen and known as the *inner cell mass*. The trophoblast (along with a maternal contribution) eventually gives rise to the placenta whilst the inner cell mass develops into the future embryo. By this time, the blastocyst has grown to about twice the size of the original ovum and the zona pellucida has become quite thin. When the blastocyst has been within the uterine cavity for two to three days, implantation occurs. The polar trophoblast invades the endometrium so that by the tenth day after ovulation the blastocyst is completely buried. Dissolution of the zona pellucida brings the secretory endometrium into direct contact with the trophoblast which undergoes rapid growth and differentiation.

The trophoblast gives rise to two layers, an inner *cytotrophoblastic layer* of mononuclear cells and an outer *syncytiotrophoblastic layer* derived by fusion of cytotrophoblastic cells to form a continuous multinucleate syncytium in which there is no internal cytoplasmic demarcation by plasma membranes. The cytotrophoblast remains as a single layer of stem cells whereas the syncytiotrophoblast becomes increasingly broad and develops finger-like projections into the endometrium. Within a short time, a sponge-like network of spaces called *lacunae* develops within the syncytiotrophoblast, initially

filled with tissue fluid and uterine secretions. Soon afterwards, invasion by the syncytiotrophoblast causes disintegration of endometrial capillaries with leakage of maternal blood into the lacunae. Progressively the syncytiotrophoblast envelops maternal capillaries expanding the lacuna network and establishing an arterial supply and venous drainage system.

By now, the syncytiotrophoblast also secretes a variety of hormones including *human chorionic gonadotrophin (HCG)*, *human placental lactogen (HPL)*, *oestrogen* and *progesterone* which are necessary to sustain the endometrial tissues. In the meantime, the blastocyst cavity becomes filled with *extraembryonic mesoderm* (mesenchyme) which completely surrounds the early embryo developing from the inner cell mass. The embryo by now comprises plates of *embryonic endoderm* and *ectoderm* on either side of which lie the *yolk sac* and *amniotic cavities* enclosed by *extraembryonic endoderm* and *extraembryonic ectoderm* respectively. Subsequently, a cavity forms within the extraembryonic mesoderm, this *extraembryonic coelom* coming to surround the developing embryo which remains attached to the trophoblast by a *connecting stalk* of extraembryonic mesoderm. The trophoblast, along with the mesodermal layer remaining beneath it, now constitutes the *chorion*.

Meanwhile the *trabeculae* of syncytiotrophoblast between the lacunae are invaded by columns of cytotrophoblastic cells called *primary chorionic villi* which grow out to the periphery and spread out over the interface between the trophoblast and endometrium forming the *cytotrophoblastic shell*. Extraembryonic mesoderm now invades the primary villi which thus develop a mesenchymal core becoming known as *secondary chorionic villi*.

By about two weeks after implantation (i.e. about 20 days after fertilisation), primitive blood vessels begin to develop in the chorionic mesoderm simultaneous with development of the primitive embryonic circulatory system, the embryo now being too large to rely on mere diffusion for its growth and metabolic requirements. When mesenchymal cores of the villi become vascularised they become known as *tertiary villi* (not illustrated).

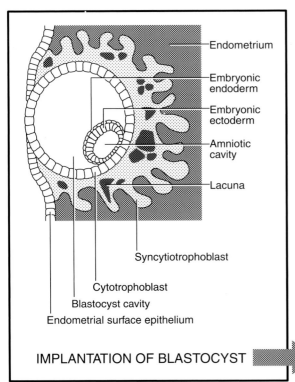

Endometrium

Embryonic
endoderm

Embryonic
ectoderm

Amniotic
cavity

Lacuna

Syncytiotrophoblast

Cytotrophoblast

Blastocyst cavity

Endometrial surface epithelium

IMPLANTATION OF BLASTOCYST

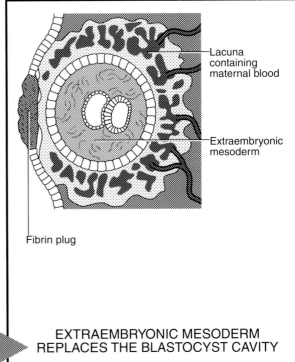

Lacuna
containing
maternal blood

Extraembryonic
mesoderm

Fibrin plug

**EXTRAEMBRYONIC MESODERM
REPLACES THE BLASTOCYST CAVITY**

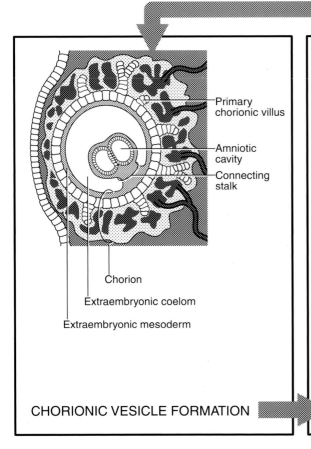

Primary
chorionic villus

Amniotic
cavity

Connecting
stalk

Chorion

Extraembryonic coelom

Extraembryonic mesoderm

CHORIONIC VESICLE FORMATION

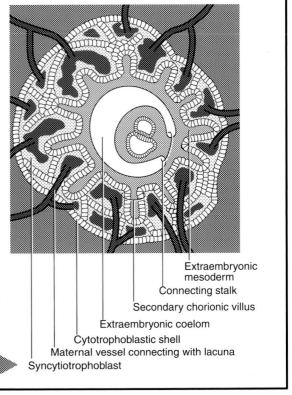

Extraembryonic
mesoderm

Connecting stalk

Secondary chorionic villus

Extraembryonic coelom

Cytotrophoblastic shell

Maternal vessel connecting with lacuna

Syncytiotrophoblast

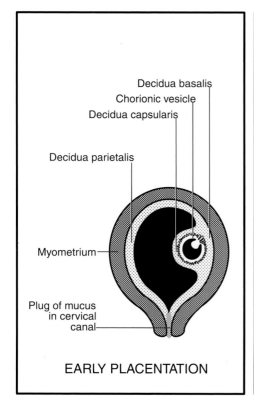

EARLY PLACENTATION

Decidua basalis
Chorionic vesicle
Decidua capsularis
Decidua parietalis
Myometrium
Plug of mucus in cervical canal

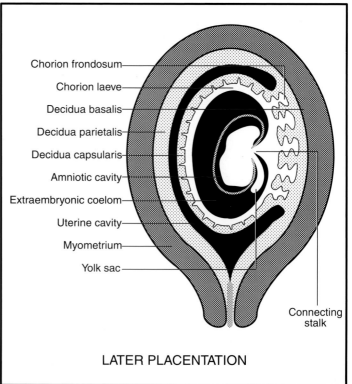

LATER PLACENTATION

Chorion frondosum
Chorion laeve
Decidua basalis
Decidua parietalis
Decidua capsularis
Amniotic cavity
Extraembryonic coelom
Uterine cavity
Myometrium
Yolk sac
Connecting stalk

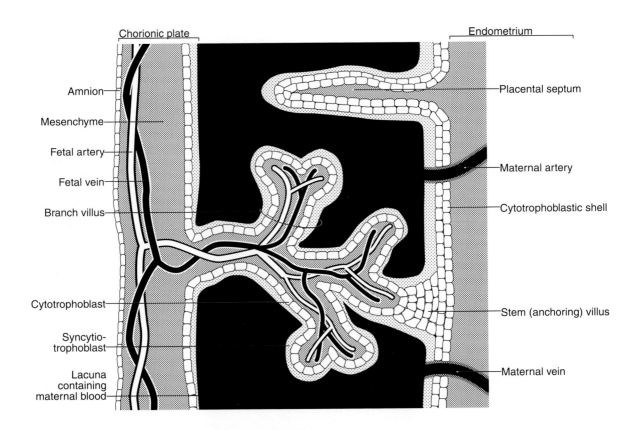

Chorionic plate
Endometrium
Amnion
Mesenchyme
Fetal artery
Fetal vein
Branch villus
Cytotrophoblast
Syncytio-trophoblast
Lacuna containing maternal blood
Placental septum
Maternal artery
Cytotrophoblastic shell
Stem (anchoring) villus
Maternal vein

Fig. 19.26 Decidua formation and early placental development *(illustrations opposite, above)*

During the process of implantation, secretion by the syncytiotrophoblast of HCG (which is functionally analogous to luteinising hormone of the anterior pituitary) interrupts the ovarian cycle. This results in growth and proliferation of stromal cells of the endometrial stratum functionalis at the implantation site into large polyhedral *decidual cells*; this change progressively extends to the whole endometrial lining of the uterus. The *decidua* beneath the developing embryo is known as the *decidua basalis* and with the trophoblast will form the future placenta; that overlying the embryo is known as the *decidua capsularis* and the decidual lining of the rest of the uterus is called the *decidua parietalis*. Ultimately, expansion of the embryo and its enveloping fluid-filled membrane system results in fusion of the opposed capsular and parietal layers of the decidua with complete obliteration of the uterine cavity.

During the first two months of embryological development the chorion, which has an increasingly villous form, grows fairly uniformly around the whole periphery of the vesicle. From the third month, the chorion in contact with the decidua basalis develops extensive frond-like villous outgrowths into the decidua becoming known as the *chorion frondosum*, whilst the superficial chorion in contact with the decidua capsularis atrophies to become the smooth *chorion laeve*. Progressively, the chorion frondosum and decidua basalis develop into the flattened placenta and the vessels connecting the chorion to the embryonic circulation become·the umbilical cord.

Fig. 19.27 Structure of placental villi *(illustration opposite, below)*

From the time maternal blood appears within the trophoblastic lacunae, the trabeculae between the lacunae become increasingly robust with *stem villi* forming anchorage points with the cytotrophoblastic shell. Side branches grow out into the lacunae, progressively forming the complex villous structure characteristic of the mature placenta. Each villus contains a mesenchymal core containing capillaries served by afferent and efferent fetal blood vessels. Between the villous capillaries and the maternal blood is a continuous layer of syncytiotrophoblast supported by a layer of proliferating cytotrophoblast cells (also known as *Langhan's cells*). From the fourth month onwards, the cytotrophoblast layer becomes less active and atrophic so that by fetal maturity it is present in as little as 20% of the villous surface. As more and more branches are added to the villous tree, the villi become smaller and smaller and the tissue barrier between fetal capillaries and maternal blood is greatly diminished.

As the placenta develops, the decidua basalis regresses so that all that remains are a number of anastomosing septa of maternal supporting tissue projecting into the cytotrophoblastic shell. When the placenta is shed immediately after childbirth, its maternal surface is seen to be divided into about 20 irregular segments called *cotyledons* demarcated from each other by the positions of the former maternal (placental) septa. The form of the placenta is essentially established by the end of the fourth month after which the placenta grows in diameter, complementing growth in the size of the uterus.

(a)

(b)

Fig. 19.28 Decidua

(H & E (a) × 100 (b) × 40)

Micrograph (a) illustrates decidual change **D** in the endometrial stroma. The decidual cells proliferate and enlarge greatly, their cytoplasm usually staining pink (eosinophilia) due to the presence of numerous mitochondria. In contrast, cells of the invading trophoblast **T** are strongly basophilic.

Micrograph (b) illustrates early gestational endometrium, the distended glands **G** being extremely rich in glycogen.

(a)

(b)

(c)

Fig. 19.29 Early placenta

(H & E (a) × 30 (b) × 150 (c) × 600)

This series of micrographs at increasing magnification shows a placenta at about 6 weeks gestational age. This can be affirmed by the presence of nucleated fetal erythrocytes in the capillary seen in micrograph (c).

At low magnification in micrograph (a), the main feature is the large numbers of villi **V** projecting into the lacuna system **L** which in vivo would be filled with maternal blood; some villi show evidence of branching.

With further magnification in micrograph (b), the villi are seen to have a highly cellular core of mesenchyme **M**. The villi are invested by trophoblast comprising inner, intensely basophilic cytotrophoblastic cells **C** and a broader, outer syncytiotrophoblastic layer **S**. In some areas, the trophoblast is thick and highly cellular representing areas of budding of the villi to produce further side branches. The specimen is a little broken up as it is derived from a curettage specimen following incomplete spontaneous abortion.

Micrograph (c) focuses on the margin of a villus at high magnification, the cellular preservation being again less than ideal due to its origin from a spontaneous abortion. The syncytiotrophoblastic layer **S** can be distinguished from the single layer of cytotrophoblastic cells **C** which are more intensely basophilic. The mesenchymal cells **M** are large with extensive branching cytoplasmic processes and the intercellular matrix is mucoid due to its high glycosaminoglycan content. Note the nucleated erythrocytes which in humans persist until 9 weeks gestational age.

Fig. 19.30 Trophoblast *(EM × 16 000)*

This micrograph shows the general ultrastructural features of the trophoblastic components; these show considerable variation from one region to another and from early to late stages of placental function.

The syncytiotrophoblast **S** typically presents vast numbers of irregular microvilli **Mv** to the maternal blood spaces **M** greatly enhancing the surface area for physiological exchange. The plasma membranes of the microvilli incorporate a wide variety of enzymes and receptors involved in membrane transfer processes as well as receptors for many hormones and growth factors. Microfilaments extend into the microvilli from a cytoskeletal network concentrated immediately below the free surface. Some areas of the syncytiotrophoblast contain rough endoplasmic reticulum whilst in others, such as shown here,

smooth endoplasmic reticulum **sER** predominates, presumably involved in steroid hormone synthesis.

The cytotrophoblast layer **C** has ultrastructural features of relatively undifferentiated stem cells exhibiting profiles of rough endoplasmic reticulum **rER**, a well defined Golgi **G**, relatively few mitochondria **Mi** and numerous polyribosomes **R** accounting for the intense cytoplasmic basophilia of light microscopy. The nucleus is typically large with dispersed chromatin and nucleoli **Nu**. The cytotrophoblast is typically tightly bound to the overlying syncytiotrophoblast by desmosomes **D** but in some areas, as in this specimen, spaces can be seen between the cell layers; the reason for this is unclear. Separating the cytotrophoblast from the underlying collagenous stroma is a relatively thick basement membrane **BM**.

(a)

(b)

(c)

Fig. 19.31 Term placenta

(H & E (a) × 60 (b) × 150 (c) × 600)

These micrographs illustrate placenta from a full term fetus.

At low magnification in micrograph (a), huge numbers of villi can be seen cut in various planes of section and varying in diameter from large main stem villi to very small terminal branch villi. Compared with early placenta shown in Figure 19.29 (a), the villous pattern is much more highly developed and the average villous diameter much less, reflecting the extensive branching growth of the villi as the placenta enlarges. Note the large vessels **V** in the biggest villi.

Micrograph (b) demonstrates the branching nature of the villi at higher magnification. Compare the marked vascularity of the villous cores with that of the much earlier placenta in Fig. 19.29 (b) and the greatly increased villous surface area exposed to the lacuna **L** filled with maternal blood.

Micrograph (c) focuses on a small branch villus and highlights the proximity of blood in fetal capillaries **C** to maternal blood in the surrounding lacuna **L**. The trophoblast is reduced to a thin layer of syncytiotrophoblast only and the capillaries tend to be located in the periphery of the core. The diffusion barrier between maternal and fetal circulations comprises five layers, namely: trophoblast, trophoblastic basement membrane, core supporting tissue, capillary endothelial basement membrane and endothelium. In many cases (as marked by the arrow), fetal capillaries are so close to the trophoblast that their basement membranes fuse, reducing the diffusion barrier to only three layers.

Fig. 19.32 Fetal membranes *(H & E × 150)*

During early development, the embryo is surrounded by the extraembryonic coelom (see Fig. 19.25) but later this becomes obliterated as the amniotic cavity expands to surround the fetus. The outer mesenchymal layer of the amnion then comes to lie in contact with (and often fuses with) the inner mesenchymal layer of the chorion forming the *chorio-amnion* or fetal membranes. The two layers are often difficult to separate from one another at birth.

The amniotic membrane **Am** comprises a single layer of epithelial cells **E** derived from extraembryonic ectoderm resting on a thick basement membrane **BM**; beneath this is a delicate avascular mesenchymal layer **M** which is a remnant of the extraembryonic mesoderm. The chorionic membrane **C** consists of three layers. A vascular collagenous inner layer **V** is also derived from extraembryonic mesoderm; the *intermediate zone* **In** seen here separating it from the amnion represents the remnant of the extraembryonic coelom and varies greatly in thickness. The trophoblast **T** of the chorion laeve is represented by the middle layer of basophilic epithelial cells and the outermost vascular collagenous layer **D** is of maternal origin representing the decidua capsularis (see Fig. 19.26).

(a)

(b)

Fig. 19.33 Umbilical cord *(H & E (a) × 7.5 (b) × 400)*

The development of the umbilical cord begins with the formation of the extraembryonic coelom which almost surrounds the early embryo and which remains attached to the chorion by the connecting stalk of mesenchyme (see Fig. 19.25). With further embryonic development, the site of attachment of the connecting stalk becomes located ventrally, just caudal to the point where the *vitello-intestinal duct* connects the *yolk sac* to the mid gut. As the embryo grows, the amniotic sac expands greatly, filling the extra embryonic coelom and compressing the vitello-intestinal duct and yolk sac remnant (surrounded by a sleeve of extraembryonic coelom) up against the connecting stalk. These structures ultimately fuse to form the umbilical cord

which now is surrounded by the amnion and amniotic cavity.

By the middle of the fifth month, the remnants of the vitello-intestinal duct, yolk sac and sheath of extraembryonic coelom atrophy and disappear. As seen in micrograph (a), all that remains are two umbilical arteries **A** and a single umbilical vein **V** embedded in mesenchyme consisting mainly of ground substance and known as *Wharton's jelly* **W**. Mesenchymal cells **M** and surface amnion **A** are shown at high magnification in micrograph (b). The umbilical arteries convey deoxygenated fetal blood to the placenta whilst the umbilical vein conveys oxygenated blood back to the fetus.

The breasts

The breasts (mammary glands) are highly modified apocrine sweat glands (see Fig. 9.16) which develop embryologically along two lines, the *milk lines*, extending from the axillae to the groins. In humans, only one gland develops on each side of the thorax although accessory breast tissue may be found anywhere along the milk lines.

The breasts of both sexes follow a similar course of development until puberty, after which the female breasts develop under the influence of pituitary, ovarian and other hormones. Until the menopause, the breasts undergo cyclical changes in activity which are controlled by the hormones of the ovarian cycle. After menopause, the breasts, like the other female reproductive tissues, undergo progressive atrophy and involution.

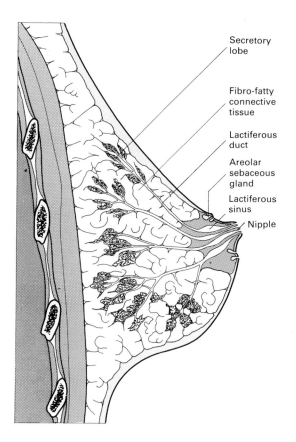

Secretory lobe

Fibro-fatty connective tissue

Lactiferous duct

Areolar sebaceous gland

Lactiferous sinus

Nipple

Fig. 19.34 Structure of the breast

This highly schematic diagram illustrates the general organisation of the breast. Each breast consists of 15 to 25 independent glandular units called *breast lobes*, each consisting of a compound tubulo-acinar gland (see Fig. 5.28). The lobes are embedded in a mass of adipose tissue which is subdivided by collagenous septa. More robust fibrous septa separate the territory of each lobe.

The lobes are arranged radially at different depths around the nipple, a single large duct, the *lactiferous duct*, draining each lobe via a separate opening on the surface of the nipple. Immediately before opening onto the surface, the duct forms a dilatation called the *lactiferous sinus*. The nipple contains bands of smooth muscle orientated parallel to the lactiferous ducts and circularly near the base; contraction of this muscle causes erection of the nipple.

Each breast lobe is divided into a variable number of *breast lobules*, each lobule consisting of a system of ducts, the *alveolar ducts*, from which large numbers of secretory alveoli develop during pregnancy. The lobules are separated by moderately dense collagenous *interlobular* tissue reminiscent of the reticular dermis of the skin (see Fig. 9.6) whereas the *intralobular* supporting tissue surrounding the ducts within each lobule is less collagenous and more cellular like the papillary dermis (see also Fig. 9.6). The skin surrounding the nipple, the *areola*, is pigmented and contains sebaceous glands which are not associated with hair follicles. The secretions of these glands probably help to protect the nipple and areola during suckling.

Fig. 19.35 Breast *(illustrations opposite; H & E (a) × 30 (b) × 60 (c) × 150 (d) × 400 (e) × 400)*

These micrographs show breast tissue from a non-pregnant woman of reproductive age. Micrograph (a) shows most of a breast lobule at low magnification. The extensive branching duct system is surrounded by relatively dense fibrous interlobular tissue **F** at the periphery of which is adipose tissue **A**. The interlacing (reticular) arrangement of the coarse collagen of the interlobular tissue is seen at higher magnification in micrograph (b) as is the arborising duct system of the lobule. Micrograph (c) focuses on a peripheral branching part of the lobule at higher magnification showing well the loose, highly vascular intralobular supporting tissue between the ducts.

The duct system is lined by cuboidal or low columnar epithelial cells **E** with oval nuclei and prominent nucleoli. In the larger ducts, as shown in micrograph (d), these often form two layers whereas in the smaller ducts shown in micrograph (e) there is only a single layer of cells. A discontinuous layer of plump myoepithelial cells **M** with unstained cytoplasm surrounds the ductal lining cells. During the reproductive years, the duct epithelium undergoes cyclical changes under the influence of ovarian hormones. Early in the cycle, the duct lumina are not clearly evident but later in the cycle the lumina become more prominent and may contain an eosinophilic secretion.

(a)

(b)

(c)

(d)

(e)

(a)

(b)

Fig. 19.36 Breast during pregnancy *(H & E (a) × 20 (b) × 128)*

Under the influence of oestrogens and progesterone produced by the corpus luteum and later by the placenta, the alveolar duct epithelium proliferates to form numerous secretory alveoli. Breast proliferation is also dependent on prolactin, human placental lactogen (a prolactin-like hormone produced by the placenta), thyroid hormone and corticosteroids.

At low magnification, the breast lobules **L** are seen to have expanded greatly at the expense of the intralobular tissue and interlobar adipose tissue although septa **S** of interlobular tissue still remain prominent.

As pregnancy progresses, the alveoli begin to secrete a protein-rich fluid called *colostrum*, the accumulation of which dilates the alveolar and duct lumina as seen in micrograph (b). Colostrum is the form of breast secretion available during the first few days after birth; it contains a laxative substance and maternal antibodies. Unlike milk, colostrum contains little lipid. Breast secretion is controlled by the hormone prolactin secreted by the anterior pituitary. During pregnancy, prolactin secretion progressively increases but its activity is suppressed by high levels of circulating oestrogens and progesterone.

(a)

(b)

Fig. 19.37 Lactating breast *(H & E (a) × 20 (b) × 128)*

After parturition, the levels of circulating progesterone and oestrogens fall, thus promoting prolactin activity. Prolactin stimulates milk production in conjunction with several other hormones.

As seen in micrograph (a), the lactating breast is composed almost entirely of alveoli distended with milk, the interlobular tissue now being reduced to thin septa **S** between the lobules. At higher magnification in (b), the alveoli are seen to be filled with an eosinophilic material containing clear vacuoles representing lipid droplets dissolved out during tissue preparation. Some individual alveoli have an appearance reminiscent of thyroid follicles; however, in most cases the irregular branching pattern of the alveoli is clear evidence of an exocrine gland.

Milk production proceeds for as long as suckling continues and can continue for some years after childbirth. The process is mediated by a neuro-hormonal reflex in which nipple stimulation by suckling causes release of prolactin from the anterior pituitary. A different neuro-hormonal reflex, also initiated by suckling, causes the release of the hormone oxytocin from the posterior pituitary. Oxytocin causes contraction of the myoepithelial cells which embrace the secretory alveoli and ducts, thus propelling milk into the lactiferous sinuses. Withdrawal of the suckling stimulus, and hence the release of pituitary hormones at weaning, results in regression of the lactating breast and resumption of the ovarian cycle.

Fig. 19.38 Lactating breast *(EM × 9000)*

This micrograph shows two secretory cells of adjacent
alveoli in a lactating breast. Their nuclei **N** are large with
prominent nucleoli. Each alveolus is bounded by a basement
membrane **BM**, the basement membranes in this example
being separated by only a shred of intralobular tissue.
Between each basement membrane and the secretory cells
are the cytoplasmic processes of myoepithelial cells **M**,
contraction of which expels milk from the gland.

The composition of milk varies somewhat during lactation
and even during each suckling episode but its main
constituents are as follows: water (88%), ions (particularly
sodium, potassium, chloride, calcium and phosphate),
protein (1.5%, mainly lactalbumin and casein),
carbohydrate (7%, mainly lactose), lipids (3.5%, mainly
triglycerides), vitamins and antibodies (of the IgA class).

The water, ions and protein are a serous secretion, the
proteins being synthesised on the rough endoplasmic
reticulum **rER**, packaged in the Golgi apparatus **G** and
secreted in vacuoles **V** by exocytosis; protein in the milk is
represented by extremely electron-dense granules. The
Golgi apparatus is extensive and the protein-containing
secretory vacuoles also contain a considerable amount of
other less electron-dense material probably lactose.

The cytoplasm of the secretory cells contains lipid
droplets **L** of various sizes not bounded by membrane; these
contain triglyceride though whether this is derived directly
from blood or synthesised in the secretory cells is uncertain.
The lipid is discharged by apocrine secretion which involves
the lipid droplet, surrounding cytoplasm and plasma
membrane being cast off into the lumen. A large lipid
droplet L_1 with thin overlying rim of cytoplasm can be seen
in the lower alveolus just prior to secretion; an even larger
droplet L_2 surrounded by a remnant of cytoplasm and
plasma membrane is seen in the lumen close by.

Vitamins and IgA are probably transported across the cell
from the bloodstream in small membranous vesicles.

20. Central nervous system

Introduction

The central nervous system, which consists of the brain and spinal cord, is composed entirely of neurones, their axons and dendrites, and the supporting cells of the CNS, the neuroglial cells; the histology of these and the meninges which invest the CNS are described in Chapter 7.

Macroscopically, sections of any part of the CNS are made up of grey matter and white matter, the grey matter containing most of the neurone cell bodies and the white matter the axons; lipid in the myelin sheaths of the axons accounts for the white appearance of the white matter. The distribution of grey matter and white matter differs greatly from one part of the brain to another as does the morphology and arrangement of the neurones. This chapter provides an outline of the histological features of the main regions of the brain and spinal cord.

The histological methods used in the study of the CNS can be divided into three groups:

- Techniques which demonstrate nuclei, cell bodies and their cytoplasmic constituents. Such methods include routine stains such as H & E and more specific methods for demonstrating particular cytoplasmic constituents such as the Nissl method for RNA. These methods show minimal detail of axons and dendrites. Moreover, since myelin (lipid) is dissolved out during preparation, white matter remains almost unstained by such methods.

- Stains which specifically demonstrate lipid. These *myelin methods*, e.g. Weigart–Pal, are particularly useful for studying the arrangement of grey matter (nuclei) and white matter in the brain stem and spinal cord (see Figs. 20.1–20.3), as well as abnormalities of myelination. With myelin methods, the white matter stains strongly, the grey matter remaining unstained.

- Heavy metal impregnation methods applied to thick tissue sections. These methods (see Fig. 20.7) demonstrate overall cell morphology and are useful for studying the distinctive shapes of neurone cell bodies in various parts of the CNS. They also outline axons and dendrites permitting study of neuronal interconnections. Such methods, which are extremely time consuming and technically exacting, were widely used around the turn of the 20th century by the great pioneers of neuroanatomy such as Cajal and Golgi from whom they take their names.

(a)

(b)

(c)

(d)

Fig. 20.1 Spinal cord *(Cat: Weigart–Pal × 10)*

(a) Cervical (b) Thoracic (c) Lumbar (d) Sacral

The structure of the spinal cord is basically similar throughout its whole length with the four main regions demonstrated in this series of micrographs.

In transverse section, the central mass of grey matter has the shape of a butterfly, the *ventral horns* **V** being most prominent and containing the cell bodies of the large lower motor neurones. The *dorsal horns* **D** are much less prominent and contain the cell bodies of small second order sensory neurones; these relay sensory information to the brain from primary afferent neurones for the modalities of temperature and pain whose cell bodies lie in the dorsal root ganglia. Small *lateral horns* **L**, which contain the cell bodies of preganglionic, sympathetic efferent neurones, are found in the thoracic and upper lumbar regions corresponding to the level of the sympathetic outflow from the cord. The volume of grey matter is much more extensive in the cervical and lumbar regions corresponding to the sensory and motor innervation of the limbs and this is reflected in the much greater diameter of the spinal cord in these areas. The *central canal* lies in the *central commissure* of grey matter; it is lined by ependymal cells and contains CSF.

The white matter of the spinal cord consists of ascending tracts of sensory fibres and descending motor tracts; passing up the spinal cord towards the brain, more and more fibres enter and leave the cord so that the volume of white matter increases progressively from the sacral to cervical regions.

Externally, the spinal cord has a deep *ventral median fissure* **F** but dorsally there is only a shallow dorsal *midline sulcus*. On each side, a *dorso-lateral sulcus* **S** marks the line of entry of the dorsal nerve roots **R** part of which can be seen in micrographs (a) and (c). The roughly triangular area of white matter between the dorsal horns represents the ascending *dorsal columns* which convey fibres for the senses of vibration, proprioception and discriminatory touch to the medulla where they synapse with second order sensory neurones in the *gracile* and *cuneate nuclei*. In the cervical region, each dorsal column is subdivided into two fascicles, the medial *fasciculus gracilis* **FG** conveying fibres from the lower limbs, and the lateral *fasciculus cuneatus* **FC** conveying fibres from the upper limbs.

Ventrolateral sulci **VS** may be discernible on each side as in micrograph (c), marking the sites of exit of the ventral nerve roots.

The ventrolateral white matter on each side is made up of various ascending and descending tracts, most notably the *lateral spinothalamic* tract (pain and temperature), *ventral spinothalamic tract* (light touch), *spinocerebellar tracts* and *corticospinal tract* (motor).

Like the brain, the spinal cord is invested by meninges, the outer surface of the dura mater being loosely connected to the periosteum of the vertebral canal by the denticulate ligaments and the intervening epidural space being filled with loose adipose tissue and an extensive venous plexus. During development, the vertebral column lengthens to a greater degree than the enclosed spinal cord and the segmental levels of the lower part of the cord therefore lie above the corresponding intervertebral foramina. Consequently, below the cervical region, the nerve roots pursue an increasingly oblique course in the subarachnoid space before passing through the intervertebral foramina; thus they can be seen adjacent to the cord particularly in the lumbar and sacral regions.

Fig. 20.2 Medulla oblongata

(Weigart–Pal × 4 (a) Upper-mid level
(b) Lower level)

The medulla oblongata, the most distal
part of the brain stem, can be roughly
divided into upper and lower parts. At
the upper medullary level shown in
micrograph (a), the fourth ventricle **V**
closes to become a narrow central canal
which continues down into the spinal
cord. Thus the medulla is often divided
into an upper, open part and a lower,
closed part. The myelin staining
method employed in these preparations
leaves grey matter relatively unstained.

The most obvious feature of the
upper half of the medulla is the *inferior
olivary nucleus* **O** with its peculiar
convoluted appearance in transverse
section; adjacent are the smaller *dorsal*
D and *medial accessory olivary nuclei* **M**
which complete the *inferior olivary
complex*. The neurones of the inferior
olivary complex relay central and spinal
afferent stimuli to the cerebellar cortex.

All of the ascending (sensory) and
descending (motor) pathways found in
the spinal cord pass through the
medulla, although their arrangement in
the medulla differs considerably from
that in the spinal cord. The most easily
recognisable features of these pathways
in the medulla are the gracile and
cuneate nuclei and fasciculi, and the
pyramids.

The dorsal white matter columns of
the spinal cord convey ascending
proprioceptive, vibration and
discriminatory touch fibres from the
lower limbs and upper limbs in the
fasciculus gracilis **FG** and *fasciculus
cuneatus* **FC** respectively. In the
similarly situated *nucleus gracilis* and
nucleus cuneatus in the dorsum of the
medulla, these fibres synapse with cell
bodies of second order neurones which
then pass upwards to the thalamus via
the *medial lemniscus* **ML** which lies
medial to the olivary complex.

Axons originating in the motor
cortex descend through the *internal
capsule*, break up into small bundles in
the *pons*, then converge again in the
medulla to form a prominent ventral
pyramid **P** on each side of the medulla;
in the pyramids, about 85% of fibres
cross to the other side in the *decussation
of the pyramids*.

The medulla also contains the
various tracts and nuclei of the eighth
to the twelfth cranial nerves as well as
the *spinal nucleus* and *tract* of the
trigeminal nerve which extends from the
pons down into the upper cervical cord.
The spinal nucleus of the trigeminal

(a)

(b)

tract **SNT** is easily recognisable
dorsolaterally throughout the medulla
with its tract of white matter lying
superficially. The *hypoglossal nucleus*
HN can also be identified in
micrograph (a). In the centre of the
lower medulla, grey matter can be seen,
still roughly resembling the
characteristic butterfly shape seen in
sections of the spinal cord; the ventral
grey matter horns contain cell bodies of
lower motor neurones running in the
spinal accessory and first cervical
nerves.

Fig. 20.3 Pons

(Weigart–Pal (a) Mid level × 3
(b) Basal pons × 480)

The pons is the middle portion of the brain stem, lying between midbrain proximally and medulla distally. In transverse section, it comprises two parts, a bulky ventral region (the *basal pons*) and a smaller dorsal (*tegmental*) region.

The basal pons consists of criss-crossed bundles of longitudinal and transverse fibres between which lie collections of neurone cell bodies known as *pontine nuclei*. Micrograph (b) shows a small area of this region at high magnification, the myelin investing the axons being stained blue; neurone cell bodies are not stained and are therefore not identifiable. The longitudinal fibres of the basal pons consist of descending fibres of two main types. Firstly, there are axons from the motor cortex passing down to synapse with lower motor neurones of the ventral horns of the spinal cord; on leaving the pons, these axons converge to form the characteristic pyramids (pyramidal tracts) of the medulla. The second group of descending fibres originate in various areas of the cortex and synapse in the pontine nuclei from which fibres then pass in the transverse bundles, crossing the mid-line to enter the cerebellum via the *middle peduncles* **M**.

The dorsal tegmentum contains the ascending spinothalamic (sensory) tracts and the nuclei of the fifth, sixth and seventh cranial nerves. On each side, the *medial lemniscus* **ML** is readily identifiable; this represents the upward continuation of proprioceptive, vibration and fine touch pathways from the gracile and cuneate nuclei of the medulla. The cerebellar peduncles are a readily recognisable feature of the pons, the middle peduncle being still present in sections through the mid pontine level as in micrograph (a); at this level the superior peduncles **SCP** are very prominent. The main bulk of the superior cerebellar peduncles is made up of fibres from the central nuclei of the cerebellum passing upwards to the thalamus and then projecting to the motor cortex.

(a)

(b)

(a)   (b)   (c)

(d)   (e)

Fig. 20.4 Cerebellum *(H & E (a) × 4 (b) × 20 (c) × 320 (d) Golgi–Cox × 320 (e) Bielschowsky/neutral red × 600)*

The cerebellum, which coordinates muscular activity and maintains posture and equilibrium, consists of a cortex of grey matter with a central core of white matter containing four pairs of nuclei. Afferent and efferent fibres pass to and from the brain stem via inferior, middle and superior cerebellar peduncles linking medulla, pons and midbrain respectively.

As seen in micrograph (a), the cerebellar cortex forms a series of deeply convoluted folds or *folia* supported by a branching central medulla **M** of white matter. At higher magnification in micrograph (b), the cortex is seen to consist of three layers. The outer *molecular layer* **ML** contains relatively few neurones and large numbers of unmyelinated fibres. The inner *granular cell layer* **GL** is extremely cellular. Between the two is a single layer of huge neurones called *Purkinje cells* **P**.

Purkinje cells **P** are seen at higher magnification in micrograph (c); they have very large cell bodies, a relatively fine axon extending down through the granular cell layer **GL**, and an extensively branching dendritic system which arborises into the outer molecular layer **ML**. This extraordinary dendritic system is best demonstrated by heavy metal methods as in micrograph (d).

The deep granular cell layer of the cortex contains numerous small neurones, the non-myelinated axons of which pass outwards to the molecular layer where they bifurcate to run parallel to the surface to synapse with the dendrites of Purkinje cells. Micrograph (e) demonstrates the course of granular cell axons in the molecular layer. The axons **A** are stained black with silver and their cell bodies in the granular cell layer **GL** are counter-stained with neutral red. In addition to the Purkinje **P** and granular cells already described, there are three other types of small neurones in the cerebellar cortex, namely *stellate cells* and *basket cells* scattered in the molecular layer **ML** and *Golgi cells* scattered in the superficial part of the granular cell layer.

In simple terms, afferent fibres enter the cerebellum from the brain stem and then pass via the white matter core to make complex connections with granular cells, Purkinje dendrites and other neurones of the cerebellar cortex; these cortical cells also make numerous interconnections with each other within the molecular layer. The only efferent fibres from the cerebellar cortex are the Purkinje cell axons which pass down through the granular cell layer into the white matter where they synapse in the central nuclei of the cerebellum.

(a)

(b)

Fig. 20.5 Substantia nigra *(H & E (a) × 100 (b) × 400)*

The substantia nigra is a large mass of grey matter extending throughout the midbrain; on each side it divides the cerebral peduncles into dorsal and ventral parts and in sections of the midbrain, as in micrograph (a), it is easily recognised by the black pigment from which its name derives. The substantia nigra has extensive connections with the cortex, spinal cord, corpus striatum and reticular formation and appears to play an important part in the fine control of motor function.

The neurones of the substantia nigra are multipolar in form and in adults the cytoplasm contains numerous granules of melanin pigment as seen in micrograph (b). The pigmented neurones of the substantia nigra contain *dopamine* which appears to act as a neurotransmitter causing inhibitory effects particularly on neurones in the corpus striatum.

DOPA (dihydroxyphenylalanine) is a precursor of dopamine and also of melanin, and the melanin of substantia nigra neurones may merely represent a residual product of normal metabolic activity; this is supported by the fact that very little melanin is present at birth with the amount increasing considerably during childhood and thereafter rising at a slower rate into old age.

Parkinson's disease, a debilitating disorder characterised by tremor, muscular rigidity and impaired speed and precision of motor functions, is associated with degeneration of neurones in the substantia nigra and a marked reduction in dopamine synthesis. Symptoms can be alleviated by the drug L-dopa, a dopamine precursor which crosses the blood–brain barrier.

Fig. 20.6 Thalamus

(H & E × 480)

The thalami are large masses of grey matter lying on each side of the third ventricle and comprising the main bulk of the *diencephalon*, the central core of the cerebrum. Functionally, the thalamus is subdivided into a large number of nuclei including reticular and motor nuclei as well as specific sensory nuclei containing the cell bodies of neurones with axons projecting to the cerebral cortex. The thalamus constitutes an extremely complex relay and integration centre for information from almost all parts of the CNS.

This micrograph shows the histological appearance of a typical thalamic nucleus consisting of a dense aggregation of neurone cell bodies criss-crossed by tracts of afferent and efferent nerve fibres.

(a)

(b)

(c)

(d)

Fig. 20.7 Cerebral cortex *(illustrations opposite; (a) Neurone cell types (b) Methylene blue × 42 (c) Golgi method × 320 (d) Nissl method × 320*

The cerebral hemispheres consist of a convoluted cortex of grey matter overlying the central medullary mass of white matter which conveys fibres between different parts of the cortex and to and from other parts of the CNS.

Histologically, the neurones of the cerebral cortex are divided into five different morphological types which are arranged in several layers. In submammalian species, the major function of the cortex concerns the sense of olfaction (smell) and the neurones are arranged into three layers. In mammals, there has evolved the so-called *neocortex* consisting of six layers of neurones. The neocortex includes the *sensory* and *motor areas* of the cortex as well as the *association cortex* and in humans constitutes about 90% of the cerebral cortex. The primitive three-layered pattern persists only in the olfactory cortex and cortical part of the limbic system in the temporal lobe.

Neurone types in the cerebral cortex
The five characteristic types of cortical neurone are shown diagrammatically in (a), the pyramidal and stellate cells being by far the most common type.

- *Pyramidal cells*, as their name implies, have pyramid-shaped cell bodies, the apex being directed towards the cortical surface. A slender axon arises from the base of the cell and passes into the underlying white matter, though in the case of small superficially-located cells, the axon may synapse in the deep layers of the cortex. From the apex, a thick branching dendrite passes towards the surface where it has an array of fine dendritic branches. In addition, short dendrites arise from the edges of the base and ramify laterally. The size of the pyramidal cells varies from small to large, the smallest tending to lie more superficially. The huge upper motor neurones of the motor cortex, known as *Betz cells*, are the largest of the pyramidal cells in the cortex.
- *Stellate (granule) cells* are small neurones with a short vertical axon and several short branching dendrites giving the cell body the shape of a star; basket and neurogliaform subtypes are also described. With routine histological methods, the cells look like small granules giving rise to their alternative name.
- *Cells of Martinotti* are small polygonal cells with a few short dendrites; the axon extends towards the surface and bifurcates to run horizontally, usually in the most superficial layer.
- *Fusiform cells* are spindle-shaped cells oriented at right angles to the surface of the cerebral cortex. The axon arises from the side of the cell body and passes superficially. Dendrites extend from each end of the cell body branching into deeper and more superficial layers.
- *Horizontal cells of Cajal* are small and spindle-shaped but oriented parallel to the surface. They are the least common cell type and are only found in the most superficial layer where their axons pass laterally to synapse with the dendrites of pyramidal cells.

In addition to neurones, the cortex contains supporting neuroglial cells, i.e. astrocytes, oligodendroglia and microglia.

Layers of the neocortex
As previously stated, the neurones in the neocortex are arranged into six layers, the layers differing in neurone morphology, size and population density. The layers merge with one another rather than being highly demarcated and vary somewhat from one region of the cortex to another depending on cortical thickness and function.

Micrograph (b) illustrates the typical layered appearance of the cerebral cortex, the more detailed characteristics of each layer being as follows:

I.   *Plexiform (molecular) layer.* This most superficial layer mainly contains dendrites and axons of cortical neurones making synapses with one another; the sparse nuclei are those of neuroglia and occasional horizontal cells of Cajal.
II. *Outer granular layer.* A dense population of small pyramidal cells and stellate cells make up this thin layer which also contains various axons and dendritic connections from deeper layers.
III. *Pyramidal cell layer.* Pyramidal cells of moderate size predominate in this broad layer, the cells increasing in size deeper in the layer.
IV. *Inner granular layer.* This layer consists mainly of densely packed stellate cells.
V.   *Ganglionic layer.* Large pyramidal cells and smaller numbers of stellate cells and cells of Martinotti make up this layer, the name of the layer originating from the huge pyramidal (ganglion) Betz cells of the motor cortex.
VI. *Multiform cell layer.* This is so named for the wide variety of differing morphological forms found in this layer. It contains numerous small pyramidal cells and cells of Martinotti, as well as stellate cells especially superficially, and fusiform cells in the deeper part.

Micrograph (c) shows part of layer V; a thick section is employed, stained with a heavy metal impregnation technique which demonstrates considerable morphological detail. Several pyramidal cells **P** are easily identifiable, the principal dendrite of each (but not the axon) being included in the plane of section. A cell of Martinotti **M** can also be identified by its polygonal shape.

Micrograph (d) also shows layer V but in this case the section is thinner and stained by a routine histological method. In this example there is little morphological detail, nevertheless most of the cells are identifiable as pyramidal cells, increasing in size in the deeper part and including several very large cells.

The synaptic interconnections within the cortex are exceedingly complex, with any one neurone synapsing with several hundred others. However, there are several basic principles of cortical organisation and function:

- Functional units are disposed vertically, corresponding to the general orientation of axons and major dendrites.
- Afferent fibres (their cell bodies lying elsewhere in the CNS) generally synapse high in the cortex with dendrites of efferent neurones, the cell bodies of which lie in deeper layers of the cortex.
- Efferent pathways, typically the axons of pyramidal cells, tend to give off branches which pass back into more superficial layers to communicate with their own dendrites via interneuronal connections involving other cortical cell types.

21. Special sense organs

Introduction

The organs of special sense are highly sophisticated sensory receptors in which the specific neural receptors are incorporated in a non-neural structure which enhances and refines the reception of incoming stimuli. The eye and audio-vestibular apparatus of the ear are the main special sense organs but the gustatory (taste) and olfactory (smell) receptors are usually also included in this category.

(a)

(b)

Fig. 21.1 Taste buds *(H & E (a) × 128 (b) × 1200)*

Taste buds, the chemoreceptors for the sense of taste (*gustation*), are in humans mainly located in the epithelium of the circumvallate papillae of the tongue (see Fig. 13.12), although they are also found scattered in other parts of the tongue, palate, pharynx and epiglottis. In the circumvallate papillae, taste buds face into the deep troughs **T** surrounding the papillae as shown in micrograph (a). Serous glands, called the glands of von Ebner, drain into the troughs where the serous secretion acts as a solvent for taste-provoking substances.

The taste bud is a barrel-shaped organ extending the full thickness of the epithelium and opening at the surface via the *taste pore* **P**. Each taste bud contains from 20 to 30 long spindle-shaped cells which extend from the basement membrane to the taste pore. Classically, two types of cell are described in the taste bud: light *gustatory cells* and dark *supporting* or *sustentacular cells*. A third cell type, the *basal cell*, is now generally recognised and may constitute the precursor of one or both of the other cell types. Both gustatory and sustentacular cells have long microvilli

extending into the taste pore which contains a glycoprotein substance thought to be secreted by the sustentacular cells.

Ultrastructural studies have shown non-myelinated nerve fibres to be associated with both cell types, but there appears to be a more intimate, synapse-like relationship between the nerve fibres and the gustatory cells. Although the so-called gustatory cells are thought to be the taste receptors, the sustentacular cells may also serve some receptor function. Like the oral epithelium, all the cells of the taste bud, which represent highly specialised epithelial cells, are renewed continuously though the gustatory and sustentacular cells are replaced at different rates.

Four taste modalities are recognised: sweet, bitter, acid and salt. Each modality tends to be principally perceived in a specific region of the tongue; however, no structural differences have been demonstrated between taste buds from different areas. The sensations of taste and smell are closely associated and loss of olfactory sense is accompanied by diminished gustatory perception.

Sustentacular microvilli   Olfactory cilia

Olfactory
nerve fibres

Sustentacular
cells

Basal
cells

Olfactory
receptor cell

(a)

(b)

Fig. 21.2 Olfactory receptors *(a) Schematic diagram (b) H & E × 720*

The receptors for the sense of smell are located in a modified form of respiratory epithelium called *olfactory epithelium* in the nasal cavity; although extensive in some mammals such as the dog, the olfactory epithelium is restricted to a small area in the roof of the nasal cavity in humans. The olfactory epithelium is very tall, pseudostratified columnar in form and contains cells of three types: olfactory receptor cells, supporting epithelial (*sustentacular*) cells and basal epithelial cells.

The *olfactory receptor cells* are true bipolar neurones (see Fig. 7.2), the cell bodies of which are located in the middle stratum of the olfactory epithelium. A single dendritic process extends from the cell body to the free surface where it terminates as a small swelling which gives rise to about a dozen extremely long modified cilia. These cilia, which contain the usual '9 plus 2' arrangement of microtubules, are non-motile and lie flattened against the epithelial surface. The cilia are thought to be the sites of interaction between odiferous substances and the receptor cells. At the basal aspect, each receptor cell gives rise to a single fine non-myelinated axon which penetrates the basement membrane to join the axons of other receptor cells. The bundles of axons pass via about 20 small holes on each side of the cribriform plate of the ethmoid bone to reach the *olfactory bulbs* of the forebrain where they synapse with second order sensory neurones.

The supporting or sustentacular cells are elongated with their tapered bases resting on the basement membrane. Many long microvilli extend from their luminal surfaces to form a tangled mat with the cilia of the receptor cells. At the luminal surface, the plasma membranes of the sustentacular and receptor cells are bound by typical junctional complexes. The functions of the sustentacular cells are poorly understood but they probably provide mechanical and physiological support for the receptor cells. The basal cells are small, conical cells which may represent epithelial stem cells although recent evidence suggests that some may represent immature receptor cells.

In histological section, it is difficult to distinguish individual cell types within the olfactory epithelium; however, the nuclei of sustentacular cells occupy the uppermost stratum, those of the receptor cells the middle stratum and the basal cells lie close to the basement membrane. Note the terminal bar **B** at the luminal surface representing junctional complexes; note also the tangled meshwork of microvilli and cilia on the surface.

The olfactory epithelium is supported by loose vascular tissue containing bundles of afferent nerve fibres **N** and numerous serous glands called *Bowman's glands* **G** which produce the watery surface secretions in which odiferous substances are dissolved.

The eye

The eye is a highly specialised organ of photoreception, a process which involves the conversion of different quanta of light energy into nerve action potentials.

The photoreceptors are modified dendrites of two types of nerve cells, *rod cells* and *cone cells*. The rods are integrated into a system which is receptive to light of differing intensity; this is perceived in a form analogous to a black and white photographic image. The cones are of three functional types receptive to the colours blue, green and red and constitute a system by which coloured images may be perceived. The rod and cone receptors and a system of integrating neurones are located in the inner layer of the eye, the *retina*. The remaining structures of the eye serve to support the retina or to focus images of the visual world upon the retina.

In addition, several accessory structures namely the *eyelids*, *lacrimal gland* and *conjunctiva* protect the eye from external damage.

Fig. 21.3 The eye *(illustration opposite)*

The eye is made up of three basic layers: the outer *corneo-scleral layer*, the intermediate *uveal layer* (*uveal tract*) and the inner *retinal layer*.

Corneo-scleral layer. The corneo-scleral layer forms a tough, fibro-elastic capsule which supports the eye. The posterior five-sixths, the *sclera*, is opaque and provides insertion for the extra-ocular muscles.

The anterior one-sixth, the *cornea*, is transparent and has a smaller radius of curvature that the sclera. The cornea is the principal refracting medium of the eye and roughly focuses an image on to the retina; the focusing power of the cornea depends mainly on the radius of curvature of its external surface. The corneo-scleral junction is known as the *limbus* and is marked internally and externally by a shallow depression.

Uveal layer. The middle layer, the uvea or uveal tract, is a highly vascular layer which is made up of three components: the *choroid, ciliary body* and the *iris*. The choroid lies between the sclera and retina in the posterior five-sixths of the eye. It provides nutritive support for the retina and is heavily pigmented, thus absorbing light which has passed through the retina. Anteriorly, the choroid merges with the ciliary body which is a circumferential thickening of the uvea lying beneath the limbus.

The ciliary body surrounds the coronal equator of the *lens* and is attached to it by the *suspensory ligament* or *zonule*. The lens is a biconvex transparent structure, the shape of which can be varied to provide fine focus of the corneal image upon the retina. The ciliary body contains smooth muscle, the tone of which controls the shape of the lens via the suspensory ligament. The lens, suspensory ligament and ciliary body partition the eye into a large posterior compartment and a smaller anterior compartment.

The iris, the third component of the uvea, forms a diaphragm extending in front of the lens from the ciliary body so as to incompletely divide the anterior compartment into two chambers; these are known by the terms *anterior* and *posterior chamber* (not to be confused with the anterior and posterior compartments mentioned above). The highly pigmented iris acts as an adjustable diaphragm which regulates the amount of light reaching the retina. The aperture of the iris is called the *pupil*.

The anterior and posterior chambers contain a watery fluid, the *aqueous humor*, which is secreted into the posterior chamber by the ciliary body and circulated through the pupil to drain into a canal at the angle of the anterior chamber, the *canal of Schlemm*. The aqueous humor is a source of nutrients for the non-vascular lens and cornea, and acts as an optical medium which is non-refractive with respect to the cornea. The pressure of aqueous humor maintains the shape of the cornea.

The large, posterior compartment of the eye contains a gelatinous mass known as the *vitreous body* consisting of transparent *vitreous humor*. The vitreous body supports the lens and retina from within as well as providing an optical medium which is non-refractive with respect to the lens. In life, the vitreous body contains a canal which extends from the exit of the optic nerve to the posterior surface of the lens; this *hyaloid canal* represents the course of the hyaloid artery which supplies the vitreous body during embryological development. The vitreous body and hyaloid canal are rarely preserved in histological preparations.

Retinal layer. The photosensitive retina forms the inner lining of most of the posterior compartment of the eye and terminates along a scalloped line, the *ora serrata*, behind the ciliary body. Anterior to the ora serrata, the retinal layer continues as a non-photosensitive epithelial layer which lines the ciliary body and the posterior surface of the iris.

The visual axis of the eye passes through a depression in the retina called the *fovea* which is surrounded by a yellow pigmented zone, the *macula lutea*. The fovea is the area of greatest visual acuity.

Afferent nerve fibres from the retina converge to form the *optic nerve* which leaves the eye through a part of the sclera known as the *lamina cribrosa*. The retina overlying the lamina cribrosa, the *optic papilla* (*optic disc*), is devoid of photoreceptors and thus represents a blind spot.

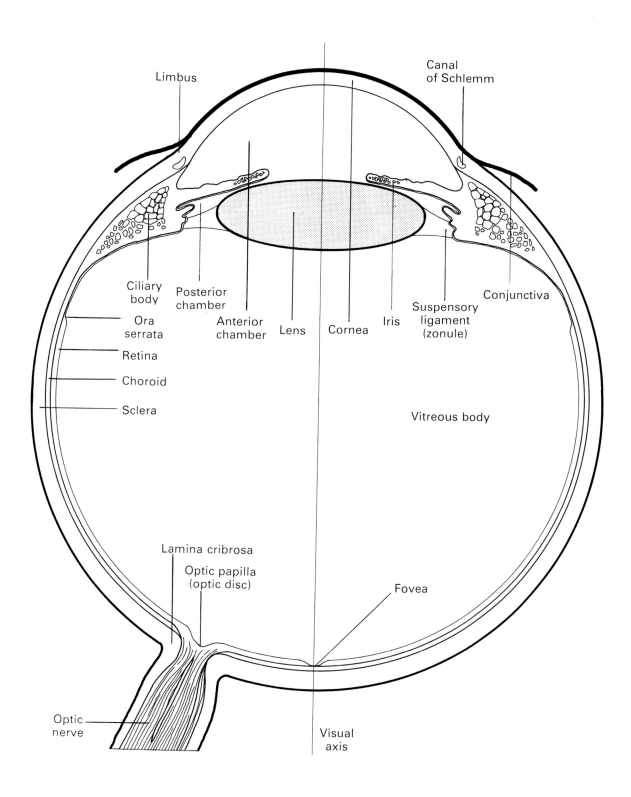

Limbus

Canal
of Schlemm

Ciliary
body

Posterior
chamber

Conjunctiva

Ora
serrata

Anterior
chamber

Lens

Cornea

Iris

Suspensory
ligament
(zonule)

Retina

Choroid

Sclera

Vitreous body

Lamina cribrosa

Optic papilla
(optic disc)

Fovea

Optic
nerve

Visual
axis

Fig. 21.4 Eye

(Monkey: H & E × 5)

This horizontal section shows the relative sizes of the components of the eye. At this magnification, the three layers comprising the wall of the globe are not readily distinguishable although in the wall of the posterior compartment, the middle layer of choroid, is recognisable by its high content of pigment.

The other uveal structures, the ciliary body **CB** and iris **I** are readily visible. The lens **L** has been artefactually distorted during preparation and the suspensory ligament by which it is attached to the ciliary body is not preserved. Note the relative thickness of the cornea **C**.

The optic nerve **O** is seen to penetrate the sclera medial to the visual axis; the fovea is not present in this plane of section.

Fig. 21.5 Wall of the eye *(H & E × 300)*

The three layers of the wall of the eye are illustrated in this micrograph.

The inner photosensitive retina is a multi-layered structure, the outermost limit of which is defined by a layer of *pigmented epithelial cells* **P**.

The choroid **C** is a layer of loose vascular supporting tissue lying between the sclera **S** externally and the retina **R** internally. The choroid and retina are separated by a membrane known as *Bruch's membrane* which probably represents the basement membrane of the pigmented epithelium. The blood supply of the uveal layer of the eye is provided by branches of the ophthalmic artery which penetrates via the sclera. Larger vessels predominate in the superficial aspect of the choroid with a rich capillary plexus in the deeper aspect providing nourishment for the outer layers of the retina by diffusion across Bruch's membrane. The choroid contains numerous large, heavily pigmented melanocytes which confer the dense pigmentation characteristic of the choroid. The pigment absorbs light rays passing through the retina and prevents interference due to light refraction.

The sclera consists of dense fibro-elastic tissue, the fibres of which are arranged in bundles parallel to the surface. This layer contains little ground substance and few fibroblasts. The sclera varies in thickness, being thickest posteriorly and thinnest at the coronal equator of the globe.

Fig. 21.6 Retina *(a) Schematic diagram (b) H & E × 640*

The retina is made up of three cell types: neurones, pigmented epithelial cells and neurone support cells. The neurones are divided into three functional groups namely photoreceptor cells (rod cells and cone cells), the cells of afferent fibres passing in the optic nerve and a group of neurones interposed between the first two types which integrate sensory input from the photoreceptors before transmission to the cerebral cortex. The integrating neurones are further subdivided into three types: *bipolar cells, horizontal cells* and *amacrine cells.*

Histologically, the retina is traditionally divided into 10 distinct histological layers as shown in the micrograph, the distribution of the different cell types being illustrated in a highly schematic manner in the diagram.

The outermost layer (1) consists of the *pigmented epithelial cells* forming a single layer resting on Bruch's membrane which separates them from the choroid. *Rod and cone processes* of the photoreceptor cells comprise the next layer (2) with a thin eosinophilic structure known as the *outer limiting membrane* (3) separating them from a layer of densely packed nuclei described as the *outer nuclear layer* (4). The outer nuclear layer contains the cell bodies of the rod and cone photoreceptors. The almost featureless layer deep to this is known as the *outer plexiform layer* (5) and contains synaptic connections between the short axons of the photoreceptor cells and integrating neurones, the cell bodies of which lie in the *inner nuclear layer* (6). In the *inner plexiform layer* (7), the integrating neurones make synaptic

connections with dendrites of neurones whose axons form the optic tract. The cell bodies of the optic tract neurones (sometimes called *ganglion cells*) comprise the *ganglion cell layer* (8). Deep to this is the layer of *afferent fibres* (9) passing towards the optic disc to form the optic nerve. Finally, the *inner limiting membrane* (10) demarcates the innermost aspect of the retina from the *vitreous body* **VB**. Note in the diagram that only bipolar cells are represented in the integrating cell layer; this layer also contains the cell bodies of the horizontal and amacrine cells as illustrated in Figure 21.8.

Towards the left of the diagram is represented an extremely elongated support cell extending between inner and outer limiting membranes and with its nucleus in the same layer as the integrating neurones. These cells, known as *Muller cells*, are analogous to the neuroglia of the CNS and have long cytoplasmic processes which embrace and sometimes even encircle the retinal neurones filling all the intervening spaces. Muller cells provide structural support and may also mediate the transfer of essential metabolites such as glucose to the retinal neurones.

The outer limiting membrane is not a true membrane but merely represents the line of intercellular junctions between Muller cells and the photoreceptor cells (shown diagrammatically in Fig. 21.7). In contrast, the inner limiting membrane represents the basement membrane of the Muller cells resting on the vitreous body.

(a)

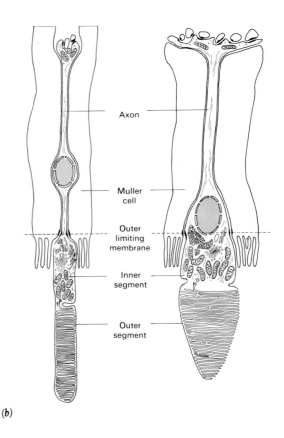

(b)

Fig. 21.7 Retinal photoreceptors *(a) H & E × 1200 (b) Schematic diagram*

The rod and cone photoreceptor layer of the retina is shown
at very high magnification in this micrograph, the cell bodies
of the rod and cone cells lying deep to the outer limiting
membrane **M**. Peripherally, the rods and cones mingle with
long microvilli extending from the pigment epithelial cells
P.

As shown in the diagram, the rod photoreceptors are long
slender bipolar cells, the single dendrite of each cell
extending beyond the outer limiting membrane as the rod
proper. The rod proper consists of *inner* and *outer segments*
connected by a thin eccentric strand of cytoplasm containing
nine microtubule doublets similar to those of a cilium but
without the inner pair of microtubules. The inner segment
contains a prominent Golgi apparatus and many
mitochondria. The outer segment has a regular cylindrical
shape and contains a stack of flattened membranous discs
which incorporate the pigment *rhodopsin* (visual purple).
The membranous discs are continuously shed from the end
of each rod and phagocytised by the pigmented epithelial
cells, the discs being continuously replaced from the inner
segment. In essence, the transduction process involves the
interaction of light with rhodopsin molecules which
promotes a configuration change within the membrane, thus
initiating an action potential. The action potential then
passes inwards along the dendrite and axon to the layer of
integrating neurones.

Cones are similar in basic structure to the rods but they
differ in several details. The outer segment of the cone is a
long conical structure about two-thirds the length of a rod
and containing a similar number of even more flattened
membranous discs. Unlike the situation in the rods however,
the disc membrane is continuous with the plasma membrane

so that, on one side, the spaces between the discs are
continuous with the extracellular environment (see
diagram). The discs are not shed although the tips of the
cones are invested by processes of pigmented epithelial cells.
The cones contain pigments similar to rhodopsin, receptive
to blue, green and red light, and the mechanism of
transduction is probably similar. The bodies of the cone
cells are generally continuous with the inner segment of the
cone proper without an intervening dendritic process and
the nuclei of cone cells thus form a row immediately deep to
the outer limiting membrane.

As seen in the micrograph, the pigmented epithelial cells
are cuboidal in shape with the nuclei located basally towards
Bruch's membrane **B**. Apically, the cells are crammed with
melanin granules, numerous mitochondria and lipofuscin, a
residual product of phagocytosis (see Fig. 1.3). The
pigmented cell microvilli which are from 5–7 µm long,
extend between the photoreceptors and, with electron
microscopy, are seen to contain membranous lamellae
similar to those in the rod outer segments; these appear to
disintegrate as they pass deeper into the pigmented cells. In
addition to phagocytosis, the pigmented epithelial cells
provide structural and metabolic support for the rods and
cones and in addition absorb light, thus preventing back
reflection.

During histological preparation, the retina frequently
becomes detached from the wall of the eye and the plane of
cleavage is usually between the rods and cones and the layer
of pigmented epithelial cells corresponding to the cavity of
the embryonic optic vesicle. This is also the plane along
which the retina cleaves in the living eye in the pathological
condition known as *retinal detachment*.

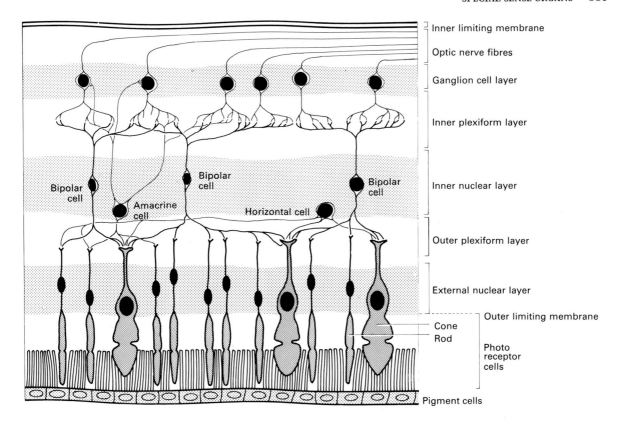

Fig. 21.8 Neuronal interconnections in the retina

This diagram demonstrates the basic pattern of neuronal interconnections between the photoreceptor cells and the afferent neurones of the optic tract. The interneurones consist of three basic cell types, bipolar cells, horizontal cells and amacrine cells, their cell bodies all being located in the inner nuclear layer (along with those of the supporting Muller cells).

Bipolar cells, the most numerous of the integrating neurones, in general make direct connections between one or more photoreceptors and one or more optic tract neurones. Horizontal cells have several short processes and one long process, the terminal branches of each making lateral connections between adjacent and more distant rods and cones in the outer plexiform layer. The amacrine cells have one or two short dendritic trunks giving rise to numerous branches which make connections with bipolar and optic tract neurones in the inner plexiform layer as well as making occasional feedback connections with photoreceptors in the outer plexiform layer.

As seen in Figure 21.7 (b) opposite, the axons of the rod photoreceptors terminate in spherical processes into which are invaginated their small number of synaptic connections. In contrast, the cone photoreceptors have a flattened pedicle which accommodates hundreds of intercellular contacts.

In all, there are more than 100 million rods and 6 million cones. The cones are particularly dense in the macula and the immediately surrounding area and, in the fovea itself, the photoreceptors are almost exclusively cones. The density of both rods and cones diminishes towards the retinal periphery. The foveal cones have an almost one to one relationship with optic tract neurones giving maximal visual discrimination. There are only about 1 million optic tract neurones and the more peripheral the photoreceptors, the greater the number of photoreceptors synapsing with each optic tract neurone. This is consistent with the main function of the more peripheral receptors (predominantly rods) which is for determination of light and dark rather than fine two-point discrimination.

Fig. 21.9 Fovea *(Masson's trichrome × 320)*

The fovea is a conical depression in the retina corresponding to the point where the visual axis of the cornea and lens meets the retina and lying about 4 mm lateral and slightly inferior to the exit of the optic nerve fibres via the optic disc. Consequently, the fovea is the area subject to the least refractory distortion. To complement this, the foveal retina is modified to obtain the maximum photoreceptor sensitivity and is thus the area of the retina with the greatest visual discrimination; however, its function is poor in conditions of low light intensity. Surrounding the fovea is an ovoid yellow area about 1 mm wide called the *macula lutea*.

As seen in this micrograph, at the fovea the inner layers of the retina are flattened laterally so as to present the least barrier to light reaching the photoreceptors. Retinal blood vessels are absent at the fovea, as can be readily seen with the ophthalmoscope, and the brownish colour of the choroidal melanin shows through the much attenuated retina. At the fovea, the photoreceptors are almost exclusively cones which are elongated and closely packed (approximately 100 000 cones are contained in the fovea). Neuronal interconnections in the bipolar cell layer provide for a one-to-one ratio of these cones to optic nerve fibres which means that each foveal photoreceptor is individually represented at the visual cortex.

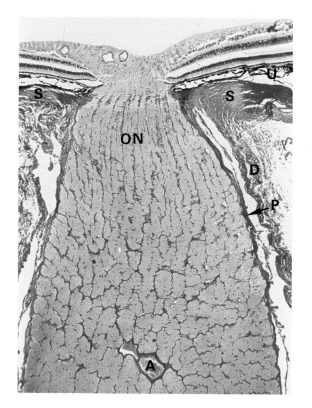

Fig. 21.10 Optic nerve

(Haematoxylin/van Gieson × 30)

The afferent fibres from the retina converge at a point medial to the fovea, the optic papilla or optic disc, fibres from the lateral quadrants sweeping above and below the macula to avoid the fovea. The fibres then penetrate the sclera **S** through the lamina cribrosa to form the optic nerve **ON**. Note the thickness of the optic tract layer overlying the disc and the absence of photoreceptor cells from the optic papilla which is thus a blind spot on the retina.

In their course across the retina, the afferent fibres are not myelinated as this would obstruct light passing to the photoreceptors. Myelination commences at the optic disc which imparts the white colour seen with the ophthalmoscope.

The optic nerve and retina develop embryologically as an outgrowth of the primitive forebrain, thus the optic nerve is invested by meninges. The dura mater **D** becomes continuous with its developmental equivalent, the sclera, while the pia-arachnoid **P** continues into the eye as the uveal tract **U**.

The main blood supply of the retina is provided by the central artery of the retina **A**, a branch of the ophthalmic artery. This divides at the optic disc into four branches supplying the quadrants of the retina. These vessels course within the optic nerve fibre layer breaking up into a rich capillary network which drains back into a venous system closely following the course of the arterial supply. The vessels are confined to the optic nerve fibre layer and more superficial layers are dependent on diffusion, the most peripheral retinal layers also being supplied likewise from the choroid.

(a)

(b)

(c)

Fig. 21.11 Ciliary body *(H & E (a) × 30 (b) × 128 (c) × 320)*

The ciliary body is a circumferential structure which bulges into the eye between the ora serrata and the limbus (see Fig. 21.3). As seen in micrograph (a), the ciliary body **CB** represents the forward continuation of the choroid layer **C** (uveal tract) of the posterior five-sixths of the wall of the eye and, like it, is highly vascular and contains a considerable amount of melanin pigment. Anteriorly, it is continuous with the third component of the uveal tract, the iris **I**, passing in front of the lens **L**.

As seen in micrograph (c), the ciliary body is lined with a double layer of cuboidal epithelium. The deep layer is highly pigmented and represents a forward continuation of the pigmented epithelial layer of the retina whilst the surface layer, which is not pigmented, is a non-photosensitive forward extension of the receptor layer of the retina.

The ciliary body is attached to the coronal equator of the lens **L** by the suspensory ligament which consists of extremely fine collagenous strands which seldom remain intact after histological preparation; a few aggregated shreds of the suspensory ligament **S** are seen in micrograph (b). Tension in the suspensory ligament tends to flatten the lens which, in the relaxed state, assumes a more globular shape. The bulk of the ciliary body consists of smooth muscle **M** arranged in such a manner that, when it contracts, tension

upon the suspensory ligament is reduced thus permitting the lens to assume a more convex shape. This mechanism permits fine focusing of images already roughly focused upon the retina by the cornea. The ciliary muscle is innervated by parasympathetic nerve fibres.

From that part of the ciliary body exposed to the angle of the posterior chamber **PC**, there project a number of branching epithelial folds called *ciliary processes* with a supporting tissue core rich in fenestrated capillaries. The ciliary processes are responsible for the continuous production of aqueous humor which then circulates into the anterior chamber via the pupil. Aqueous humor is continuously reabsorbed into the canal of Schlemm **CS** seen at the angle of the anterior chamber in micrograph (a).

Aqueous humor is a clear, watery fluid somewhat similar in composition to CSF and hypotonic with respect to plasma. The production of aqueous humor is presumed to be an active process mediated by the two epithelial layers lining the ciliary processes. Balanced rates of secretion and reabsorption of aqueous humor result in the maintenance of a constant intra-ocular pressure of about 15 mm of mercury which stabilises the lens and cornea. The flow of aqueous humor also provides for a continuous exchange of metabolites with the cells of the avascular cornea and lens.

(a)

(b)

Fig. 21.12 Iris *(H & E (a) × 20 (b) × 80)*

The iris is the most anterior part of the uveal layer of the eye. It arises from the ciliary body and forms a diaphragm in front of the lens, so dividing the anterior compartment of the eye into posterior **PC** and anterior chambers **AC** which communicate via the pupil. The pupillary edge of the iris rests on the anterior edge of the lens in life.

The main mass of the iris consists of loose, highly vascular tissue which is pigmented due to the presence of numerous melanocytes scattered in the stroma. The anterior surface of the iris is irregular and consists of a discontinuous layer of fibroblasts and melanocytes; in the fetus the surface is lined by endothelial cells but these become absent during early childhood. In contrast, the posterior surface is relatively smooth and is lined by epithelium which is derived embryologically as a continuation of the two layers which line the surface of the ciliary body. The surface layer, non-pigmented in the ciliary body, becomes heavily pigmented in the iris such that the individual cells are completely

obscured. The deep layer, pigmented in the ciliary body, is transformed in the iris into lightly pigmented myoepithelial cells which constitute the radially orientated *dilator pupillae* muscle **DP** of the iris. Even at high magnification, these myoepithelial cells are difficult to distinguish.

The *constrictor muscle of the pupil (constrictor pupillae)* **CP** consists of a band of circumferentially oriented smooth muscle fibres situated in the stroma near to the free edge of the iris. Like the smooth muscle of the ciliary body, the constrictor pupillae is innervated by the parasympathetic nervous system whereas the myoepithelial cells of the dilator pupillae are innervated by the sympathetic nervous system.

The colour of the iris depends on the amount of pigment in the stroma, the amount of pigment in the posterior epithelial layer being relatively constant between individuals. Blue eyes contain little stromal pigment whereas brown eyes have much stromal pigment.

Fig. 21.13 Canal of Schlemm *(H & E × 75)*

The canal of Schlemm **CS** is a circumferential canal lined by endothelium which is situated in the inner aspect of the corneal margin **C** immediately adjacent to the angle of the anterior chamber **AC**. At the angle of the anterior chamber, there is a meshwork of fine collagenous trabeculae **T** lined by endothelium; aqueous humor percolates through the spaces between the trabeculae before reaching the canal of Schlemm. There is no direct communication between the trabecular spaces and the canal of Schlemm, thus reabsorption of aqueous humor involves passage across two layers of endothelium and intervening supporting tissue. The mechanism of transport is not understood; disruption of this process leads to increased intra-ocular pressure as in the disease known as *glaucoma*. The canal of Schlemm drains via minute channels through the sclera into the episcleral venous system, a pressure gradient being maintained to prevent reflux of blood. Note the close relationship of the root of the iris **I** with the canal of Schlemm.

(a)   (b)   (c)   (d)

Fig. 21.14 The lens and its development *(H & E (a) × 64 (b) × 150 (c) × 50 (d) × 50)*

The lens is an elastic biconvex structure which, although transparent and apparently amorphous, is almost entirely composed of living cells. The lens cells are highly modified epithelial cells derived embryologically from ectoderm which forms a depression, the *lens pit*, overlying the embryonic *optic vesicle*.

With further development, the lens pit becomes deeper, its margins fusing to form the *lens vesicle* which becomes detached from the surface and sinks deeper to become enveloped by the growing optic vesicle; at this stage the lens vesicle merely consists of a single layer of epithelial cells.

The posterior cells of the lens vesicle now become greatly elongated antero-posteriorly filling the central cavity of the vesicle. This stage of development is shown in micrograph (a), the arrowhead marking the junction between posterior and anterior cells of the former lens vesicle. Note the developing cornea **C** and retina **R**. The lens cells in the central antero-posterior axis then undergo maturation as seen in micrograph (b) losing their nuclei to become known as *lens fibres*. Proliferation of the cells at the lens equator **E** adds further fibres to the central mass, the growth process continuing at a slow rate even into old age.

When fully developed, the lens substance consists of two to three thousand anucleate fibres, each stretching between anterior and posterior poles of the lens. The fibres have the shape of extremely elongated six-sided prisms, the more peripheral fibres curving to follow the antero-posterior surface contour of the lens. The fibres contain a crystalline protein and the cell membranes of adjacent fibres are fused, leaving little intervening extracellular substance.

The anterior lens surface is covered by a single layer of cuboidal cells which retain their nuclei, this layer merging with the residual proliferative cells at the equatorial margin of the lens. The whole lens is enveloped by a thick epithelial basement membrane forming the *lens capsule* which is connected via the suspensory ligament to the ciliary body.

Micrograph (c) shows part of the mature lens including the anterior cuboidal epithelium **A** and lens capsule **C**. The lens substance is particularly prone to artefactual distortion during histological preparation. Micrograph (d) shows the equatorial region of the lens and nearby ciliary processes **CP**. Note the anterior epithelial layer **A** and nuclei **N** in the more recently formed peripheral fibres.

Fig. 21.15 Cornea *(H & E × 80)*

The cornea is the thick transparent portion of the corneo-scleral layer enclosing the anterior one-sixth of the eye. The relatively fixed convexity of the external surface provides the principal mechanism for focusing images upon the retina.

The cornea is an avascular structure consisting of five layers. The outer surface is lined by stratified squamous epithelium **Ep** about five cells thick which is not normally keratinised. This epithelium is supported by a specialised basement membrane known as *Bowman's membrane* **BM** which is particularly prominent in humans. The bulk of the cornea, the *substantia propria* **SP**, consists of a highly regular form of dense collagenous tissue forming thin lamellae. Fibroblasts and occasional leucocytes are scattered in the ground substance between the lamellae. The inner surface of the cornea is lined by a layer of flattened endothelial cells **En** which are supported by a very thick elastic basement membrane known as *Descemet's membrane* **DM**. The corneal endothelium is highly active in pumping fluid from the substantia propria preventing excessive hydration which would result in the cornea becoming opaque.

The cornea is sustained by diffusion of metabolites from the aqueous humor and the blood vessels of the limbus; some oxygen is derived directly from the external environment.

Fig. 21.16 Conjunctiva

(Haematoxylin/van Gieson × 128)

The conjunctiva is the epithelium which covers the exposed part of the sclera and inner surface of the eyelids. It is stratified columnar in form and for a stratified epithelium is unusual in that it contains goblet cells in the surface layers. The conjunctival mucous secretions contribute to the protective layer on the exposed surface of the eye.

Beneath the conjunctival epithelium is loose vascular supporting tissue.

Fig. 21.17 Lacrimal gland

(H & E × 150)

The lacrimal gland is responsible for the secretion of tears, a watery fluid containing the antibacterial enzyme *lysozyme* and electrolytes of similar concentration to that of plasma.

Histologically, the lacrimal glands are similar to the salivary glands in lobular structure and compound tubulo-acinar form of the secretory units. The secretory cells have the typical appearance of serous (protein-secreting) cells with basally located nuclei and strongly stained granular cytoplasm.

Each gland drains via a dozen or more small ducts into the superior fornix. Tears drain to the inner aspect of the eye and then into the nasal cavity via the nasolacrimal duct.

Fig. 21.18 Eyelid *(H & E × 16)*

Each eyelid consists of a dense fibro-elastic plate, the *tarsus* **T**, covered externally by thin, highly-folded skin **S** and on the internal aspect by smooth conjunctiva **C**. The skin contains scattered fine hair follicles **F** and the underlying supporting tissue is extremely loose and devoid of fat.

Skeletal muscle **M** of *orbicularis oculi* (and *levator palpebrae* in the upper eyelid) lies immediately superficial to the tarsal plate and is separated from it by a layer of supporting tissue **A** which, in the upper lid, represents a forward continuation of the sub-aponeurotic layer of the scalp. The clinical importance of this is that blood or inflammatory exudates collecting above the scalp aponeurosis may track forward into the superficial planes of the eyelid; being extremely lax, this area may become markedly swollen. This supporting tissue layer also contains the sensory nerves of the eyelid.

Within the tarsal plate lie some 12–30 *tarsal (Meibomian) glands* **G** oriented vertically and opening at the free margin of the eyelid via minute foramina. These glands are modified sebaceous glands each consisting of a long central duct into which open numerous sebaceous acini. Associated with the eyelashes **E** are sebaceous glands known as the *glands of Zeis* and modified apocrine sweat glands known as the *glands of Moll*. Together, the glands of the eyelid produce an oily layer which is thought to cover the tear layer, thereby preventing evaporation of the tears.

The ear

The ear or vestibulo-cochlear apparatus has the dual sensory function of maintenance of equilibrium and hearing (stato-acoustic system).

Structurally the system may be divided into three parts, the *external ear*, the *middle ear* and the *internal ear*. The specific sensory receptors for both movement and sound are situated in a membranous structure located in the internal ear while the external and middle ear are concerned with reception, transmission and amplification of incoming sound waves.

Fig. 21.19 The ear *(illustration opposite)*

The main structural elements of the vestibulo-cochlear apparatus are illustrated in this diagram.

External ear

The external ear is responsible for reception of sound waves which are funnelled onto the ear drum (*tympanic membrane*). It consists of the auricle (*pinna*), a modified horn-shaped structure composed of elastic cartilage covered by skin, which converges onto the *external auditory meatus (canal)*. Elastic cartilage also forms the wall of the outer third of the canal whilst the inner two-thirds of the canal lie in the petrous part of the temporal bone. The canal is lined by hairy skin containing sebaceous glands and modified apocrine sweat glands which secrete a waxy material called *cerumen*.

Middle ear

The middle ear is an air-filled cavity located in the petrous temporal bone and is separated from the external auditory canal by the tympanic membrane. Sound waves impinging on the tympanic membrane are converted into mechanical vibrations which are then amplified by a system of levers made up of three small bones called *ossicles* (the *malleus, incus* and *stapes*) and transmitted to the fluid-filled inner ear cavity. The ossicles articulate with one another via synovial joints and the malleus and incus pivot on tiny ligaments which are attached to the wall of the middle ear cavity. Small slips of muscle, the *tensor tympani* and *stapedius*, pass to the mid point of the tympanic membrane and stapes bone respectively and damp down excessive vibrations which might otherwise damage the delicate auditory apparatus. The middle ear cavity communicates anteriorly with the nasopharynx via the *auditory (Eustachian) tube* which permits equalisation of pressure changes with the external environment. Posteriorly, the middle ear cavity communicates with numerous interconnected air spaces which lighten the mass of the mastoid part of the temporal bone. The whole of the middle ear and mastoid cavities are lined by simple squamous or cuboidal epithelium.

Internal ear

The internal ear consists of an interconnected fluid-filled *membranous labyrinth* lying within a labyrinth of spaces of complementary shape in the temporal bone (the *osseous labyrinth*). The membranous labyrinth is bound down to the walls of the osseous labyrinth in various places but in the main is separated from the bony walls by a fluid-filled space. The fluid within the membranous labyrinth is known as *endolymph* and the fluid in the surrounding peri-membranous space is known as *perilymph*. The peri-membranous space is directly connected with the subarachnoid space and, like the latter, is crossed by delicate fibrous strands and lined by flat squamous epithelium; the perilymphatic fluid is thus similar in composition to CSF. In contrast, the membranous labyrinth is a closed system with a sac, the *endolymphatic sac*, lying in the subdural space of the underlying brain. The membranous labyrinth is lined by a simple epithelium except in the endolymphatic sac where the cells are columnar with morphological features suggesting that this is the site of endolymph absorption.

The osseous labyrinth may be divided into three main areas:

1. **The vestibule.** The central space of the osseous labyrinth is called the *vestibule*; it gives rise to three *semicircular canals* posteriorly, and the *cochlear* anteriorly. The vestibule contains two components of the membranous labyrinth namely the *utricle* and the *saccule*, which are connected by a short, Y-shaped duct from which arises the endolymphatic duct. The walls of the utricle and saccule each contain a specialised area of sensory receptor cells known as a *macula* (see Fig. 21.27) from which axons pass into the *vestibular nerve* as part of the sensory input for maintenance of equilibrium. Laterally, the vestibule is separated from the middle ear cavity by a thin bony plate containing two fenestrations, one oval and the other round in shape. The *oval window* is occluded by the base of the stirrup-shaped stapes bone and its surrounding *annular ligament* whereby vibrations are transmitted to the perilymph from the tympanic membrane via the ossicle chain. The *round window* is closed by a membrane similar to the tympanic membrane and it is thus sometimes described as the *secondary tympanic membrane*. This membrane permits vibrations which have passed to sensory receptors for sound to be dissipated (see later).

2. **The semicircular canals.** Three semicircular canals arise from the posterior aspect of the vestibules, two being disposed in vertical planes at right angles to one another and the other in a near horizontal plane. Within each semicircular canal is a semicircular membranous duct filled with endolymph and continuous at both ends with the utricle; near one end of each semicircular membranous duct is a dilated area called the *ampulla*. In each ampulla, there is a ridge called the *crista ampullaris* (see Fig. 21.8) containing sensory receptors with axons converging on the vestibular nerve. Together with the receptors of the maculae of the utricle and saccule, these receptors form the sensory afferents for the maintenance of balance and equilibrium.

3. **The cochlear.** The cochlear occupies a conical, spiral-shaped space in the temporal bone extending from the anterior aspect of the vestibule; the space is roughly similar in shape to that inside the shell of a cone-shaped snail or shellfish. The membranous component of the cochlear arises from the saccule and spirals upwards with its blind end attached at the apex of the osseous space. The membranous canal is triangular in cross-section and attached to the bony walls of the cochlear in such a manner as to divide the osseous space into three spiral compartments (see Fig. 21.24). The middle compartment, the *scala media*, contains endolymph and the upper and lower compartments contain perilymph. At the base of the cochlear, the upper perilymph compartment is directly continuous with the perilymph of the vestibule and via this space, called the *scala vestibuli*, vibrations pass through the perilymph towards the apex of the cochlear. At the apex, the scala vestibuli becomes continuous with the lower perilymphatic space of the cochlear spiral via a minute hole called the *helicotrema*. This lower space terminates at the secondary tympanic membrane covering the round window and 'spent' vibrations are thus dissipated; the lower perilymphatic space is therefore known as the *scala tympani*. The sensory receptors for sound are located in a spiral-shaped structure known as the *organ of Corti* shown in detail in Figure 21.25.

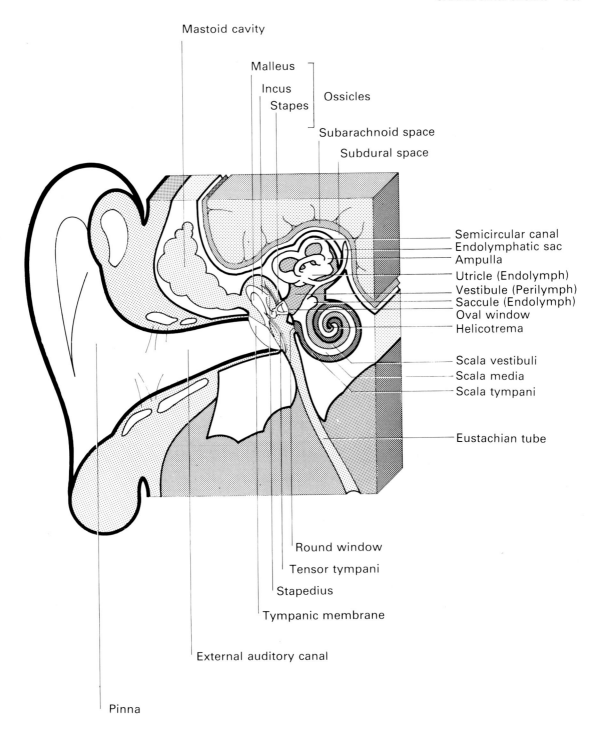

Mastoid cavity

Malleus

Incus

Stapes

Ossicles

Subarachnoid space

Subdural space

Semicircular canal
Endolymphatic sac
Ampulla
Utricle (Endolymph)
Vestibule (Perilymph)
Saccule (Endolymph)
Oval window
Helicotrema

Scala vestibuli
Scala media
Scala tympani

Eustachian tube

Round window

Tensor tympani

Stapedius

Tympanic membrane

External auditory canal

Pinna

Fig. 21.20 The ear *(H & E × 8)*

This micrograph shows a horizontal section through the vestibulo-cochlear apparatus which lies within the temporal bone **B**. The tympanic membrane **TM** can be seen stretched between the tympanic plate of the temporal bone anteriorly and the lateral part of the petrous temporal bone posteriorly, dividing the external auditory meatus **EAM** from the cavity of the middle ear **ME**. Part of one of the ossicles **O**, the handle of the malleus, can be seen attached to the inner aspect of the tympanic membrane. From the anterior aspect of the middle ear chamber, the auditory canal **AC** (Eustachian canal) passes forwards towards the nasopharynx; in the mastoid part of the temporal bone there are numerous irregular mastoid air spaces **MAS**.

Near the centre of the field is the vestibule of the inner ear **V** containing two delicate membranous structures, the utricle **U** and saccule **S** more anteriorly. Two of the semicircular canals **SC** can be identified deep in the posterior part of the petrous temporal bone. Immediately posterior to the middle ear cavity, the facial nerve **FN** is seen in transverse section as it passes inferiorly; just medial to it lies the stapedius muscle **SM**.

Anterior to the vestibule, the conical spiral of the cochlear **C** has been cut in longitudinal section through its central bony axis. From the base of the cochlear, the vestibulo-auditory nerve **VAN** passes towards the brain stem **BS**, behind which the cerebellum is easily recognisable.

Fig. 21.21 External auditory meatus
(H & E × 100)

The external auditory meatus is the canal leading from the auricle to the tympanic membrane. The wall of the outer third is formed by elastic cartilage whereas the inner two-thirds is formed by the temporal bone. The canal is lined by skin which is devoid of the usual dermal papillae and closely bound down to the underlying cartilage or bone by a dense collagenous dermis. The skin of the outer third (as shown here) has fine hairs and the dermis contains numerous coiled tubular *ceruminous glands* **G** which secrete wax (cerumen) and which represent specialised apocrine sweat glands (see Fig. 9.16). The ceruminous glands open directly onto the skin surface or into the sebaceous glands associated with hair follicles **F**. The meatal hairs provide protection from foreign bodies whilst the cerumen protects the skin of the external meatus from moisture and infection.

Fig. 21.22 Tympanic membrane and ossicle

(H & E × 20)

The tympanic membrane (ear drum) is a thin fibrous membrane separating the external auditory canal from the cavity of the middle ear. With the exception of a small triangular area superiorly, the *pars flaccida*, the membrane is tense (*pars tensa*), being firmly attached to the surrounding bone by a fibrocartilaginous ring. The handle of the malleus is attached to the centre of the membrane, the chain of ossicles pulling the membrane slightly inwards.

The tympanic membrane is made up of three layers: an external *cuticular layer*, an intermediate *fibrous layer* and an inner *mucous layer*. The cuticular layer **C** consists of thin hairless skin, the epidermis being only about 10 cells thick and the basal layer being flat and devoid of the usual epidermal ridges. The thin dermis contains plump fibroblasts and a fine vascular network.

The intermediate fibrous layer **F** consists of an outer layer of fibres radiating from the centre of the membrane towards the circumference and an inner layer of fibres disposed circumferentially at the periphery. These fibres have long been assumed to be collagen associated with a fine meshwork of elastin; however, recent evidence suggests that the fibres are of a unique composition especially adapted for the function of the tympanic membrane.

The inner mucous layer **M** represents a continuation of the modified respiratory-type mucous membrane lining the middle ear cavity but in this situation it is merely a single layer of cuboidal cells devoid of cilia and goblet cells. The underlying lamina propria is thin with a blood supply separate from that of the dermis of the cuticular layer. A similar modified respiratory-type mucosa invests the ossicles, small muscles and nerves exposed to the middle ear cavity.

The ossicles consist of compact bone formed by endochondral ossification which accounts for the cartilage **Ca** seen in this specimen from a kitten. Note also the tensor tympani muscle **Mu**.

Fig. 21.23 Auditory (Eustachian) canal

(H & E × 320)

The auditory canal connects the cavity of the middle ear with the nasopharynx and allows for equalisation of air pressure between the middle ear and the external environment. From the middle ear, the tube first passes through bone but towards the pharynx, the wall is supported on two sides by cartilage and on the remaining two sides by fibrous tissue.

The tube is lined by typical pseudostratified respiratory epithelium with numerous goblet cells particularly towards the pharyngeal end. The *salpingo-pharyngeus, tensor palati* and *levator veli palati* muscles are connected to the fibrocartilaginous part of the tube causing it to dilate during swallowing.

(a)

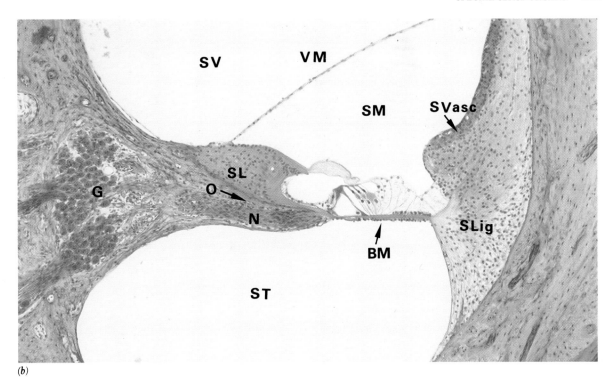

(b)

Fig. 21.24 Cochlear *(illustration (a) opposite; H & E (a) × 20 (b) × 96)*

The cochlear is the component of the internal ear which contains the auditory sense organ. The conical spiral-shaped form of the cochlear can be visualised in micrograph (a) which shows a cochlear cut in a plane of section which includes its long bony axis. Note that the cavity in the petrous temporal bone is reminiscent of the space inside a conical snail shell. The cochlear has two-and-a-half full turns and in this section, therefore, five separate cross-sections of the cochlear can be seen, each turn of the spiral being separated from the next by a thin plate of bone. A corkscrew-like bony structure, the *modiolus*, forms the central axis of the cochlear.

Each turn of the cochlear canal can be seen to be divided into three compartments, shown at higher magnification in micrograph (b). The central compartment, the *scala media* **SM**, is roughly triangular in cross-section, with the apex attached to a spicule of bone spiralling outwards from the modiolus and known as the *osseous spiral lamina* **O**. Above the free edge of the osseous spiral lamina is a thickened mass of tissue known as the *spiral limbus* **SL**. The base of the scala media is thickened and attached to the outer wall of the cochlear. The membrane making up the walls of the scala media represents that part of the membranous labyrinth extending up into the cochlear from the saccule, and the scala media is thus filled with endolymph.

Above the scala media is the *scala vestibuli* **SV** originating in the vestibule near the oval window and base of stapes; vibrations are conducted towards the apex of the cochlear in the perilymph of the scala vestibuli. Below the scala media is the perilymphatic space which spirals down from the apex to

the secondary tympanic membrane, the *scala tympani* **ST**.

The membrane separating the scala media and the scala tympani, known as the *basilar membrane* **BM**, supports the *organ of Corti* which contains the auditory receptor cells; the organ of Corti is described in detail in Figure 21.25. The cells of the organ of Corti are derived from the simple epithelium lining the membranous labyrinth which embryologically is of ectodermal origin. The basilar membrane is composed of fibrous tissue. Axially, it is attached to the osseous spiral lamina and laterally to the *spiral ligament* **SLig** which consists of a marked thickening of the endosteum of the lateral wall of the cochlear canal. The thickened outer wall of the scala media is highly vascular and lined by a stratified epithelium; this area, known as the *stria vascularis* **SVasc**, is responsible for maintaining the correct ionic composition of endolymph.

The membrane between the scala media and scala vestibuli, the *vestibular (Reissner's) membrane* **VM**, is composed of extremely delicate fibrous tissue lined by simple squamous epithelium on both sides. The scala vestibuli and scala tympani are lined by a simple unspecialised squamous epithelium of mesodermal origin.

In micrograph (b) bundles of afferent nerve fibres **N** can be seen arising from the base of the organ of Corti and converging towards the *spiral ganglion* **G** in the modiolus at the base of the spiral lamina. These ganglion cells represent the cell bodies of bipolar sensory neurones, and their proximal axons form the auditory component of the eighth cranial nerve (see Fig. 21.26).

(a)

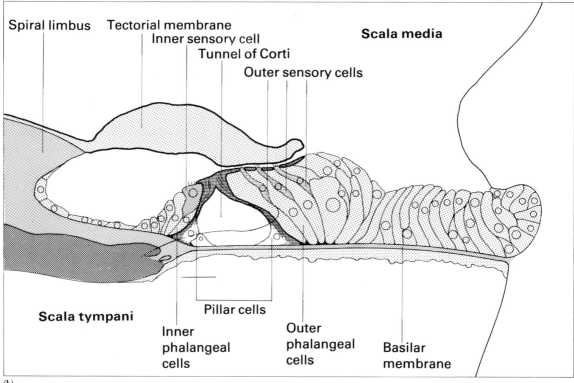

Spiral limbus   Tectorial membrane   Scala media

Inner sensory cell

Tunnel of Corti

Outer sensory cells

Scala tympani

Pillar cells

Inner phalangeal cells

Outer phalangeal cells

Basilar membrane

(b)

Fig. 21.25 Organ of Corti *(illustrations opposite; (a) H & E × 480 (b) Schematic diagram)*

The organ of Corti is a highly specialised epithelial structure containing receptor cells which convert (transduce) mechanical energy in the form of vibrations into electrochemical energy resulting in excitation of auditory sensory receptors.

The organ of Corti lies in the scala media **SM** supported on the basilar membrane. The basilar membrane consists of a thin sheet of fibrous tissue stretched between the osseous spiral lamina **O** of the modiolus and the spiral ligament **SLig** laterally; its under surface, exposed to the scala tympani, is lined by a simple epithelium. The basilar membrane is thinnest at the base of the cochlear and becomes progressively thicker as it spirals towards the apex.

The organ of Corti consists of two basic types of cells, *sensory (hair) cells* and *support cells* of several different types. At the centre of the organ is a triangular-shaped canal, the *inner tunnel* or *tunnel of Corti* **T**, bounded on each side by a single row of tall columnar cells called *pillar cells*. Each pillar cell contains a dense bundle (pillar) of microtubules and the pillars on either side of the tunnel of Corti converge at the surface and then curve laterally to form a thin, hood-like structure containing small fenestrations. The cell bodies of the pillar cells lie in the acute angles formed by the pillars and the basilar membrane at the floor of the tunnel.

On the inner aspect of the inner row of pillar cells is a single row of flask-shaped cells called *inner phalangeal cells* which support a single row of *inner sensory (hair) cells*. The phalangeal cells contain microtubules, some of which support the base of the hair cells while others extend to the free surface around the hair cells. Beyond the outer row of pillar cells there are three to five rows of *outer phalangeal cells* which support the same number of rows of *outer sensory (hair) cells*. Cytoplasmic extensions of the phalangeal cells extend to the surface between and around the hair cells and their microtubules support the fenestrated hood-like structure formed by the pillar cells. Through the fenestrations project the free ends of the sensory cells. A variety of other specialised epithelial cells provides the remaining support for the organ of Corti.

The sensory cells are known as hair cells because numerous sterocilia, i.e. very long microvilli (see Fig. 5.17), project from their free ends. As previously described, the spiral ganglion of the cochlear contains bipolar cell bodies of first order sensory neurones. From here, axons pass towards the base of the rows of hair cells, those going to the outer hair cells traversing the tunnel of Corti as shown in the diagram. The end of each fibre ramifies into a number of dendrites which make synaptic contact with several hair cells; each sensory cell may synapse with dendrites of several different sensory neurones. In addition, inhibitory neurones arising in the brain stem send fibres which also synapse with the sensory cells and exert a suppressive effect.

From the layer of *border cells* which cover the spiral limbus **SL**, there extends a flap-like mass of glycosaminoglycans called the *tectorial membrane* **TM** which overlies the sensory cells and into which the tips of the stereocilia of the sensory cells are embedded.

Function of the organ of Corti

Details of the exact physiological processes for the sense of hearing remain to be discovered. However, in brief, the mechanism is as follows. Sound waves are funnelled into the external auditory meatus and impinge on the tympanic membrane which vibrates at the appropriate frequency. These vibrations are transmitted to the stapes bone via the malleus and incus and, in the process, their amplitude is enhanced about tenfold. The base of the stapes, which lies in the oval window, conducts the vibrations into the perilymph of the vestibule of the inner ear and pressure waves pass from here into the scala vestibuli of the cochlear. These pressure waves are probably conducted directly to the endolymph of the scala media across the delicate vestibular membrane from which vibrations are induced in the basilar membrane upon which rests the organ of Corti. From here, 'spent' vibrations are transmitted into the perilymph of the scala tympani and dissipated at the secondary tympanic membrane over the round window.

The basilar membrane is thinnest at the base of the cochlear and thickest at the apex. It appears that, at every point on the spiral, the membrane is 'tuned' to vibrate to a particular frequency of sound waves reaching the ear; the overall range of frequencies encompassed is of the order of 11 octaves with the highest frequencies (pitch) being sensed towards the base of the cochlear and progressively lower frequencies being sensed along the spiral towards the apex. For any given sound frequency, only one specific point of the basilar membrane and organ of Corti is thought to vibrate and thereby activate the appropriate receptor cells to initiate afferent sensory impulses which then pass to the auditory cortex of the brain. The process of transduction of mechanical energy into electro-chemical energy probably results from deformation of the stereocilia of the sensory cells.

The sensory input from the cochlear is integrated in the brain stem and auditory cortex from which efferent suppressor pathways can modulate receptor activity to enhance auditory acuity.

Fig. 21.26 Spiral ganglion

(H & E × 320)

The spiral ganglion is a spiral-shaped mass of nerve cell bodies lying in a canal at the extremity of the osseous spiral lamina of the modiolus.

As seen in this micrograph, the ganglion cells **G** have the typical appearance of somatic ganglion cells (see Fig. 7.17) and represent the cell bodies of bipolar sensory neurones relaying information from the receptors of the organ of Corti to the brain.

Note the afferent fibres **A** entering the ganglion from the organ of Corti and numerous bundles of efferent fibres **E** which pass to the centre of the modiolus to form the *cochlear nerve*, the auditory component of the eighth cranial nerve; the cochlear nerve is readily seen in Figure 21.24(a).

Fig. 21.27 Receptor organs of the saccule and utricle *(illustrations opposite)*

(a) H & E × 480 (b) H & E × 600 (c) Scanning EM × 5000 (d) Schematic diagram

The saccule and utricle are two dilated regions of the membranous labyrinth lying within the vestibule of the inner ear and filled with endolymph. The walls of each are composed of a fibrous membrane which is bound down in places to the periosteum of the vestibule and in other areas attached to the periosteum by fibrous strands, the intervening space being filled with perilymph. Internally, the saccule and utricle are lined by simple cuboidal epithelium but in each there is a region of highly specialised epithelium called the *macula*, shown in micrographs (a) and (b), containing receptor cells which contribute part of the sensory input to that part of the brain responsible for maintaining balance and equilibrium. The macula of the utricle is oriented at right angles to that of the saccule.

The maculae are made up of two basic cell types, *sensory cells* and *support cells*. The support cells are tall and columnar with basally-located nuclei and microvilli at their free surface. The receptor cells lie between the support cells, with their larger nuclei placed more centrally. Each receptor cell has a single eccentrically-located cilium of typical conformation (see Fig. 5.15) and many stereocilia (long microvilli) projecting from its surface giving rise to the name *hair cells*. The 'hairs' are embedded in a thick, gelatinous plaque of glycoprotein probably secreted by the supporting cells; this is lost during histological preparation. At the surface of the glycoprotein layer is a mass of crystals mainly composed of calcium carbonate and known as *otoliths*. These are shown in micrograph (c).

There are two different forms of sensory cells. The first type is bulbous in shape and stains poorly, its nuclei tending to lie at a lower level than those of the second type which are more slender in shape. The bulbous receptor cells (goblet cells) are invested by a meshwork of dendritic processes of afferent sensory neurones whereas the slender (columnar) receptors have only small dendritic processes at their bases. The receptor cells also have synaptic connections with modulatory (inhibitory) neurones from the CNS.

Function of the maculae

The function of the maculae relates mainly to the maintenance of balance by providing sensory information about the static position of the head in space. This is of particular importance when the eyes are closed, or in the dark or under water, and the maculae are consequently more developed in animals other than humans.

When the head is moved from a position of equilibrium, the otolithic membrane tends to move with respect to the receptor cells, thus bending their stereocilia. When the stereocilia are bent in the direction of the cilium, the receptor cell undergoes excitation and, when the relative movement is in the opposite direction, excitation is inhibited.

The neural pathways of the balance and equilibrium mechanism are extremely complex and the sensory input from the maculae is integrated with that of proprioceptors, muscle spindles etc. to elicit reflex responses directed towards the maintenance of postural equilibrium.

(a)

(b)

(c)

(d)

Otoliths

Glycoprotein layer

Cilium

Stereocilia

Hair cells:
Goblet cell
Columnar cell

Supporting cell

Sensory dendrites

Nerve fibre

(a)

Fig. 21.28 Receptor organs of the semicircular canals

(a) Masson's trichrome × 200 (b) Schematic diagram (opposite)

Three semicircular canals arise from the vestibule of the inner ear, each containing a membranous semicircular duct which opens at both ends into the utricle. At one end of each duct is a dilated portion, the ampulla, which contains a receptor organ called the *crista ampullaris*.

Each crista ampullaris is an elongated epithelial structure situated on a ridge of supporting tissue arising from the membranous wall of the ampulla and oriented at right angles to the direction of flow of the endolymph in the semicircular canal. Structurally, the cristae ampullares bear many similarities to the maculae of the utricle and saccule (see Fig. 21.27). The receptor cells are of two morphological forms, one globular and the other more slender, the former being invested by a basket of sensory dendrites and the latter having small dendritic endings at its base only. The receptor cells are supported by a single layer of columnar cells which is continuous with the simple cuboidal epithelium lining the rest of the membranous labyrinth.

Like those of the maculae, the receptor cells of the cristae have numerous stereocilia and a single cilium, the cilium being situated at the margin of the cell nearest to the utricle. The stereocilia and the cilia of the sensory receptors are embedded in a ridge of gelatinous glycoprotein which is tall and cone-shaped in cross-section giving rise to the term *cupula*. In contrast to the macula, the cupula does not contain otolithic crystals.

Function of the crista ampullaris

When the head is moved in the plane of a particular semicircular canal, the inertia of the endolymph acts so as to deflect the cupula in the opposite direction. The stereocilia of the sensory cells are then deflected towards or away from the cilia, resulting in excitation or inhibition respectively.

In each ear there are three semicircular canals, two in vertical planes and one in a near-horizontal plane. Each is paired with a semicircular canal in the other ear, the members of each pair being oriented in parallel. The sensory input from the cristae ampullares mainly concerns changes in the direction and rate of movement of the head. Afferent impulses pass via bipolar sensory neurones with cell bodies in the vestibular ganglion which lies at the base of the internal auditory meatus. Afferent fibres pass via the vestibular part of the eighth cranial nerve to the brain stem, cerebellum and cerebral cortex where sensory information from various other sources is integrated for the maintenance of balance, position sense and equilibrium.

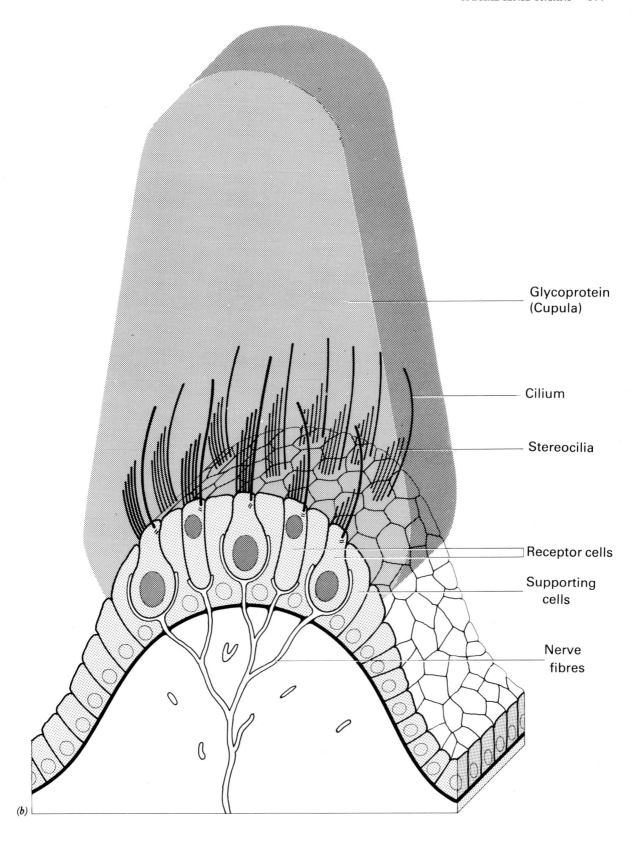

Glycoprotein
(Cupula)

Cilium

Stereocilia

Receptor cells

Supporting
cells

Nerve
fibres

(b)

Notes on staining techniques

● **Haematoxylin and eosin (H & E)**

This is the most commonly used technique in animal histology and routine pathology. The basic dye, haematoxylin, stains acidic structures a purplish blue. Nuclei, ribosomes and rough endoplasmic reticulum have a strong affinity for this dye owing to their high content of DNA and RNA respectively. In contrast, eosin is an acidic dye which stains basic structures red or pink. Most cytoplasmic proteins are basic and hence cytoplasm usually stains pink or pinkish red. In general, when the H & E staining technique is applied to animal cells, nuclei stain blue and cytoplasm stains pink or red.

● **Periodic acid-Schiff reaction (PAS)**

Staining techniques which specifically stain components of cells and tissues are called histochemical staining techniques. Such techniques are invaluable for the understanding of cell and tissue structure and function, and for making a diagnosis on diseased tissues. The PAS reaction stains complex carbohydrates a deep red colour, traditionally described as magenta. The mucin produced by goblet cells of the gastrointestinal and respiratory tracts stains magenta with this technique (and is therefore termed PAS positive). Basement membranes and the brush borders of kidney tubules and the small and large intestines are also PAS positive, as is cartilage and to some extent collagen. Glycogen, the intracellular storage form of carbohydrate found in cells such as hepatocytes and muscle cells, is also PAS positive.

● **Masson's trichrome**

This technique is a so-called connective tissue technique since it is used to demonstrate supporting tissue elements, principally collagen. As its name implies, the staining technique produces three colours: nuclei and other basophilic structures are stained blue, collagen is stained green or blue depending on which variant of the technique is used, and cytoplasm, muscle, erythrocytes and keratin are stained bright red.

● **Alcian blue**

Alcian blue is a mucin stain which may be used in conjunction with other staining methods such as H & E or van Gieson (see below). Certain types of mucin, but not all, are stained blue by the Alcian blue method, as is cartilage. When the technique is combined with van Gieson, the Alcian blue colour becomes green.

● **Van Gieson**

This is another connective tissue method in which collagen is stained red, nuclei are blue and erythrocytes and cytoplasm yellow. When used in combination with an elastic stain, elastin is stained blue/black in addition to the results described above. This staining technique is particularly useful for blood vessels and skin.

● **Reticulin stain**

This method demonstrates the reticulin fibres of supporting tissue which are stained blue/black by this technique. Nuclei may be counterstained blue with haematoxylin or red with the dye, neutral red.

● **Azan**

This technique is traditionally classed as a connective tissue method but is excellent for demonstrating fine cytological detail, especially in epithelium. Nuclei are stained bright red; collagen, basement membrane and mucin are stained blue; muscle and red blood cells are stained orange to red.

● **Giemsa**

This technique is a standard method for staining blood cells and other smears of cells, e.g. bone marrow. Nuclei are stained dark blue to violet, background cytoplasm pale blue and erythrocytes pale pink.

● **Toluidine blue**

This is a basic stain which stains acidic components various shades of blue. It is commonly employed on very thin, resin embedded specimens. Some tissue components are able to turn the blue dye red, a phenomenon known as metachromasia.

● **Silver and gold methods**

These methods were extremely popular at the end of the nineteenth century and are occasionally used today to demonstrate such fine structures as cell processes, e.g. in neurones, motor end-plates and intercellular junctions. Depending on the method used, the end product is either black, brown or golden.

● **Chrome alum/haematoxylin**

This method is rarely used and is similar to the H & E method in principle, in that nuclei are stained blue and cytoplasm is stained red. Empirically this method demonstrates the glucagon-secreting cells of the pancreas pink and the insulin-secreting cells blue.

● **Isamine blue/eosin**

This method is also similar to the H & E method but the blue component is rather more intense.

● **Nissl and methylene blue methods**

These techniques use a basic dye to stain the rough endoplasmic reticulum found in neurones; when this is seen as clumps it is called Nissl substance.

● **Sudan black and osmium**

These dyes stain lipid-containing structures such as myelin a brownish-black colour.

Index